PREFACE

Veterinary Technicians, being the unsung heroes of animal healthcare are notable for their vast activities behind the scenes. The journey towards becoming a Veterinary Technician can be very challenging but on the flip side can most importantly be rewarding.

A careful study of this Guide by Alice Fraley; as an intending Veterinary Technician is a significant step in achieving your Veterinary Technician goal seeing as this guide is a blend of "straight forward language" with occasional "Veterinary Professional Terminologies" resulting in a balanced technical detail with readability.

This guide also serves as a manual for all Veterinary Professionals because it cuts across the important domains of the practice (which includes anatomy, physiology, pharmacology, pathology etc.), giving the information required to form the basis for the practice and also ensuring to carefully relate the necessary detailed information about these domains to the real time practice of Veterinary professionals.

This guide contains a vast number of clinical questions and answers which do not only aim at evaluating the readers' understanding of the key domains in the profession but also to educate the readers on the reasons (physiological or pathological) that gave rise to such results.

The book followed the Global Standards set for animals and pet care by renowned bodies because our aim is to ensure the continuous relevance of this guide regardless of the continuous evolving veterinary medical field due to the emergence of advancements in medical practices. We made sure to create room for periodic updates in the guide.

Being opportune to take part in the review of this guide, I can confidently recommend this guide as a must have for individuals interested in the Veterinary Professional field as it covers the basic knowledge for Veterinary professionals which include Veterinary technicians, Veterinary Doctors, Veterinary Behaviorists and others within the Veterinary field.

Dr. Miracle Ekeoma Ohanwe
Doctor of Veterinary Medicine

MYRA VETERINARY SOLUTIONS
Email: ohanwemiracle@gmail.com

VTNE Exam Mastery Guide
© Copyright 2025 by Alice Fraley
All rights reserved

This document is geared towards providing exact and reliable information with regards to the topic and issue covered. The publication is sold with the idea that the publisher is not required to render accounting, officially permitted, or otherwise, qualified services. If advice is necessary, legal or professional, a practiced individual in the profession should be ordered.

In no way is it legal to reproduce, duplicate, or transmit any part of this document in either electronic means or in printed format. Recording of this publication is strictly prohibited and any storage of this document is not allowed unless with written permission from the publisher. All rights reserved.

The information provided herein is stated to be truthful and consistent, in that any liability, in terms of inattention or otherwise, by any usage or abuse of any policies, processes, or directions contained within is the solitary and utter responsibility of the recipient reader. Under no circumstances will any legal responsibility or blame be held against the publisher for any reparation, damages, or monetary loss due to the information herein, either directly or indirectly.

Respective authors own all copyrights not held by the publisher.

The information herein is offered for informational purposes solely, and is universal as so. The presentation of the information is without contract or any type of guarantee assurance.

The trademarks that are used are without any consent, and the publication of the trademark is without permission or backing by the trademark owner. All trademarks and brands within this book are for clarifying purposes only and are the owned by the owners themselves, not affiliated with this document.

TABLE OF CONTENTS

CHAPTER 1: UNDERSTANDING THE VTNE LANDSCAPE 1

Overview of the VTNE 1

Exam Structure and Format 2

Registration Process and Requirements 3

Scoring and Results Interpretation 4

Common Pitfalls and How to Avoid Them 6

CHAPTER 2: VETERINARY TECHNICIAN PROFESSION INSIGHTS 8

Roles and Responsibilities 8

Career Pathways and Opportunities 9

Ethical Considerations in Practice 10

Professional Development and Continuing Education 11

Real-life Case Studies from Veterinary Technicians 13

CHAPTER 3: MASTERING VETERINARY ANATOMY AND PHYSIOLOGY 15

Introduction to Animal Anatomy 15

Understanding Physiological Systems 16

Pathophysiology in Veterinary Medicine 18

Comparative Anatomy: Domestic Animals 19

Clinical Relevance of Anatomy and Physiology 20

CHAPTER 4: DEEP DIVE INTO PHARMACOLOGY 22

Principles of Pharmacology 22

Common Veterinary Medications 23

Drug Interactions and Side Effects 25

Dosage Calculations and Administration 26

Pharmacokinetics and Pharmacodynamics 27

Legal and Ethical Considerations in Pharmacology 28

CHAPTER 5: SURGICAL NURSING AND ANESTHESIA 31

Preoperative Care and Assessment 31

Surgical Instruments and Techniques 32

Anesthesia Types and Administration 33

Monitoring and Postoperative Care 34

Pain Management in Veterinary Practice 36

CHAPTER 6: DIAGNOSTIC IMAGING TECHNIQUES 38

Basics of Radiography 38

Ultrasound Utilization 39

Advanced Imaging: CT and MRI 40

Interpretation of Diagnostic Images 41

Safety Protocols and Best Practices 42

CHAPTER 7: LABORATORY PROCEDURES AND TECHNIQUES 44

Sample Collection and Handling 44

Hematology and Blood Chemistry 45

Microbiology and Parasitology 46

Urinalysis and Cytology 47

Quality Control in Veterinary Laboratories 48

CHAPTER 8: DENTISTRY AND ORAL HEALTH IN ANIMALS 50

Anatomy of the Oral Cavity 50

Common Dental Diseases 51

Dental Prophylaxis and Treatments 52

Tools and Techniques in Veterinary Dentistry 53

Client Education on Oral Health 54

CHAPTER 9: UNDERSTANDING ANIMAL BEHAVIOR 56

Fundamentals of Animal Behavior 56

Behavioral Disorders and Treatments 57

Techniques for Behavior Modification 58

Human-Animal Bond and Its Implications 59

Case Studies in Veterinary Behavior 61

CHAPTER 10: PRACTICE MANAGEMENT FOR VETERINARY TECHNICIANS 63

Fundamentals of Practice Management 63

Client Communication and Customer Service 64

Inventory and Financial Management 66

Legalities in Veterinary Practice 67

Strategies for Effective Team Collaboration 68

CHAPTER 11: EFFECTIVE STUDY TECHNIQUES AND EXAM PREPARATION 71

Time Management Strategies 71

Stress Reduction Techniques 72

Memory Enhancement: WAKEUPMEMORY 73

Exam Day Tips and Tricks 75

CHAPTER 12: FULL PRACTICE TESTS 77

Full Test 1 with Detailed Explanations 77

Full Test 2 with Detailed Explanations 109

Full Test 3 with Detailed Explanations 142

Full Test 4 with Detailed Explanations 173

Full Test 5 with Detailed Explanations 205

Full Test 6 with Detailed Explanations 231

Full Test 7 with Detailed Explanations 263

Full Test 8 with Detailed Explanations 295

EXTRA CONTENTS 328

Audiobook	328
Digital Flashcards	328
WAKEUPMEMORY Technique	328
6 Online Tests	328

CHAPTER 1
UNDERSTANDING THE VTNE LANDSCAPE

Overview of the VTNE

The Veterinary Technician National Exam (VTNE) stands as a pivotal milestone for aspiring veterinary technicians, serving as a comprehensive assessment of the skills and knowledge required to excel in this dynamic and rewarding field. Understanding the landscape of the VTNE is essential for candidates to approach their preparation with confidence and clarity, ensuring that they are well-equipped to tackle the challenges posed by the exam.

The VTNE is administered by the American Association of Veterinary State Boards (AAVSB) and is a standardized examination designed to evaluate the competency of veterinary technicians across various domains. This exam is recognized by most states and provinces in North America as a critical step in the licensure process, making it a crucial component of a veterinary technician's career path. The exam itself is meticulously structured to cover a broad range of topics that are vital to the practice of veterinary medicine.

Candidates approaching the VTNE must first familiarize themselves with the exam's structure and content areas. The VTNE is composed of 170 multiple-choice questions, of which 150 are scored, and the remaining 20 are pilot questions used to develop future exams. The exam is divided into nine distinct domains, each representing a key aspect of veterinary technology. These domains include pharmacy and pharmacology, surgical nursing, dentistry, laboratory procedures, animal care and nursing, diagnostic imaging, anesthesia, emergency medicine, and pain management, and the final domain encompasses questions related to the veterinary technician's role in public health and safety.

Each domain is weighted differently, with certain areas like animal care and nursing, and anesthesia, comprising a larger portion of the exam. This distribution reflects the practical realities of veterinary practice, where certain skills and knowledge areas are more frequently applied. Understanding this distribution is crucial for candidates to prioritize their study efforts effectively, focusing more on high-weight domains while ensuring a solid foundation across all areas.

Preparation for the VTNE involves a strategic approach that encompasses a variety of study methods and resources. Candidates often begin by reviewing the official VTNE Candidate Handbook, which provides comprehensive information about the exam format, content areas, and sample questions. This handbook serves as a valuable starting point, offering insights into the types of questions candidates can expect and the critical topics that must be mastered.

In addition to utilizing written resources, many candidates benefit from enrolling in review courses or joining study groups. These collective environments provide opportunities for interactive learning, where candidates can engage in discussions, share study tips, and clarify doubts. Review courses are particularly beneficial as they are often led by experienced instructors who provide expert guidance and insights into the nuances of the exam. Furthermore, study groups foster a sense of camaraderie and motivation, encouraging candidates to remain committed to their preparation efforts.

A pivotal aspect of exam preparation involves the practical application of knowledge through practice exams. Simulated exams allow candidates to familiarize themselves with the timing and pressure of the actual VTNE, helping to build confidence and reduce anxiety. Practice exams also serve as diagnostic tools, identifying areas of weakness that require further study. By taking multiple practice exams, candidates can track their progress over time and tailor their study strategies to address specific gaps in knowledge.

Time management during the exam is another critical factor for success. With 170 questions to answer in a three-hour period, candidates must pace themselves to ensure that they can thoughtfully consider each question without feeling rushed. Developing a time management strategy during practice exams can help candidates refine their approach, striking a balance between speed and accuracy.

In the weeks leading up to the exam, candidates should focus on refining their study techniques and maintaining a positive mindset. This period is crucial for reinforcing knowledge and building confidence, ensuring that candidates are mentally and emotionally prepared for the exam day. Stress management techniques, such as mindfulness exercises and relaxation practices, can be beneficial in reducing anxiety and promoting a calm state of mind.

On the day of the exam, candidates should arrive at the testing center well-prepared and equipped with the necessary materials, such as valid identification. It is important to be aware of the testing center's rules and regulations to avoid any last-minute complications. A good night's sleep before the exam and a nutritious breakfast on the day of the exam can also contribute to optimal performance.

The VTNE is not merely a hurdle to overcome; it is a comprehensive evaluation that ensures veterinary technicians possess the requisite knowledge and skills to provide high-quality care to animals. By understanding the exam's landscape, candidates can approach their preparation with strategic insight, maximizing their chances of success and paving the way for a fulfilling career in veterinary medicine.

This overview of the VTNE underscores the importance of thorough preparation, strategic planning, and a positive mindset. By embracing these principles, candidates can confidently navigate the challenges of the exam, ultimately achieving their goal of becoming skilled and compassionate veterinary technicians.

Exam Structure and Format

The Veterinary Technician National Exam (VTNE) is a crucial step for aspiring veterinary technicians, providing a comprehensive assessment of the essential skills and knowledge required in the field. The exam's structure and format are meticulously designed to evaluate candidates' proficiency across multiple domains, ensuring they are well-prepared for the diverse responsibilities that come with the profession.

The VTNE consists of 170 multiple-choice questions, which candidates must complete within a three-hour timeframe. Of these questions, 150 are scored, while the remaining 20 are unscored pilot questions used to develop future exam iterations. This blend of scored and unscored questions is a standard practice in standardized testing, allowing exam administrators to continually refine and update the exam based on evolving industry standards and practices.

Understanding the breakdown of the exam's domains is critical for effective preparation. The VTNE is divided into nine primary domains, each representing a key area of veterinary technology. These domains include pharmacy and pharmacology, surgical nursing, dentistry, laboratory procedures, animal care and nursing, diagnostic imaging, anesthesia, emergency medicine and pain management, and public health and safety. Each domain is weighted differently, reflecting its importance in veterinary practice. For instance, animal care and nursing, along with anesthesia, typically carry a higher weight due to their frequent application in clinical settings.

Familiarity with the types of questions within these domains is also essential. Questions are designed to test not only the recall of factual knowledge but also the application of that knowledge in practical scenarios. This approach ensures that candidates are not only knowledgeable but also capable of critical thinking and problem-solving in real-world situations. It is not uncommon for questions to present a clinical scenario, requiring candidates to determine the most appropriate course of action based on their understanding of veterinary principles.

The exam also incorporates a range of question formats to assess different cognitive skills. Candidates may encounter straightforward recall questions that test their knowledge of specific facts, such as drug classifications or anatomical structures. More complex questions might require the application of knowledge to diagnose a condition or develop a treatment plan. These questions are often scenario-based and may include distractors—incorrect options that are plausible but ultimately incorrect. This format challenges candidates to critically analyze the information presented and apply their understanding effectively.

In preparing for the VTNE, it is beneficial for candidates to simulate the exam environment as closely as possible. Practice exams are an invaluable tool for this purpose, providing insights into the pacing and pressure of the actual exam. They allow candidates to experience the mental stamina required to maintain focus over a three-hour period, as well as the strategic thinking necessary to manage time effectively across all domains.

Effective time management during the exam is crucial. With approximately one minute allocated per question, candidates must balance speed with accuracy, ensuring that they do not linger too long on any single question. Developing a time management strategy during practice exams can help candidates refine their pacing, allowing for a more confident and composed approach on the exam day.

Another key consideration is the use of the process of elimination. This technique is particularly useful when faced with difficult questions. By systematically eliminating clearly incorrect options, candidates can increase their chances of selecting the correct answer, even if they are initially uncertain. This method not only enhances accuracy but also helps to conserve valuable time for more challenging questions.

Preparation for the VTNE should also involve a thorough review of the official VTNE Candidate Handbook. This handbook provides detailed information on the exam format, content areas, and sample questions, serving as an essential resource for candidates. It outlines the competencies required in each domain and offers guidance on what examiners are looking for in terms of knowledge and skills.

In addition to the handbook, candidates may benefit from utilizing a variety of study materials, including textbooks, review courses, and online resources. These materials offer a comprehensive overview of the topics covered in the exam and provide opportunities for targeted practice. Review courses, in particular, can be beneficial as they often include expert instruction and insights from experienced veterinary professionals.

While the technical aspects of the exam are paramount, candidates should also be mindful of their mental and emotional preparation. The importance of a positive mindset cannot be overstated, as it can significantly impact performance. Techniques such as visualization, positive affirmations, and stress-reduction exercises can be effective in cultivating a calm and focused state of mind.

On the day of the exam, candidates should arrive at the testing center equipped with the necessary materials, such as valid identification, and be familiar with the testing center's rules and procedures. It is advisable to arrive early to allow time to settle in and mentally prepare for the exam ahead.

Ultimately, the VTNE is a comprehensive evaluation designed to ensure that veterinary technicians possess the essential skills and knowledge to excel in their roles. By understanding the exam's structure and format, candidates can approach their preparation with a strategic mindset, maximizing their chances of success and paving the way for a fulfilling career in veterinary medicine. The journey to becoming a veterinary technician is both challenging and rewarding, and mastering the VTNE is a significant step towards achieving that goal.

Registration Process and Requirements

Embarking on the journey to become a certified veterinary technician involves navigating the registration process for the Veterinary Technician National Exam (VTNE). Understanding the steps and requirements for registration is critical to ensure a smooth and stress-free experience. The VTNE is administered by the American Association of Veterinary State Boards (AAVSB), and their guidelines must be meticulously followed to secure your place in the exam.

The first step in the registration process is ensuring eligibility. Candidates must have graduated from, or be in the final stages of graduating from, an accredited veterinary technology program. Accreditation is typically provided by the American Veterinary Medical Association (AVMA), and it is essential to confirm that your program meets these standards. Some states may have additional requirements, such as specific coursework or clinical hours, so it's crucial to verify these details with both your educational institution and the regulatory board in the state where you plan to practice.

Once eligibility is confirmed, the next step is to create an account with the AAVSB. This account will serve as your portal for all exam-related activities, including registration, accessing study materials, and receiving exam results. Creating an account is straightforward, requiring personal information, educational background, and, in some cases, documentation to verify your eligibility. It's important to ensure that all information provided is accurate and up-to-date to avoid any delays in the registration process.

After setting up your account, you can proceed with the exam application. This involves selecting your preferred testing window, which the AAVSB offers three times a year: spring, summer, and fall. Each testing window spans approximately one month, providing flexibility in scheduling your exam. It's advisable to select a date that allows ample time for preparation while also considering personal and professional commitments.

The application process also requires payment of the exam fee. The fee is non-refundable and must be paid in full at the time of application. It's essential to budget for this expense as part of your overall exam preparation plan. Some candidates may qualify for financial assistance through their educational institution or professional organizations, so it's worth exploring these options if needed.

Once your application and payment are submitted, the AAVSB will review your materials to ensure all requirements are met. Upon successful review, you will receive an Authorization to Test (ATT) letter. This letter is a crucial document, as it contains your unique candidate identification number and instructions for scheduling your exam at a designated testing center. It's important to keep this letter safe and accessible, as you will need it on the day of the exam.

With the ATT letter in hand, the next step is to schedule your exam. The AAVSB partners with Prometric, a leading provider of testing services, to administer the VTNE at testing centers across North America. Scheduling can be done online through the Prometric website or by phone, and it's advisable to book your appointment as soon as possible to secure your preferred date and location. Testing centers can fill up quickly, especially during peak periods, so early scheduling is recommended.

On the day of the exam, candidates must arrive at the testing center with the ATT letter and valid government-issued identification. This ID must match the name on your ATT letter exactly, so ensure that there are no discrepancies. The testing center will have specific rules and regulations, such as prohibited items and conduct, which candidates must adhere to. Familiarizing yourself with these guidelines in advance can help reduce stress and ensure a smooth testing experience.

In addition to the general registration process, candidates should be aware of any state-specific requirements. Some states may require additional documentation, such as proof of residency or a background check, as part of their licensure process. It's essential to research these requirements early in your preparation to allow sufficient time to gather and submit any necessary materials.

Preparation for the VTNE extends beyond meeting the technical requirements of registration. It also involves cultivating a positive mindset and developing effective study habits. The registration process can be a source of anxiety for many candidates, but approaching it with confidence and organization can alleviate much of this stress. Creating a checklist of tasks and deadlines can help keep you on track and ensure that no detail is overlooked.

Networking with peers and mentors can provide valuable support and insights during the registration process. Fellow students and instructors from your veterinary technology program can offer advice based on their own experiences, while professional organizations can provide resources and guidance. Engaging with a community of like-minded individuals can also boost motivation and morale, reminding you that you are not alone on this journey.

In summary, understanding the registration process and requirements for the VTNE is a vital step in your path to becoming a licensed veterinary technician. By ensuring eligibility, creating an AAVSB account, submitting your application and fee, receiving your ATT letter, and scheduling your exam, you are setting the foundation for success. With careful planning and preparation, you can confidently navigate this process and focus on preparing for the exam itself, knowing that you have met all necessary requirements.

Scoring and Results Interpretation

Navigating the intricacies of the Veterinary Technician National Exam (VTNE) requires not only understanding its structure but also mastering the art of interpreting the results. The scoring system of the

VTNE is designed to assess the readiness of candidates to enter the veterinary technology field, ensuring they possess the necessary knowledge and skills to perform effectively on the job.

The VTNE is a computer-based exam, and its scoring methodology is both precise and systematic. Each of the 150 scored questions contributes to a candidate's final score, while the 20 unscored questions are included for research purposes to test their validity for future exams. These unscored questions are indistinguishable from the scored ones, which necessitates that candidates approach each question with equal seriousness.

The exam employs a scaled scoring system, where the raw score (the number of questions answered correctly) is converted to a scaled score ranging from 200 to 800. This conversion is crucial as it accounts for varying levels of difficulty across different versions of the exam. By standardizing scores, the AAVSB ensures that all candidates are assessed equitably, irrespective of the specific questions they encounter. To pass the VTNE, candidates must achieve a scaled score of at least 425. This benchmark reflects a level of proficiency deemed necessary for competent practice in veterinary technology.

Understanding how this score translates into practical implications requires insight into the areas of strength and weakness. The score report provided to candidates post-exam is an invaluable tool in this regard. It not only indicates the overall score but also breaks down performance across the nine domains of the VTNE. This domain-specific feedback is particularly beneficial for candidates who do not pass the exam, as it highlights areas requiring further study and improvement.

Candidates should approach their score report with a strategic mindset. By analyzing the breakdown of scores, they can identify patterns in their performance. For instance, consistently high scores in certain domains may indicate a strong grasp of those areas, while lower scores in others suggest a need for more focused study. This targeted approach to exam review can inform future preparation strategies, allowing candidates to allocate their study time and resources more efficiently.

For those who do not achieve a passing score, it is important to view the experience as an opportunity for growth and learning. The VTNE is a challenging exam, and not passing on the first attempt is not uncommon. Many candidates find that the experience of taking the exam provides valuable insights into their strengths and areas for development. By leveraging the detailed feedback from the score report, candidates can refine their study techniques and build a more robust understanding of the material.

It's also worth noting that the AAVSB allows candidates to retake the VTNE up to five times, with a mandatory waiting period between attempts. This policy provides ample opportunity for candidates to improve their knowledge and skills before reattempting the exam. However, repeated attempts should be approached with a strategic plan in place. Candidates are encouraged to seek additional resources, such as review courses or tutoring, to address specific areas of difficulty.

In preparation for interpreting the results, candidates should familiarize themselves with the statistical concepts underlying the scoring process. Understanding terms like "scaled score," "percentile rank," and "domain performance" can enhance a candidate's ability to contextualize their results. For instance, knowing that a scaled score accounts for exam difficulty can alleviate concerns about lower-than-expected raw scores, while understanding percentile rank can provide insight into how a candidate's performance compares to that of their peers.

In addition to individual score reports, candidates should be aware of the broader implications of their results. A passing score on the VTNE is a critical step towards obtaining licensure as a veterinary technician. However, state-specific requirements must also be met. Candidates should ensure they understand the licensing process in their state, as additional steps such as jurisprudence exams or background checks may be required.

For candidates who pass the VTNE, interpreting the results involves a sense of accomplishment and readiness to advance in their careers. Achieving a passing score validates the hard work and dedication invested in their education and exam preparation. It signifies a readiness to enter the workforce as a competent and capable veterinary technician, equipped to provide high-quality care to animals and support to veterinary teams.

However, the journey does not end with passing the VTNE. Continuous professional development is essential in the ever-evolving field of veterinary medicine. Newly certified veterinary technicians are encouraged to seek opportunities for further education and specialization, whether through continuing education courses, workshops, or advanced certifications. This commitment to lifelong learning not only enhances career prospects but also ensures the delivery of the highest standard of care to patients.

In summary, the scoring and results interpretation of the VTNE are integral components of the exam process. By understanding the scoring methodology and effectively analyzing the score report, candidates can gain valuable insights into their performance and areas for improvement. Whether celebrating a passing score or preparing for a retake, candidates are encouraged to view their results as a stepping stone towards a fulfilling and impactful career in veterinary technology. With determination and strategic planning, the VTNE becomes not just an exam, but a pivotal moment in the journey to becoming a skilled veterinary professional.

Common Pitfalls and How to Avoid Them

Navigating the complexities of the Veterinary Technician National Exam (VTNE) can be a daunting task, and even the most prepared candidates may encounter challenges along the way. Understanding common pitfalls and learning how to avoid them is crucial for success. By identifying potential stumbling blocks and implementing proactive strategies, candidates can enhance their preparation and approach the exam with greater confidence.

One of the most prevalent pitfalls is inadequate time management during the exam. With 170 questions to answer in just three hours, candidates must balance speed with accuracy to ensure they have ample time to address each question. Many candidates fall into the trap of spending too much time on challenging questions, which can lead to rushed answers later in the exam. To avoid this, it's essential to develop a time management strategy during practice exams. Candidates should learn to quickly identify questions they are unsure about and make a strategic decision to move on, marking them for review if time permits.

Another common issue is over-reliance on rote memorization. While factual knowledge is important, the VTNE also assesses critical thinking and the ability to apply knowledge in practical scenarios. Candidates who focus solely on memorizing facts may struggle with questions that require problem-solving and clinical reasoning. To circumvent this, candidates should incorporate scenario-based learning into their study routine. This approach involves working through case studies and clinical scenarios, which helps to develop the application skills necessary for the exam.

Test anxiety is a significant challenge for many candidates, affecting performance and concentration. The pressure of taking a high-stakes exam can lead to stress and anxiety, which can impede cognitive function. To mitigate test anxiety, candidates should practice relaxation techniques such as deep breathing, visualization, or mindfulness exercises. These techniques can help calm nerves and maintain focus during the exam. Additionally, creating a realistic study schedule that allows for breaks and relaxation can prevent burnout and reduce overall anxiety.

A lack of familiarity with the exam format is another pitfall that candidates should address. The VTNE's computer-based format and the nature of multiple-choice questions can be unfamiliar to some, leading to confusion and errors. Familiarizing oneself with the format through practice exams and review of sample questions is crucial. This familiarity helps candidates become comfortable with the testing environment and the types of questions they will encounter.

Neglecting weaker areas during preparation can also hinder success. It's natural to gravitate towards subjects one feels confident in, but neglecting weaker areas can result in an imbalanced preparation. Candidates should use their performance on practice exams to identify domains where they need more focus. A targeted study plan that addresses these weaker areas can improve overall performance and increase the likelihood of passing the exam.

Procrastination and lack of organization are pitfalls that can derail even the most diligent candidates. The VTNE requires a comprehensive understanding of a wide range of topics, and last-minute cramming is unlikely to be effective. Candidates should create a structured study schedule well in advance of the exam date, allocating time for each domain based on their strengths and weaknesses. Regular review sessions and consistent study habits can prevent the need for frantic, last-minute preparation.

Misinterpreting questions is another common issue that can lead to incorrect answers. The VTNE often presents questions that are intentionally designed to test a candidate's understanding and critical thinking skills. Misreading or misunderstanding the question can lead to selecting the wrong answer. To avoid this, candidates should carefully read each question and all answer options before making a selection. Paying attention to keywords and phrases can also help in understanding the question's intent.

Ignoring the importance of self-care during the preparation period is a pitfall that can impact both physical and mental well-being. Studying for the VTNE is undoubtedly demanding, but neglecting self-care can lead to burnout and decreased performance. Candidates should prioritize healthy habits such as regular exercise, adequate sleep, and a balanced diet. Taking time for hobbies and relaxation activities can also provide a mental break and recharge energy levels.

Finally, underestimating the importance of support networks can be detrimental. Preparing for the VTNE can be an isolating experience, but candidates do not have to navigate it alone. Engaging with peers, mentors, and professional networks can provide valuable support, encouragement, and insights. Study groups, online forums, and professional organizations offer opportunities for collaborative learning and shared experiences.

In summary, by recognizing and addressing these common pitfalls, candidates can enhance their preparation and approach the VTNE with greater confidence and competence. Developing effective time management strategies, incorporating scenario-based learning, and addressing test anxiety are key components of a successful preparation plan. Additionally, maintaining a balanced approach that includes self-care and support from peers and mentors can contribute to a positive and successful exam experience. With careful planning and determination, candidates can navigate the challenges of the VTNE and embark on a rewarding career as a veterinary technician.

CHAPTER 2
VETERINARY TECHNICIAN PROFESSION INSIGHTS

Roles and Responsibilities

The profession of a veterinary technician is a dynamic and multifaceted one, requiring a diverse skill set to meet the demands of an evolving veterinary landscape. These professionals play a crucial role in veterinary healthcare teams, supporting veterinarians in delivering high-quality care to animals. To truly understand the breadth of a veterinary technician's responsibilities, it's important to delve into the various roles they undertake within clinical and non-clinical settings.

At the heart of a veterinary technician's duties lies animal care and nursing. This core responsibility involves monitoring the health and well-being of animals under their care, ensuring that they receive the appropriate treatment and attention. From administering medications and vaccines to providing post-operative care, veterinary technicians serve as the frontline caregivers. They are often the first to notice changes in an animal's condition, making their observations critical for early intervention and treatment adjustments.

In surgical settings, veterinary technicians take on the role of surgical nurses. They are responsible for preparing animals for surgery, which includes tasks such as shaving and disinfecting the surgical site, as well as ensuring that all necessary equipment and instruments are sterilized and ready for use. During the procedure, they assist the veterinarian by passing instruments, monitoring anesthesia, and maintaining a sterile environment. Their expertise in aseptic techniques is crucial in preventing infections and ensuring successful surgical outcomes.

Diagnostic testing and laboratory procedures are another key area where veterinary technicians excel. They are trained to perform a variety of tests, including blood work, urinalysis, and fecal examinations. These tests provide valuable information that aids in diagnosing medical conditions and formulating treatment plans. Veterinary technicians must be adept at using laboratory equipment and interpreting test results accurately, as this data often guides clinical decisions.

In addition to technical skills, veterinary technicians are often tasked with client communication and education. They serve as a bridge between the veterinarian and the pet owner, explaining complex medical information in a way that is understandable and relatable. This role requires excellent interpersonal skills, as technicians must be able to convey empathy and understanding while addressing concerns and questions. Educating clients on topics such as nutrition, preventive care, and post-treatment home care is essential to ensuring the health and longevity of their pets.

Emergency and critical care scenarios call for veterinary technicians to act swiftly and decisively. In these high-pressure situations, they must be able to perform tasks such as resuscitation, wound care, and fluid therapy with precision and accuracy. Their ability to remain calm under pressure and think critically can make a significant difference in the outcome of emergency cases. Veterinary technicians in emergency settings must also be prepared to work irregular hours, as animals can require urgent care at any time.

Beyond the confines of clinical practice, veterinary technicians have the opportunity to specialize in various fields, expanding their roles and responsibilities even further. Specializations such as anesthesia, dentistry, and behavior offer technicians the chance to focus on specific areas of interest and expertise. For example, a veterinary technician specializing in anesthesia will have advanced knowledge in anesthetic protocols, pain management, and monitoring techniques, making them an invaluable asset in surgical teams.

In research and laboratory settings, veterinary technicians contribute to scientific advancements by assisting with experiments and data collection. Their responsibilities may include handling laboratory animals, administering treatments, and recording observations. The meticulous nature of this work requires a keen eye for detail and adherence to ethical standards, as the welfare of research animals is of utmost importance.

Veterinary technicians may also find fulfilling roles in wildlife and exotic animal care. Working in zoos, aquariums, or wildlife rehabilitation centers, they apply their skills to a diverse range of species, each with unique needs and behaviors. This role demands adaptability and a willingness to continually learn, as caring for exotic animals often involves unconventional methods and approaches.

In conclusion, the roles and responsibilities of veterinary technicians are vast and varied, encompassing a wide range of tasks and specialties. Their contributions to veterinary medicine are invaluable, as they ensure the smooth operation of clinical practices and the well-being of animals in their care. By embracing the diverse opportunities available within the profession, veterinary technicians can carve out fulfilling careers that align with their passions and strengths. Whether in clinical practice, research, education, or public health, these professionals are integral to the advancement and success of veterinary medicine.

Career Pathways and Opportunities

The journey of a veterinary technician is a gateway to a myriad of career pathways, each offering unique opportunities to impact the field of veterinary medicine. This profession, defined by its diversity and adaptability, invites individuals to explore roles that align with their passions and strengths. From clinical practice to specialized fields, the career possibilities for veterinary technicians are as expansive as they are rewarding.

Clinical practice is often the starting point for many veterinary technicians, providing a foundational experience in animal care. Within a veterinary clinic or hospital, technicians perform a variety of tasks that are critical to patient care. This environment offers exposure to a broad range of medical cases, from routine check-ups to complex surgical procedures. For those who enjoy direct animal interaction and thrive in a fast-paced setting, clinical practice is both challenging and fulfilling.

Beyond the general veterinary clinic, there are specialized practices that cater to specific types of animals or medical specialties. Some technicians choose to work in equine clinics, where they focus on the care of horses. This role requires knowledge of equine anatomy and common health issues, and often involves working outdoors or traveling to stables and farms. Similarly, technicians interested in aquatic life may find their niche in practices that specialize in fish and marine animals, contributing to the health and care of these unique species.

Emergency and critical care is another specialized field that offers dynamic and high-intensity work. Veterinary technicians in this area are integral to emergency response teams, providing urgent care to animals in life-threatening situations. The ability to think quickly and remain composed under pressure is essential. Emergency settings require technicians to expand their skill set, often involving advanced procedures such as resuscitation, wound management, and intensive monitoring.

For those with a passion for wildlife and conservation, working in zoos, wildlife rehabilitation centers, or conservation organizations presents an exciting opportunity. Veterinary technicians in these settings care for a diverse array of species, each with unique needs and behaviors. This role often involves collaboration with zoologists and conservationists, contributing to research and public education efforts aimed at preserving biodiversity and protecting endangered species.

The realm of research and academia offers another pathway for veterinary technicians interested in scientific inquiry and education. In research facilities, technicians assist with studies that advance veterinary medicine and animal health. Their responsibilities may include handling research animals, conducting experiments, and collecting data. This role demands meticulous attention to detail and adherence to ethical standards for animal welfare.

Education and training roles allow veterinary technicians to share their knowledge and experience with aspiring professionals. By teaching in veterinary technology programs or conducting workshops and seminars, technicians can inspire and educate the next generation of veterinary professionals. This career pathway not only contributes to the growth of the profession but also offers personal fulfillment through mentorship and leadership.

Veterinary technicians with an interest in business and management may explore opportunities in practice management or sales. As practice managers, they oversee the operations of a veterinary practice, handling tasks such as scheduling, budgeting, and staff management. In sales, technicians can leverage their expertise to promote veterinary products and services, working for pharmaceutical companies or equipment manufacturers. These roles require strong communication and organizational skills, as well as an understanding of the veterinary industry.

The field of veterinary technology also offers avenues for further specialization and certification. Advanced certifications are available in areas such as anesthesia, dentistry, behavior, and nutrition, allowing technicians to deepen their expertise and enhance their career prospects. Pursuing specialization can lead to roles that focus on specific areas of interest, providing opportunities for professional growth and recognition.

Public health is an emerging field where veterinary technicians can make a significant impact. In roles that bridge veterinary medicine and public health, technicians contribute to disease prevention and control efforts, focusing on zoonotic diseases that affect both animals and humans. Their work may involve surveillance, education, and policy development, highlighting the interconnectedness of animal and human health.

In addition to specific career pathways, the profession of veterinary technology offers flexibility and adaptability. Technicians may choose to work part-time or pursue freelance opportunities, providing services such as pet care consulting or veterinary writing. This flexibility allows individuals to balance their professional aspirations with personal commitments, creating a career that is both sustainable and rewarding.

Regardless of the chosen path, continuous professional development is essential for veterinary technicians to stay current with advancements in the field. Engaging in continuing education, attending conferences, and participating in professional organizations are valuable ways to enhance skills and knowledge. By embracing lifelong learning, technicians can adapt to changes in the industry and maintain a high standard of care for their patients.

The career pathways and opportunities available to veterinary technicians are vast and varied, reflecting the dynamic nature of the profession. Whether working in clinical practice, research, education, or public health, these professionals are united by their commitment to animal welfare and their dedication to advancing veterinary medicine. By exploring the diverse options available, veterinary technicians can forge fulfilling careers that align with their passions and contribute to the well-being of animals and communities. With determination and a willingness to explore new opportunities, veterinary technicians can make a lasting impact in the field and achieve personal and professional fulfillment.

Ethical Considerations in Practice

Ethical considerations are at the heart of the veterinary technician profession, guiding decision-making processes and ensuring the welfare of animals under their care. Navigating ethical dilemmas requires a firm understanding of the principles that govern veterinary practice, as well as the ability to balance the interests of animals, clients, and the veterinary team. As veterinary technicians often find themselves on the front lines of animal care, they must be equipped to handle complex situations with integrity and professionalism.

One of the primary ethical responsibilities of veterinary technicians is to advocate for the welfare of animals. This duty involves ensuring that animals receive appropriate care, treatment, and respect throughout their interactions with veterinary professionals. Veterinary technicians must prioritize the well-being of their patients, even in scenarios where clients may have differing opinions or financial constraints. Advocating for an animal's best interest might mean discussing alternative treatment options or, in some cases, making difficult recommendations regarding euthanasia when quality of life is severely compromised.

Informed consent is another crucial ethical consideration in veterinary practice. Veterinary technicians play a pivotal role in facilitating communication between veterinarians and pet owners, ensuring that clients fully understand the implications of proposed treatments or procedures. This process involves providing clear, accurate, and comprehensive information, allowing clients to make informed decisions about their pets' care. Ethical practice demands transparency and honesty, as well as respect for the client's autonomy in decision-making.

Confidentiality is an ethical cornerstone that veterinary technicians must uphold. Just as in human healthcare, protecting the privacy of client and patient information is imperative. This responsibility extends to maintaining the confidentiality of medical records and any personal information shared by clients. Ethical breaches in confidentiality can erode trust between clients and veterinary professionals, underscoring the importance of discretion and professionalism at all times.

The issue of affordability and access to veterinary care presents an ethical challenge that veterinary technicians frequently encounter. Many pet owners face financial constraints that limit their ability to provide optimal care for their animals. In such situations, veterinary technicians must navigate the delicate balance between delivering high-quality care and respecting the financial limitations of clients. This challenge often requires creativity in finding feasible solutions, such as exploring payment plans, offering preventative care advice, or discussing alternative treatment options that align with the client's budget.

Ethical considerations also arise in the context of professional boundaries. Veterinary technicians, driven by a passion for animal welfare, may feel compelled to go above and beyond in their roles. However, it is essential to recognize and respect the boundaries of the technician's scope of practice. Performing tasks or making decisions that fall outside of their expertise or authority can have serious ethical and legal implications. Maintaining professional boundaries ensures that technicians work collaboratively within the veterinary team, relying on veterinarians for guidance and direction when necessary.

The use of animals in research and education is another area where ethical considerations are paramount. Veterinary technicians involved in research must adhere to strict ethical guidelines that prioritize the welfare of research animals. This responsibility involves ensuring humane treatment, minimizing suffering, and implementing appropriate care protocols. In educational settings, technicians must balance the need for hands-on learning experiences with ethical considerations related to the use of live animals in teaching.

Euthanasia, while often necessary in veterinary practice, presents profound ethical challenges. Veterinary technicians must approach this sensitive issue with compassion and empathy, recognizing the emotional toll it takes on clients and themselves. Ethical practice requires technicians to support clients in making informed decisions about euthanasia, providing guidance and emotional support throughout the process. Additionally, technicians must be mindful of their own well-being, seeking support when needed to cope with the emotional impact of euthanasia.

Professional integrity is a fundamental ethical principle that underpins all aspects of veterinary practice. Veterinary technicians must adhere to established codes of ethics, demonstrating honesty, accountability, and respect in their interactions with colleagues, clients, and patients. Ethical practice involves acknowledging and addressing conflicts of interest, avoiding actions that may compromise professional judgment, and upholding the reputation of the veterinary profession.

In conclusion, ethical considerations are integral to the veterinary technician profession, shaping the way technicians interact with animals, clients, and the veterinary team. By adhering to ethical principles and prioritizing animal welfare, veterinary technicians uphold the values of integrity, compassion, and professionalism. Through continuous education and a commitment to ethical practice, technicians can navigate the challenges of their profession with confidence and ensure the well-being of the animals in their care.

Professional Development and Continuing Education

The path of a veterinary technician is not static; it is a journey of continual learning and growth. Professional development and continuing education are essential components that contribute to the competence and success of veterinary technicians. As the field of veterinary medicine evolves, staying abreast of new advancements, techniques, and knowledge is imperative for providing the highest standard of care to animals and ensuring personal career advancement.

Professional development encompasses a wide range of activities and opportunities that enhance a veterinary technician's skills, knowledge, and abilities. Engaging in professional development allows technicians to refine their existing competencies and acquire new ones, fostering a culture of lifelong learning. This may involve attending workshops, seminars, and conferences where experts share insights on the latest trends and innovations in veterinary medicine. Such events provide invaluable networking opportunities, allowing technicians to connect with peers, mentors, and industry leaders who can offer guidance and support.

Continuing education is a critical aspect of maintaining licensure and certification for veterinary technicians. Most regulatory bodies require technicians to complete a certain number of continuing education credits within a specified period to remain in good standing. This requirement ensures that technicians remain informed about the latest developments in the field, including new treatments, diagnostic tools, and best practices. By fulfilling continuing education requirements, technicians demonstrate their commitment to professional excellence and ethical standards.

Online platforms have revolutionized access to continuing education, making it more convenient than ever for veterinary technicians to enhance their knowledge. Webinars, virtual courses, and online certifications offer flexibility, allowing technicians to learn at their own pace and according to their schedules. These digital resources cover a diverse array of topics, from specialized medical procedures to client communication and practice management, catering to the varied interests and needs of the veterinary community.

Specialization is another avenue for professional development that enables veterinary technicians to focus on specific areas of interest. By pursuing advanced certifications in fields such as anesthesia, dentistry, behavior, or emergency and critical care, technicians can deepen their expertise and expand their career opportunities. Specialization not only enhances the individual's skill set but also contributes to the overall quality of care provided by veterinary teams. Technicians with specialized knowledge become valuable assets, often taking on leadership roles and contributing to the training and mentorship of their peers.

Mentorship plays a vital role in the professional development of veterinary technicians. Experienced mentors can provide guidance, share valuable insights, and offer support as technicians navigate their careers. Establishing a mentoring relationship can be mutually beneficial, as mentors also gain fresh perspectives and the satisfaction of contributing to the growth of the profession. Whether formal or informal, mentorship fosters a collaborative environment where knowledge is shared and professional bonds are strengthened.

In addition to formal education and training, self-directed learning is a powerful tool for professional development. Veterinary technicians are encouraged to seek out resources such as textbooks, journals, and online forums to stay informed about new research and emerging practices. Engaging in self-directed study not only enhances knowledge but also cultivates critical thinking and problem-solving skills, which are essential for adapting to the ever-changing landscape of veterinary medicine.

Participation in professional organizations is another effective way for veterinary technicians to engage in continuous learning and development. Organizations such as the National Association of Veterinary Technicians in America (NAVTA) provide members with access to educational resources, professional development programs, and networking opportunities. Membership in such organizations also allows technicians to contribute to the advancement of the profession by participating in advocacy efforts, research initiatives, and policy development.

Leadership development is a key component of professional growth for veterinary technicians seeking to advance their careers. Leadership skills are valuable not only for those aspiring to managerial positions but also for technicians who wish to influence positive change within their teams and organizations. Leadership training programs and workshops equip technicians with the skills needed to effectively communicate, motivate, and inspire others, fostering a collaborative and productive work environment.

Reflective practice is an often-overlooked aspect of professional development that encourages veterinary technicians to critically evaluate their experiences and identify areas for improvement. By reflecting on their actions, decisions, and interactions, technicians gain insights into their strengths and weaknesses, enabling them to set goals for personal and professional growth. Reflective practice fosters self-awareness and accountability, essential qualities for maintaining high standards of care and ethical conduct.

Balancing professional development with personal well-being is crucial for sustaining a long and rewarding career in veterinary medicine. Veterinary technicians must prioritize self-care and work-life balance to prevent burnout and maintain their passion for the profession. Setting realistic goals, managing time effectively, and seeking support from peers and mentors can help technicians navigate the demands of continuing education while maintaining a healthy and fulfilling personal life.

Professional development and continuing education are integral components of a veterinary technician's career journey. By embracing opportunities for growth and learning, technicians can enhance their skills, advance their careers, and contribute to the advancement of veterinary medicine. Through dedication to lifelong learning, veterinary technicians uphold the values of excellence and professionalism, ensuring the well-being of the animals they care for and the success of the veterinary teams they are a part of.

Real-life Case Studies from Veterinary Technicians

The world of veterinary technicians is filled with diverse challenges and rewarding experiences that shape their professional journeys. Real-life case studies provide invaluable insights into the complexities and nuances of this profession, highlighting the skills and dedication required to navigate a variety of situations. Through these narratives, we gain a deeper understanding of the vital role veterinary technicians play in animal healthcare and the profound impact they have on the lives of both animals and their owners.

One notable case involves a veterinary technician named Laura, who worked in a bustling emergency clinic. Late one night, a frantic owner rushed in with a dog named Max, who had been hit by a car. Max was in critical condition, suffering from multiple fractures and internal injuries. Laura's quick response and calm demeanor were crucial as she immediately initiated triage, assessing Max's vital signs and stabilizing him for further treatment. Her ability to remain composed under pressure allowed the veterinary team to perform life-saving surgery. Throughout the night, Laura monitored Max's condition, administering pain relief and fluids, while providing emotional support to his distraught owner. Her dedication and expertise were instrumental in Max's recovery, underscoring the critical role veterinary technicians play in emergency care.

In another instance, a technician named Sarah found herself faced with a challenging behavioral case. A cat named Whiskers, known for his aggressive tendencies, was brought in for a routine dental cleaning. Understanding the importance of reducing stress for both the animal and the staff, Sarah worked closely with the veterinarian to develop a strategy that prioritized Whiskers' comfort. She employed her knowledge of animal behavior to create a calming environment, using pheromone diffusers and gentle handling techniques. Her empathetic approach and patience not only facilitated a successful procedure but also helped Whiskers to feel more at ease during future visits. This case highlights the importance of understanding animal behavior and the positive impact of compassionate care.

A different kind of challenge arose when Mark, a veterinary technician at a wildlife rehabilitation center, was tasked with caring for an injured bald eagle. The majestic bird had suffered a fractured wing and required specialized treatment. Mark's extensive knowledge of avian anatomy and rehabilitation techniques was put to the test as he assisted the veterinarian in designing a recovery plan. He meticulously managed the eagle's care, ensuring that its wing was properly immobilized and that it received a balanced diet tailored to its nutritional needs. Mark's attention to detail and commitment to the eagle's rehabilitation ultimately led to its successful release back into the wild. This case exemplifies the diverse knowledge and skills required of veterinary technicians working with wildlife.

In a more routine setting, Emily, a technician at a small animal clinic, encountered a case that tested her communication skills. A young couple brought in their new puppy, Daisy, for her first wellness exam. As first-time pet owners, they were eager but overwhelmed by the responsibilities of pet care. Emily recognized the importance of educating them about preventive care, nutrition, and training. She took the time to patiently explain each aspect of Daisy's care, using relatable analogies and encouraging questions. Her approachable demeanor and thorough guidance empowered the couple to confidently care for Daisy, strengthening the bond between them and their new pet. This case underscores the significant role veterinary technicians play in client education and support.

Another illustrative case involves a technician named James, who worked in a research facility conducting studies on feline nutrition. One of the cats under his care developed a sudden allergic reaction, presenting symptoms of swelling and difficulty breathing. James' immediate recognition of the signs and prompt action in administering antihistamines were crucial in averting a more severe reaction. His vigilance and ability to act swiftly ensured the cat's safety and allowed the research to continue without interruption. This scenario highlights the importance of keen observation and quick decision-making in research settings.

These case studies offer a glimpse into the varied and rewarding experiences of veterinary technicians. Each scenario showcases the diverse skills and qualities that define the profession, from emergency response and patient care to communication and education. Veterinary technicians are often the unsung heroes of animal healthcare, working tirelessly behind the scenes to ensure the well-being of their patients.

In addition to technical expertise, these cases emphasize the importance of collaboration and teamwork within veterinary settings. Veterinary technicians are integral members of the healthcare team, working closely with veterinarians, fellow technicians, and support staff to provide comprehensive care. Their ability to communicate effectively and work collaboratively enhances the overall efficiency and success of veterinary practices.

Furthermore, these narratives highlight the personal fulfillment and sense of purpose that veterinary technicians derive from their work. The opportunity to make a tangible difference in the lives of animals and their owners is a powerful motivator, driving technicians to continually refine their skills and expand their knowledge. Whether in clinical practice, research, or wildlife rehabilitation, veterinary technicians are united by their passion for animal welfare and their dedication to advancing the field of veterinary medicine.

In conclusion, real-life case studies from veterinary technicians reveal the depth and breadth of this dynamic profession. Through their stories, we gain a deeper appreciation for the challenges and triumphs that define their daily work. Veterinary technicians are not only skilled professionals but also compassionate caregivers and educators, making a lasting impact on the animals and communities they serve. As the field of veterinary medicine continues to evolve, the contributions of veterinary technicians will remain indispensable, shaping the future of animal healthcare and enhancing the lives of countless animals and their owners.

CHAPTER 3
MASTERING VETERINARY ANATOMY AND PHYSIOLOGY

Introduction to Animal Anatomy

Understanding animal anatomy is foundational for anyone pursuing a career in veterinary medicine. It serves as the starting point from which all veterinary knowledge branches out, providing the essential framework for diagnosing ailments and developing treatment plans. By grasping the intricacies of animal structure, veterinary technicians can deliver more precise and effective care, enhancing both their confidence and competence in various clinical settings.

Animal anatomy, while complex, is fascinating in its detail and diversity. Each species possesses unique anatomical features that have evolved to suit their environments and lifestyles. For instance, the elongated neck of a giraffe enables it to reach high foliage, while the streamlined body of a fish allows efficient navigation through water. These adaptations are not merely superficial; they are intricately linked to the animal's internal structure and biological functions.

One of the primary systems to explore in animal anatomy is the skeletal system. This framework provides support and shape to the body, protecting vital organs and enabling movement. In mammals, the skeleton is composed of two main parts: the axial skeleton, which includes the skull, vertebral column, and rib cage, and the appendicular skeleton, comprising the limbs and girdles. Understanding the skeletal variations across species is crucial, as it impacts everything from mobility to surgical interventions.

The muscular system works in tandem with the skeletal system to facilitate movement. Muscles contract and relax, pulling on bones to produce motion. Veterinary technicians must familiarize themselves with the major muscle groups and their functions, as this knowledge is vital for assessing injuries and implementing rehabilitation protocols. The arrangement of muscles can vary significantly between species, influencing factors such as speed, strength, and endurance.

The circulatory system is another critical aspect of animal anatomy. It is responsible for the transport of nutrients, oxygen, and waste products throughout the body. A comprehensive understanding of the heart, blood vessels, and blood composition is essential for monitoring cardiovascular health and administering treatments such as intravenous fluids. The circulatory system's efficiency can differ greatly among species, with adaptations that support specific metabolic demands.

The respiratory system's primary function is gas exchange, supplying oxygen to the body and expelling carbon dioxide. Knowledge of the respiratory anatomy, including the trachea, bronchi, and lungs, is crucial for evaluating breathing issues and providing appropriate interventions. In species such as birds, the respiratory system is highly specialized, featuring air sacs that allow continuous airflow through the lungs, a unique adaptation for sustained flight.

Digestive anatomy varies widely across species, reflecting their dietary habits and nutritional needs. Herbivores, carnivores, and omnivores each have distinct digestive structures that enable them to process different types of food efficiently. Understanding these differences is vital for developing appropriate dietary plans and diagnosing gastrointestinal disorders. For example, ruminants like cows possess a complex, multi-chambered stomach that facilitates the breakdown of fibrous plant material.

The nervous system orchestrates the body's responses to internal and external stimuli, making it a central component of animal anatomy. It comprises the brain, spinal cord, and peripheral nerves, all of which work together to regulate bodily functions and behaviors. Veterinary technicians must be adept at recognizing neurological signs and symptoms, as they often provide critical clues for diagnosing conditions that affect the nervous system.

The integumentary system, which includes the skin, hair, feathers, and nails, serves as the body's first line of defense against environmental threats. It plays a significant role in thermoregulation, sensation, and protection. Familiarity with the integumentary system is essential for diagnosing and treating dermatological issues, as well as understanding species-specific adaptations, such as the insulating fur of polar animals or the water-repellent feathers of aquatic birds.

The reproductive system is integral to the continuation of species and varies widely across the animal kingdom. A thorough understanding of reproductive anatomy is necessary for managing breeding programs, diagnosing reproductive disorders, and assisting with birthing processes. Veterinary technicians often play a crucial role in reproductive health, particularly in settings such as farms and zoos.

Practical application of anatomical knowledge extends beyond the classroom or textbook. It requires hands-on experience and continuous learning. Veterinary technicians should seize every opportunity to participate in dissections, observe surgeries, and engage with real-world cases. These experiences reinforce theoretical knowledge and enhance technical skills, preparing technicians for the diverse challenges they will encounter in their careers.

The study of animal anatomy is not an isolated task but a collaborative endeavor. It involves working alongside veterinarians, fellow technicians, and other professionals to provide comprehensive care. Open communication and teamwork are essential, as they foster an environment where knowledge can be shared, and insights gained through collective experience.

For those dedicated to mastering veterinary anatomy, the rewards are immense. A deep understanding of animal structure and function enables technicians to excel in their roles, providing high-quality care and making informed decisions that impact animal health and welfare. As veterinary medicine continues to advance, the foundation of anatomical knowledge remains a constant, guiding professionals in their pursuit of excellence and compassion in animal care.

Understanding Physiological Systems

Understanding physiological systems is essential for anyone involved in veterinary medicine. These systems are the intricate networks that allow animals to survive, grow, and thrive, each one performing vital functions that sustain life. By comprehending how these systems operate and interact, veterinary technicians can better diagnose issues, implement treatments, and ensure the overall well-being of their patients.

The circulatory system is a cornerstone of animal physiology, responsible for transporting nutrients, gases, and waste products throughout the body. It comprises the heart, blood vessels, and blood, each playing a critical role in maintaining homeostasis. The heart acts as a pump, propelling oxygen-rich blood through arteries to tissues and organs. After delivering oxygen and nutrients, blood returns through veins to the heart, where it is pumped to the lungs for re-oxygenation. Veterinary technicians must understand the nuances of this system to assess cardiovascular health and administer interventions such as fluid therapy or emergency resuscitation.

Closely linked to the circulatory system is the respiratory system, which facilitates gas exchange. The process begins as air enters through the nose or mouth, traveling down the trachea into the lungs. Here, oxygen diffuses into the bloodstream, while carbon dioxide, a metabolic waste product, is expelled. This exchange is vital for cellular respiration, which produces the energy required for bodily functions. Technicians need to recognize normal and abnormal respiratory patterns, as well as understand the mechanisms of diseases like pneumonia or asthma, to provide effective care.

The digestive system breaks down food into nutrients that the body can absorb and utilize. It starts with ingestion, where food is taken in through the mouth. Mechanical and chemical digestion occurs in the stomach and intestines, breaking food into simpler molecules. These nutrients are absorbed into the bloodstream and transported to cells for energy, growth, and repair. The digestive system also involves waste elimination, with undigested material excreted as feces. Understanding this system aids in diagnosing issues such as obstructions, infections, or malabsorption disorders, allowing technicians to suggest dietary adjustments or treatments.

The nervous system is the command center of the body, coordinating voluntary and involuntary actions. It consists of the central nervous system, comprised of the brain and spinal cord, and the peripheral nervous system, which includes nerves extending throughout the body. The nervous system processes sensory information, controls muscles, and regulates bodily functions. Recognizing signs of neurological disorders, such as seizures or paralysis, requires a solid grasp of this system. Veterinary technicians often assist in neurological examinations and monitoring, contributing to accurate diagnoses and effective treatments.

The endocrine system is a network of glands that produce hormones, chemical messengers that regulate physiological processes. Hormones influence growth, metabolism, reproduction, and stress responses. Key endocrine glands include the pituitary, thyroid, and adrenal glands, each releasing specific hormones into the bloodstream. Imbalances in hormone levels can lead to conditions like diabetes or hyperthyroidism. Veterinary technicians play a role in monitoring these conditions, collecting samples for analysis and administering medications.

The urinary system is responsible for filtering blood and removing waste products through urine. It includes the kidneys, ureters, bladder, and urethra. The kidneys filter blood, reabsorbing essential nutrients and excreting waste products and excess fluid. This process maintains electrolyte balance and blood pressure. Technicians need to understand the urinary system to identify signs of kidney disease, infections, or blockages, often performing tasks such as urine collection and analysis.

The immune system defends the body against pathogens and foreign substances. It consists of various cells, tissues, and organs, including white blood cells, lymph nodes, and the spleen. The immune system identifies and destroys harmful invaders, preventing illness and infection. Veterinary technicians must recognize symptoms of immune-related diseases, administer vaccines, and assist in diagnostic testing to ensure effective immune function.

The integumentary system, encompassing the skin, hair, and nails, serves as a barrier against environmental threats. It plays a role in thermoregulation, sensation, and protection. Technicians need to understand this system to identify dermatological issues, such as infections, allergies, or parasites, and to administer treatments like topical medications or baths.

The reproductive system varies widely among species and is crucial for the propagation of life. It includes organs involved in producing gametes, facilitating fertilization, and supporting embryonic development. Veterinary technicians often assist in reproductive health management, performing tasks related to breeding, pregnancy, and neonatal care.

The skeletal and muscular systems work together to provide structure, protection, and movement. The skeleton supports the body and protects internal organs, while muscles contract to produce movement. Understanding these systems helps technicians assess injuries, support rehabilitation, and implement exercise regimens for recovery or maintenance of physical health.

Integrating knowledge of these physiological systems allows veterinary technicians to provide comprehensive care. Each system is interconnected, and a disruption in one can affect others. By understanding these connections, technicians can better anticipate complications, implement holistic treatment plans, and contribute to the well-being of their patients.

Hands-on experience is crucial for mastering physiological systems. Engaging in clinical practice, observing surgeries, and participating in case studies reinforce theoretical knowledge and enhance practical skills. Collaboration with veterinarians and other technicians fosters an environment of learning and support, promoting a deeper understanding of complex physiological processes.

The study of physiological systems is a dynamic and rewarding pursuit. It empowers veterinary technicians with the knowledge and skills necessary to excel in their roles, making a tangible difference in the lives of animals and their owners. Through dedication, curiosity, and a commitment to excellence, technicians can contribute to the advancement of veterinary medicine and enhance the field's understanding of animal physiology.

Pathophysiology in Veterinary Medicine

Pathophysiology in veterinary medicine is the study of how normal physiological processes are altered by disease or injury in animals. This field is crucial for veterinary technicians to grasp, as it bridges the gap between understanding healthy physiological systems and recognizing the manifestations of disease. By mastering pathophysiology, technicians can better assist veterinarians in diagnosing conditions, monitoring treatments, and improving patient outcomes.

The onset of disease often begins with subtle changes at the cellular level. Cells may be damaged by various factors, including pathogens, toxins, or trauma, leading to cellular dysfunction or death. This cellular response is the foundation of pathophysiological changes and can result in inflammation, necrosis, or fibrosis. Recognizing these changes is vital for identifying the underlying causes of disease and predicting its progression. For instance, an understanding of cellular damage is essential when dealing with conditions like dermatitis, where external irritants lead to inflammation and skin lesions.

Inflammation is a common pathophysiological response to injury or infection, characterized by redness, heat, swelling, pain, and loss of function. It is the body's natural defense mechanism, aiming to eliminate harmful stimuli and initiate healing. However, chronic inflammation can contribute to disease development, such as arthritis or inflammatory bowel disease. Veterinary technicians need to identify signs of inflammation and understand its role in disease processes to provide appropriate interventions and support healing.

The immune system plays a critical role in pathophysiology, protecting the body from infections and foreign substances. However, dysregulation of the immune response can lead to autoimmune diseases, where the body attacks its own tissues, or immunodeficiency, where the body is unable to mount an adequate defense. Understanding immune-mediated pathophysiology is crucial for managing conditions like lupus or feline immunodeficiency virus (FIV). Technicians often assist in diagnostic testing and monitoring immune responses to ensure effective management of these diseases.

Cardiovascular pathophysiology involves changes in heart and blood vessel function, leading to conditions such as heart failure, hypertension, or arrhythmias. These disorders can result from structural abnormalities, electrical disturbances, or impaired blood flow. Recognizing the signs of cardiovascular disease, such as coughing, exercise intolerance, or syncope, is essential for timely intervention. Technicians play a key role in monitoring vital signs, administering medications, and educating owners on managing chronic heart conditions.

Respiratory pathophysiology encompasses disorders that affect the airways, lungs, or pleura, leading to impaired gas exchange and breathing difficulties. Conditions such as asthma, pneumonia, or pleural effusion can alter normal respiratory function. Veterinary technicians must be adept at assessing respiratory rate, effort, and sounds, as well as providing oxygen therapy and supporting ventilation. Early recognition of respiratory distress is crucial to prevent severe complications and improve patient outcomes.

Gastrointestinal pathophysiology involves disruptions in digestion, absorption, or motility, leading to conditions like gastritis, pancreatitis, or intestinal obstructions. These disorders can manifest as vomiting, diarrhea, or abdominal pain. Understanding the pathophysiology of gastrointestinal diseases allows technicians to assist in diagnostic procedures, such as radiography or endoscopy, and implement dietary modifications or supportive care to alleviate symptoms.

Renal pathophysiology encompasses disorders of the kidneys or urinary tract, leading to conditions such as acute kidney injury, chronic kidney disease, or urinary tract infections. These disorders can result in electrolyte imbalances, dehydration, or toxin accumulation. Recognizing signs of renal dysfunction, such as polyuria, polydipsia, or azotemia, is essential for early intervention. Technicians often assist in fluid therapy, monitoring renal function, and educating owners on long-term management strategies.

Endocrine pathophysiology involves imbalances in hormone production or action, leading to conditions like diabetes mellitus, hyperthyroidism, or Cushing's disease. These disorders can result from glandular dysfunction, receptor defects, or feedback disruptions. Recognizing signs of endocrine disorders, such as weight changes, polyphagia, or lethargy, is crucial for timely diagnosis and treatment. Technicians play a vital role in monitoring blood glucose levels, administering medications, and providing dietary advice to manage these conditions effectively.

Neurological pathophysiology encompasses disorders of the brain, spinal cord, or peripheral nerves, leading to conditions like epilepsy, intervertebral disc disease, or peripheral neuropathy. These disorders can manifest as seizures, ataxia, or paresis. Understanding the pathophysiology of neurological diseases allows technicians to assist in diagnostic imaging, such as MRI or CT scans, and support rehabilitation efforts to improve neurological function and quality of life.

Oncological pathophysiology involves the uncontrolled growth of abnormal cells, leading to benign or malignant tumors. Cancer can affect any organ or tissue, with potential for local invasion or metastasis. Recognizing signs of cancer, such as unexplained weight loss, masses, or changes in behavior, is essential for early detection and intervention. Technicians play a crucial role in administering chemotherapy, managing pain, and providing palliative care to support patients and their families.

The complexity of pathophysiological processes underscores the importance of continuous learning and collaboration in veterinary medicine. Veterinary technicians must stay informed about the latest research and advancements in disease mechanisms to provide the highest standard of care. Engaging in professional development opportunities, such as workshops or conferences, allows technicians to expand their knowledge and refine their skills.

Mastering pathophysiology in veterinary medicine empowers technicians to make informed decisions, improving patient outcomes and advancing the field of animal healthcare. Through dedication, curiosity, and a commitment to excellence, veterinary technicians can navigate the complexities of disease processes, providing compassionate and effective care to animals and their owners. The study of pathophysiology is a dynamic and rewarding pursuit, offering opportunities for growth, discovery, and the chance to make a meaningful impact on animal health and welfare.

Comparative Anatomy: Domestic Animals

Comparative anatomy provides a fascinating lens through which to view the structural differences and similarities among various domestic animals. This field of study is essential for veterinary technicians, as it enables them to understand how anatomical variations influence the health, behavior, and care of different species. By comparing the anatomy of domestic animals, technicians can tailor medical treatments, dietary plans, and care routines to suit each species' unique needs.

The skeletal system is a prime example of anatomical diversity among domestic animals. Consider the elongated spine and flexible vertebrae of a cat, which provide agility and enable it to land on its feet after a fall. Contrast this with the sturdy, fused vertebrae of a horse adapted for strength and endurance in running. Understanding these differences is crucial when assessing injuries or planning rehabilitation programs. In dogs, the variation in skull shapes, from the elongated snout of a Greyhound to the flat face of a Bulldog, affects not only appearance but also breathing and dental health.

The muscular system also varies significantly, tailored to the specific functions and lifestyles of different species. Horses, for instance, have well-developed hindquarters, enabling powerful propulsion, crucial for galloping. Cats possess a higher proportion of fast-twitch muscle fibers, facilitating sudden bursts of speed and agility, essential for hunting. Recognizing these muscular adaptations allows technicians to better understand species-specific exercise needs and potential muscular disorders.

The digestive system offers another area ripe for comparison. Ruminants like cows and sheep possess a complex, multi-chambered stomach designed for breaking down fibrous plant material through fermentation. This contrasts sharply with the simple, single-chambered stomach of carnivores like dogs and cats, which are adapted to digest protein-rich diets efficiently. Understanding these differences is vital for developing appropriate feeding regimens and diagnosing gastrointestinal issues. For instance, feeding high-fiber diets to carnivores can lead to digestive upset, while insufficient fiber in a ruminant's diet can cause serious health problems.

The respiratory system exhibits notable variations, particularly in how different animals have adapted to their environments. Birds, though not typically classified as domestic animals, provide an interesting comparison with their highly efficient respiratory system, featuring air sacs that allow continuous airflow through the lungs. This adaptation supports the high metabolic demands of flight. In contrast, dogs, especially brachycephalic breeds, may experience restricted airflow due to their shortened skull structure, leading to breathing difficulties. Understanding these respiratory variations is crucial for identifying and managing conditions like brachycephalic obstructive airway syndrome in certain dog breeds.

The cardiovascular system, while generally similar across species, has adaptations that reflect specific physiological needs. For example, the large hearts of athletic species like horses are well adapted to pump significant volumes of blood, supporting high levels of physical exertion. Dogs, especially working breeds, also have robust cardiovascular systems to endure prolonged activity. Recognizing these differences aids in assessing cardiovascular health and fitness, allowing for tailored exercise and conditioning programs.

The nervous system, responsible for controlling and coordinating bodily functions, shows both similarities and differences among species. Domestic animals like dogs and cats share a similar brain structure, but the size and complexity of certain brain regions can vary, influencing behavior and sensory perception. For instance, dogs have a highly developed olfactory system, underscoring their reliance on scent for communication and navigation. Understanding these neurological differences helps technicians interpret behavior and identify potential neurological disorders.

The reproductive system also presents intriguing differences among domestic animals. The estrous cycles, gestation periods, and reproductive anatomy vary significantly, influencing breeding and management practices. Horses, for instance, are seasonal breeders with a lengthy gestation period, while rabbits can breed year-round with a much shorter gestation. Recognizing these reproductive variations is essential for managing breeding programs and ensuring the health and welfare of both the mother and offspring.

The integumentary system, encompassing the skin, hair, and nails, also varies, reflecting adaptations to different environments and lifestyles. Dogs and cats have fur that provides insulation and protection, with variations in coat length and type among breeds. Horses have a thicker skin and a mane, offering protection and aiding in thermoregulation. Understanding these differences helps in diagnosing dermatological issues and managing skin and coat health.

A deeper understanding of comparative anatomy extends beyond structural differences to encompass physiological adaptations. For instance, the metabolic rate of different species can influence everything from diet to medication dosages. Cats, with their unique liver enzyme pathways, require careful consideration when prescribing medications, as they metabolize drugs differently than dogs. Recognizing these physiological nuances is critical for ensuring safe and effective treatment.

Comparative anatomy offers a rich and rewarding field of study, providing veterinary technicians with the insights needed to tailor care to the unique needs of each species. By understanding the anatomical and physiological differences among domestic animals, technicians can deliver more effective and compassionate care, improving the health and well-being of their patients. Through dedication, curiosity, and a commitment to excellence, veterinary technicians can harness the power of comparative anatomy to make a meaningful impact in the lives of animals and their caretakers.

Clinical Relevance of Anatomy and Physiology

The clinical relevance of anatomy and physiology in veterinary medicine cannot be overstated. These foundational sciences are the bedrock upon which all diagnostic and therapeutic decisions are made. A thorough understanding of anatomy and physiology allows veterinary technicians to interpret clinical signs accurately, assist in surgical procedures, and contribute significantly to the overall health management of animals.

Consider the scenario of a dog brought into a clinic with lameness in one of its hind legs. A technician well-versed in anatomy can quickly narrow down potential issues by understanding the complex interplay of bones, joints, muscles, tendons, and nerves in the limb. Knowing the anatomical landmarks, such as the femur, tibia, and patella, helps in identifying possible fractures or dislocations. Similarly, understanding the physiology of the canine musculoskeletal system enables the technician to consider conditions like arthritis or ligament tears, such as a cranial cruciate ligament (CCL) rupture.

In the realm of diagnostics, anatomy and physiology play a pivotal role. For instance, when performing radiographs, technicians must position the animal correctly to capture clear images of the area of interest. This requires a detailed understanding of anatomical structures to ensure that the images are diagnostically useful. Additionally, interpreting these images requires knowledge of normal anatomy to differentiate between healthy and pathological conditions.

Surgical procedures are another area where anatomy and physiology are indispensable. During surgery, technicians assist veterinarians by providing instruments, monitoring anesthesia, and ensuring aseptic conditions. Knowledge of anatomical layers, such as skin, fascia, and muscle, is crucial for efficient and safe surgical assistance. Moreover, understanding the physiological responses to anesthesia, such as changes in heart rate and blood pressure, allows technicians to monitor and respond to the animal's needs throughout the procedure.

In critical care and emergency settings, a deep understanding of anatomy and physiology can be life-saving. For example, in cases of trauma, technicians must quickly assess the animal's condition and prioritize interventions. Recognizing signs of shock, such as pale mucous membranes or rapid breathing, requires an understanding of the cardiovascular and respiratory systems. Administering intravenous fluids or oxygen therapy effectively hinges on this foundational knowledge.

Anatomy and physiology also inform the development and implementation of treatment plans. In managing chronic conditions like diabetes or kidney disease, technicians rely on their understanding of endocrine and renal physiology to monitor the animal's response to treatment. This includes interpreting laboratory results, such as blood glucose levels or kidney function tests, and adjusting care plans accordingly.

The relevance of anatomy and physiology extends beyond individual patient care to encompass public health and disease prevention. Technicians play a crucial role in vaccination programs, parasite control, and biosecurity measures. Understanding the anatomy and physiology of pathogens, such as viruses and bacteria, informs strategies to prevent and control outbreaks. For instance, knowledge of how diseases like rabies affect the nervous system underscores the importance of vaccination and quarantine protocols.

Client education is another critical aspect where anatomy and physiology are essential. By explaining the anatomical and physiological basis of a pet's condition, technicians can help owners understand the importance of recommended treatments and preventative measures. This educational role empowers clients to make informed decisions about their animal's care and fosters a collaborative approach to health management.

Anatomy and physiology also underpin the ethical and humane treatment of animals. Understanding the sensory and emotional capacities of different species informs practices that minimize stress and pain. For example, recognizing signs of fear or discomfort during handling allows technicians to employ techniques that ensure the animal's well-being while facilitating necessary medical procedures.

Ultimately, the clinical relevance of anatomy and physiology is reflected in the improved quality of life for animals and their owners. Veterinary technicians, by leveraging their expertise in these foundational sciences, play a pivotal role in the health and well-being of the animals they serve. Through dedication, curiosity, and a commitment to excellence, technicians harness the power of anatomy and physiology to make a meaningful impact in the field of veterinary medicine.

CHAPTER 4
DEEP DIVE INTO PHARMACOLOGY

Principles of Pharmacology

Pharmacology, the science of drugs and their effects on living organisms, is a cornerstone of veterinary medicine. Understanding the principles of pharmacology is essential for veterinary technicians, as it enables them to assist veterinarians in selecting appropriate medications, calculating accurate dosages, and monitoring patients for therapeutic efficacy and adverse effects. By mastering these principles, technicians contribute to the safe and effective use of pharmaceuticals in animal care.

The journey of a drug through the body can be described through four primary pharmacokinetic processes: absorption, distribution, metabolism, and excretion. Absorption is the process by which a drug enters the bloodstream from its site of administration. Factors affecting absorption include the route of administration, the drug's formulation, and the animal's physiological state. For instance, oral medications may be absorbed more slowly than intravenous ones due to the need to pass through the gastrointestinal tract. Veterinary technicians must be familiar with these factors to anticipate how quickly a drug will take effect.

Once absorbed, the drug is distributed throughout the body. Distribution depends on blood flow, the permeability of cell membranes, and the drug's affinity for tissue binding. Lipid-soluble drugs, for example, may accumulate in fatty tissues, whereas water-soluble drugs are more likely to remain in the bloodstream. Understanding these distribution patterns helps technicians predict where a drug will exert its effects and identify potential sites of toxicity.

Metabolism, primarily occurring in the liver, involves the chemical alteration of a drug to facilitate its excretion. This process often transforms active drugs into inactive metabolites, although some drugs are metabolized into active forms. Species-specific differences in liver enzyme activity can significantly affect drug metabolism. For instance, cats have limited capacity to metabolize certain drugs due to lower levels of specific liver enzymes. Technicians must be aware of these species differences to avoid adverse drug reactions.

Excretion is the removal of drugs and their metabolites from the body, primarily through the kidneys in urine or the liver in bile. Impaired renal or hepatic function can lead to drug accumulation and toxicity. Monitoring an animal's organ function is crucial for adjusting dosages and ensuring safe drug elimination. Technicians play a vital role in collecting samples for laboratory testing and interpreting results to guide medication adjustments.

Pharmacodynamics, the study of how drugs exert their effects, is another critical principle. Drugs interact with specific receptors, enzymes, or ion channels to produce therapeutic effects or side effects. The relationship between drug concentration and effect is often characterized by the dose-response curve, illustrating the drug's potency and efficacy. Technicians must understand these interactions to anticipate therapeutic outcomes and manage adverse effects effectively.

The therapeutic index is a key concept in pharmacology, representing the ratio between a drug's effective dose and its toxic dose. A narrow therapeutic index indicates a small margin of safety, requiring precise dosing and careful monitoring. Drugs like digoxin, used in heart failure management, exemplify this concept. Technicians must ensure accurate dosing and watch for signs of toxicity, such as gastrointestinal distress or arrhythmias, to prevent adverse outcomes.

Drug interactions can alter the effects of medications, either enhancing or diminishing their efficacy. These interactions can be pharmacokinetic, affecting absorption, distribution, metabolism, or excretion, or pharmacodynamic, influencing the drug's action at its site of effect. Understanding potential interactions is crucial when administering multiple medications, as they can lead to unexpected side effects or reduced therapeutic benefits. Technicians should maintain accurate medication records and communicate any changes to the veterinary team.

Routes of drug administration vary widely, each with its advantages and limitations. Common routes include oral, intravenous, intramuscular, subcutaneous, and topical. The choice of route depends on factors such as the drug's formulation, the desired speed of effect, and the animal's condition. Intravenous administration provides rapid effects, ideal for emergencies, while oral administration is more convenient for long-term therapy. Technicians must be proficient in administering medications through various routes, ensuring proper technique and adherence to aseptic protocols.

Dosage calculations are a critical skill for veterinary technicians, ensuring that animals receive the correct amount of medication. These calculations often involve considering the animal's weight, the drug's concentration, and the prescribed dosage. Accurate calculations prevent underdosing, which may lead to treatment failure, and overdosing, which can cause toxicity. Technicians must double-check their calculations and consult with veterinarians when in doubt.

Monitoring and managing adverse drug reactions are essential components of pharmacology. Adverse reactions can range from mild, such as gastrointestinal upset, to severe, such as anaphylaxis. Technicians must be vigilant in observing animals for signs of adverse effects and report any concerns promptly. Providing supportive care, such as administering antihistamines or fluids, may be necessary to manage these reactions.

Patient compliance is a crucial factor in the success of pharmacological treatments. Technicians play a key role in educating clients on administering medications, emphasizing the importance of adherence to prescribed regimens. Demonstrating techniques, providing written instructions, and addressing client concerns can enhance compliance and improve treatment outcomes.

Mastering the principles of pharmacology empowers veterinary technicians to make informed decisions, improving patient outcomes and advancing the field of animal healthcare. Through dedication, curiosity, and a commitment to excellence, technicians harness the power of pharmacology to make a meaningful impact in the lives of animals and their caretakers. The study of pharmacology is a dynamic and rewarding pursuit, offering opportunities for growth, discovery, and the chance to make a positive difference in veterinary medicine.

Common Veterinary Medications

Veterinary medicine relies on a diverse array of medications to treat, manage, and prevent diseases in animals. Understanding common veterinary medications is vital for veterinary technicians, as it enables them to assist veterinarians in prescribing and administering these drugs effectively. Familiarity with these medications, their uses, and potential side effects ensures that technicians can provide safe and compassionate care to animal patients.

Antibiotics are a cornerstone of veterinary medicine, used to treat bacterial infections in various species. Drugs like amoxicillin, enrofloxacin, and cephalexin are frequently prescribed for conditions ranging from skin infections to respiratory diseases. Veterinary technicians must understand the importance of completing the full course of antibiotics and educating clients about the risks of antibiotic resistance. Recognizing signs of adverse reactions, such as gastrointestinal upset or allergic responses, is critical for patient safety.

Antiparasitic medications are another essential category, combating internal and external parasites that can significantly affect an animal's health. Ivermectin, fenbendazole, and praziquantel are commonly used to treat parasites like heartworms, intestinal worms, and tapeworms. Technicians play a crucial role in administering these medications and ensuring adherence to preventive schedules. Understanding the life cycles of parasites helps in advising clients on environmental control measures to prevent reinfestation.

Anti-inflammatory medications, including corticosteroids and non-steroidal anti-inflammatory drugs (NSAIDs), are frequently used to manage pain and inflammation in animals. Drugs like prednisone, carprofen, and meloxicam are effective for conditions such as arthritis, allergies, and post-surgical pain. Technicians should be aware of the potential side effects, such as gastrointestinal ulcers or renal impairment, and monitor patients closely. Educating clients on proper dosing and monitoring for adverse effects enhances treatment outcomes.

Analgesics are vital for managing pain, ensuring animal comfort, and improving quality of life. Opioids like buprenorphine and tramadol are potent pain relievers used in acute and chronic pain management. Veterinary technicians must understand the importance of pain assessment and the appropriate use of analgesics to prevent under-treatment or overuse. Monitoring for side effects such as sedation or respiratory depression is crucial when administering these medications.

Vaccines play a pivotal role in preventive medicine, protecting animals from infectious diseases. Rabies, distemper, parvovirus, and feline leukemia are among the diseases commonly prevented through vaccination. Veterinary technicians are responsible for administering vaccines, maintaining vaccination records, and educating clients on the importance of keeping vaccinations up to date. Understanding vaccine protocols and potential side effects, such as mild fever or injection site reactions, is essential for effective immunization programs.

Endocrine medications are used to manage hormonal imbalances and related conditions. Insulin is a critical medication for diabetic animals, requiring precise dosing and monitoring. Levothyroxine addresses hypothyroidism in dogs, while methimazole treats hyperthyroidism in cats. Technicians must be adept at teaching clients how to administer these medications and recognize signs of improper dosing, such as lethargy or changes in appetite.

Anticonvulsants like phenobarbital and potassium bromide are used to manage seizures in animals with epilepsy. Veterinary technicians play a crucial role in monitoring therapeutic drug levels and adjusting dosages as needed. Educating clients on the importance of consistent medication administration and recognizing breakthrough seizures is vital for effective seizure management.

Antiemetic medications, such as maropitant and metoclopramide, are used to control nausea and vomiting in animals with gastrointestinal disturbances. These drugs can significantly improve the quality of life for animals undergoing chemotherapy or suffering from motion sickness. Veterinary technicians must be familiar with these medications and their appropriate use, as well as potential side effects like diarrhea or lethargy.

Cardiovascular medications, including diuretics, ACE inhibitors, and beta-blockers, are used to manage heart diseases in animals. Furosemide, enalapril, and atenolol are commonly prescribed to control symptoms such as edema, hypertension, and arrhythmias. Technicians must understand the pharmacology of these medications to monitor for side effects like electrolyte imbalances or hypotension and educate clients on the importance of adherence to prescribed treatment plans.

Behavioral medications, such as fluoxetine and clomipramine, are used to address anxiety and behavioral disorders in animals. These drugs can help manage conditions like separation anxiety or compulsive behaviors. Veterinary technicians play a key role in educating clients about the gradual onset of effects, potential side effects like changes in appetite, and the importance of behavioral modification techniques in conjunction with medication.

Antifungal medications, including ketoconazole and itraconazole, are used to treat fungal infections like ringworm or systemic mycoses. Veterinary technicians must be aware of the importance of monitoring liver function during treatment and recognizing signs of adverse reactions, such as jaundice or gastrointestinal upset.

Fluid therapy is an integral part of veterinary medicine, used to treat dehydration, electrolyte imbalances, and shock. Understanding the different types of fluids, such as crystalloids and colloids, and their appropriate use is essential for effective fluid management. Veterinary technicians are responsible for calculating fluid rates, monitoring infusion sites, and assessing the animal's response to therapy.

Understanding common veterinary medications empowers veterinary technicians to make informed decisions, improving patient outcomes and advancing the field of animal healthcare. Through dedication, curiosity, and a commitment to excellence, technicians harness the power of pharmacology to make a meaningful impact in the lives of animals and their caretakers. The study of veterinary medications is a dynamic and rewarding pursuit, offering opportunities for growth, discovery, and the chance to make a positive difference in veterinary medicine.

Drug Interactions and Side Effects

Navigating the landscape of drug interactions and side effects is a critical aspect of veterinary pharmacology. Understanding how different medications interact and the potential side effects they may cause is essential for ensuring the safety and well-being of animal patients. Veterinary technicians play a pivotal role in this process, helping veterinarians manage and mitigate the risks associated with pharmacotherapy.

Drug interactions occur when the effects of one drug are altered by the presence of another. These interactions can be pharmacokinetic, affecting the absorption, distribution, metabolism, or excretion of a drug, or pharmacodynamic, where the drugs influence each other's effects at their sites of action. Recognizing these interactions is crucial for preventing adverse effects and ensuring therapeutic efficacy.

Pharmacokinetic interactions often arise when drugs compete for the same metabolic pathways. For instance, non-steroidal anti-inflammatory drugs (NSAIDs) and certain antibiotics may compete for liver enzymes, potentially leading to increased levels of one or both drugs. This can result in toxicity or reduced effectiveness. Veterinary technicians must be vigilant in identifying such potential interactions, especially when animals are prescribed multiple medications.

Pharmacodynamic interactions can lead to additive, synergistic, or antagonistic effects. An example of an additive effect is the combined use of two analgesics, such as acetaminophen and an opioid, which together provide enhanced pain relief. Conversely, the concurrent use of diuretics and non-steroidal anti-inflammatory drugs may lead to antagonistic effects, as NSAIDs can reduce the efficacy of diuretics by decreasing renal blood flow. Understanding these interactions helps technicians and veterinarians make informed decisions about medication regimens.

Herbal supplements and over-the-counter medications can also interact with prescribed veterinary drugs. St. John's Wort, a common herbal remedy, can induce liver enzymes, potentially reducing the effectiveness of other medications. Veterinary technicians should take thorough medication histories, including any supplements or non-prescription drugs, and educate clients about the potential risks of drug interactions.

Side effects are unintended and often undesirable effects of medications. These can range from mild, such as transient gastrointestinal upset, to severe, such as anaphylaxis. Recognizing and managing side effects is a crucial responsibility for veterinary technicians. Identifying early signs of adverse reactions and communicating these to the veterinary team is essential for prompt intervention.

Gastrointestinal side effects are among the most common in veterinary medicine. Many medications, including antibiotics and NSAIDs, can cause nausea, vomiting, diarrhea, or appetite changes. Veterinary technicians should advise clients to administer medications with food when appropriate and monitor animals for any signs of gastrointestinal distress. In cases of severe or persistent symptoms, discontinuing the medication or adjusting the dose may be necessary, under veterinary guidance.

Hepatotoxicity, or liver damage, is a potential side effect of several medications, including certain anticonvulsants and antibiotics. Veterinary technicians should monitor liver function tests in animals receiving these drugs and watch for clinical signs of liver dysfunction, such as jaundice or lethargy. Prompt recognition and management of hepatotoxicity can prevent further liver damage and improve outcomes.

Nephrotoxicity, or kidney damage, is another significant concern, particularly with medications like aminoglycoside antibiotics and certain chemotherapeutic agents. Veterinary technicians should ensure that animals on potentially nephrotoxic drugs are adequately hydrated and monitor renal function tests regularly. Identifying early signs of renal impairment allows for timely intervention, such as dose adjustment or discontinuation of the drug.

Allergic reactions to medications can vary from mild skin rashes to life-threatening anaphylaxis. Veterinary technicians must be prepared to recognize and respond to signs of allergic reactions, such as swelling, hives, or difficulty breathing. Administering antihistamines or corticosteroids and providing supportive care may be necessary to manage these reactions. Educating clients about the signs of allergic reactions and advising them to seek immediate veterinary assistance if they occur is crucial.

Long-term medication use can lead to cumulative side effects, such as osteoporosis with prolonged corticosteroid use or hypothyroidism with certain anticonvulsants. Veterinary technicians should monitor animals on long-term medications for signs of chronic side effects and communicate any concerns to the veterinary team. Regular follow-up appointments and laboratory testing are essential components of managing long-term medication therapy.

Patient-specific factors, such as age, breed, and underlying health conditions, can influence the risk of drug interactions and side effects. Puppies and kittens, for instance, have immature liver and kidney function, affecting drug metabolism and excretion. Certain breeds, like Collies, may have genetic sensitivities to specific drugs, such as ivermectin. Veterinary technicians must consider these factors when assisting with medication management and educate clients about any breed-specific risks.

Understanding drug interactions and side effects empowers veterinary technicians to make informed decisions, improving patient outcomes and advancing the field of animal healthcare. Through dedication, curiosity, and a commitment to excellence, technicians harness the power of pharmacology to make a meaningful impact in the lives of animals and their caretakers. The study of veterinary pharmacology is a dynamic and rewarding pursuit, offering opportunities for growth, discovery, and the chance to make a positive difference in veterinary medicine.

Dosage Calculations and Administration

Dosage calculations and administration are fundamental skills in veterinary pharmacology, requiring precision and a deep understanding of pharmacokinetics. These skills ensure that animals receive accurate doses of medication, maximizing therapeutic benefits while minimizing the risk of adverse effects. Veterinary technicians play a crucial role in this process, assisting veterinarians in calculating, preparing, and administering medications safely and effectively.

Accurate dosage calculations begin with understanding the basic formula: Dose = (Weight × Dosage)/Concentration. Weight is typically measured in kilograms, dosage is expressed as milligrams per kilogram (mg/kg), and concentration is given as milligrams per milliliter (mg/mL) or milligrams per tablet. This calculation provides the amount of medication required for a specific animal based on its weight and the prescribed dosage.

Consider a scenario where a dog requires an antibiotic at a dosage of 10 mg/kg, and the dog weighs 20 kg. If the antibiotic is available in a concentration of 50 mg/mL, the calculation would be: Dose = (20 kg × 10 mg/kg) / 50 mg/mL = 4 mL. This means the dog should receive 4 mL of the antibiotic. Understanding this calculation process is essential for ensuring accurate dosing.

It is vital to consider species-specific differences when calculating dosages. Different animals metabolize drugs at varying rates, meaning that a dosage appropriate for one species may be harmful to another. For example, cats often require lower dosages than dogs due to their unique liver metabolism. Veterinary technicians must be aware of these differences and consult species-specific guidelines when calculating dosages.

Pediatric and geriatric patients present additional challenges in dosage calculations. Puppies, kittens, and older animals may have altered pharmacokinetics due to immature or declining organ function, necessitating adjusted dosages. Veterinary technicians should monitor these animals closely for signs of under- or overdosing and communicate any concerns to the veterinary team.

Once the correct dosage is calculated, veterinary technicians must prepare and administer the medication accurately. Oral medications can come in various forms, including tablets, capsules, and liquids. For tablets and capsules, technicians may need to split or crush them to achieve the correct dose. However, caution is required, as altering the form of some medications can affect their absorption or efficacy. Liquids should be measured using appropriate syringes or droppers to ensure precision.

Injectable medications require aseptic technique and knowledge of different injection routes, such as intramuscular (IM), subcutaneous (SC), or intravenous (IV). Each route has specific anatomical landmarks and techniques to ensure proper administration. For instance, IM injections are typically given in the quadriceps or lumbar muscles, while SC injections are administered in the loose skin over the shoulders. Veterinary technicians must be proficient in these techniques to minimize discomfort and prevent complications.

Topical medications, including creams, ointments, and patches, require careful application to ensure proper absorption. Technicians should wear gloves to prevent contamination and apply the medication evenly over the affected area. In some cases, the area may need to be shaved or cleaned before application to enhance absorption.

Transdermal patches, used for medications like fentanyl, require special attention to ensure they adhere properly and are not accidentally removed or ingested by the animal. Veterinary technicians should educate clients on monitoring the patch and preventing other animals or children from coming into contact with it.

Calculating and administering medications also involves understanding the potential for drug interactions and contraindications. Veterinary technicians must maintain accurate medication records and communicate any changes or additions to the veterinary team. This ensures that all team members are aware of the animal's current medication regimen and can make informed decisions about future treatments.

Monitoring animals after medication administration is crucial for assessing therapeutic efficacy and identifying any adverse effects. Veterinary technicians should observe animals for changes in behavior, appetite, or clinical signs and report any concerns promptly. Regular follow-up appointments and laboratory tests may be necessary to evaluate the animal's response to treatment and adjust dosages as needed.

Understanding dosage calculations and administration empowers veterinary technicians to make informed decisions, improving patient outcomes and advancing the field of animal healthcare. Through dedication, curiosity, and a commitment to excellence, technicians harness the power of pharmacology to make a meaningful impact in the lives of animals and their caretakers. The study of dosage calculations and administration is a dynamic and rewarding pursuit, offering opportunities for growth, discovery, and the chance to make a positive difference in veterinary medicine.

Pharmacokinetics and Pharmacodynamics

Pharmacokinetics and pharmacodynamics are the twin pillars of pharmacology, each playing a crucial role in understanding how drugs exert their effects on the body. Veterinary technicians, by mastering these concepts, enhance their ability to assist veterinarians in designing effective treatment plans and monitoring therapeutic outcomes.

Pharmacokinetics refers to the journey a drug takes through the body and encompasses four primary processes: absorption, distribution, metabolism, and excretion. Absorption is the process by which a drug enters the bloodstream from its site of administration. The route of administration—oral, intravenous, intramuscular, or topical—greatly influences the speed and efficiency of absorption. For instance, intravenous administration delivers a drug directly into the bloodstream, resulting in rapid onset of action. In contrast, oral drugs must navigate the gastrointestinal tract, where factors like gastric pH and motility can affect absorption rates.

Once absorbed, a drug is distributed throughout the body. Distribution depends on blood flow, tissue permeability, and the drug's affinity for binding with plasma proteins. Lipid-soluble drugs, such as diazepam, readily cross cell membranes and may accumulate in fatty tissues, potentially prolonging their effects. Water-soluble drugs, like gentamicin, tend to remain in the extracellular fluid and are often cleared more quickly. Understanding these distribution dynamics helps technicians predict where a drug will exert its primary effects and identify potential sites of toxicity.

Metabolism, primarily occurring in the liver, involves the chemical alteration of a drug to prepare it for excretion. This often transforms active drugs into inactive metabolites, but some drugs, such as prednisone, are converted into active forms. Species-specific differences in liver enzyme activity can significantly impact drug metabolism. Cats, for example, have limited capacity to metabolize certain drugs due to lower levels of specific liver enzymes. Veterinary technicians must be aware of these differences to avoid adverse drug reactions and ensure appropriate dosing.

Excretion is the final phase, where drugs and their metabolites are eliminated from the body, primarily through the kidneys in urine or the liver in bile. Impaired renal or hepatic function can lead to drug accumulation and toxicity. Monitoring an animal's organ function is crucial for adjusting dosages and ensuring safe drug elimination. Technicians play a vital role in collecting samples for laboratory testing and interpreting results to guide medication adjustments.

Pharmacodynamics, on the other hand, focuses on how drugs interact with their targets to produce therapeutic effects or side effects. This involves the drug's mechanism of action, such as binding to specific receptors, inhibiting enzymes, or altering ion channel activity. The relationship between drug concentration and effect is often depicted by the dose-response curve, illustrating the drug's potency and efficacy. For example, a low dose of an antihistamine may relieve mild allergies, while higher doses provide sedation.

Receptor binding is a key aspect of pharmacodynamics. Drugs may act as agonists, activating receptors to produce a response, or antagonists, blocking receptors to prevent a response. Beta-blockers like propranolol, for instance, act as antagonists at beta-adrenergic receptors, reducing heart rate and blood pressure. Technicians must understand these interactions to anticipate therapeutic outcomes and manage adverse effects effectively.

The therapeutic index is a critical concept in pharmacodynamics, representing the ratio between a drug's effective dose and its toxic dose. A narrow therapeutic index indicates a small margin of safety, requiring precise dosing and careful monitoring. Drugs like digoxin, used in heart failure management, exemplify this concept. Technicians must ensure accurate dosing and watch for signs of toxicity, such as gastrointestinal distress or arrhythmias, to prevent adverse outcomes.

Drug interactions can alter the effects of medications, either enhancing or diminishing their efficacy. These interactions can be pharmacokinetic, affecting absorption, distribution, metabolism, or excretion, or pharmacodynamic, influencing the drug's action at its site of effect. Understanding potential interactions is crucial when administering multiple medications, as they can lead to unexpected side effects or reduced therapeutic benefits. Technicians should maintain accurate medication records and communicate any changes to the veterinary team.

Patient-specific factors, such as age, breed, and underlying health conditions, can influence pharmacokinetics and pharmacodynamics. Puppies and kittens, for instance, have immature liver and kidney function, affecting drug metabolism and excretion. Certain breeds, like Greyhounds, may have genetic sensitivities to specific drugs, such as thiopental. Veterinary technicians must consider these factors when assisting with medication management and educate clients about any breed-specific risks.

Understanding pharmacokinetics and pharmacodynamics empowers veterinary technicians to make informed decisions, improving patient outcomes and advancing the field of animal healthcare. Through dedication, curiosity, and a commitment to excellence, technicians harness the power of pharmacology to make a meaningful impact in the lives of animals and their caretakers. The study of these principles is a dynamic and rewarding pursuit, offering opportunities for growth, discovery, and the chance to make a positive difference in veterinary medicine.

Legal and Ethical Considerations in Pharmacology

Navigating the legal and ethical landscape of pharmacology is paramount for veterinary technicians who play a critical role in the safe and effective use of medications. Understanding the regulations governing the prescription, dispensing, and administration of drugs is essential for maintaining professional integrity and ensuring the welfare of animal patients.

The foundation of legal considerations in pharmacology lies in the regulation of drug approval and usage by governmental agencies. In the United States, the Food and Drug Administration (FDA) oversees veterinary medications, ensuring they meet rigorous safety and efficacy standards before approval. Veterinary technicians must be familiar with these regulations to understand which medications are legally available for use in animals and under what circumstances.

Prescription medications require a valid veterinarian-client-patient relationship (VCPR), a legal framework that mandates a veterinarian's oversight in diagnosing and prescribing treatment. Veterinary technicians play a supportive role in maintaining this relationship by facilitating communication between veterinarians and clients and ensuring that treatment plans are followed accurately. Adhering to the VCPR is crucial for legal compliance and for fostering trust between clients and the veterinary team.

Dispensing medications involves strict adherence to labeling and record-keeping requirements. Labels must include the drug name, dosage instructions, expiration date, and the prescribing veterinarian's information. Veterinary technicians are responsible for ensuring that these labels are accurate and legible, minimizing the risk of medication errors. Maintaining comprehensive records of all dispensed medications not only supports legal compliance but also aids in monitoring treatment outcomes and managing potential adverse reactions.

Compounding, the process of altering or combining drugs to meet specific patient needs, is subject to additional legal considerations. While compounding can be invaluable for creating tailored treatments, it must be done in accordance with state and federal regulations to ensure patient safety. Veterinary technicians must be aware of the limitations and requirements of compounding, such as using FDA-approved ingredients and adhering to established guidelines for preparation and storage.

Controlled substances, which have a high potential for abuse, are subject to stringent regulations under the Controlled Substances Act. These drugs must be stored securely, and their use must be meticulously documented. Veterinary technicians involved in handling controlled substances must be diligent in following protocols for inventory management, administration, and disposal. Failure to comply with these regulations can result in severe legal repercussions for both the individual and the practice.

Ethical considerations in pharmacology revolve around the principles of beneficence, non-maleficence, autonomy, and justice. Beneficence and non-maleficence guide veterinary professionals to provide treatments that benefit the animal while minimizing harm. This requires careful consideration of the risks and benefits of any medication, as well as ongoing monitoring for adverse effects.

Autonomy respects the client's right to make informed decisions about their animal's care. Veterinary technicians can facilitate this by providing clear, accurate information about treatment options, potential side effects, and expected outcomes. Ensuring that clients understand this information empowers them to make choices that align with their values and preferences.

Justice involves the fair and equitable distribution of veterinary care resources. Veterinary technicians should be mindful of the ethical implications of treatment decisions, ensuring that all animals receive appropriate care regardless of their owner's financial or social status. This may involve advocating for cost-effective treatment options or exploring alternative resources for clients facing financial constraints.

Informed consent is a cornerstone of ethical veterinary practice, requiring that clients are fully informed about the nature, risks, and benefits of proposed treatments before giving their consent. Veterinary technicians play a key role in this process by providing information, answering questions, and ensuring that clients feel supported in their decision-making. Documenting informed consent discussions in the patient's medical record is essential for both legal and ethical accountability.

Confidentiality is another critical ethical consideration, as veterinary professionals must protect client and patient information. Veterinary technicians should be aware of confidentiality policies and ensure that sensitive information is shared only with authorized individuals. Maintaining confidentiality fosters trust between clients and the veterinary team, which is essential for effective communication and collaboration.

Understanding legal and ethical considerations in pharmacology empowers veterinary technicians to make informed decisions, improving patient outcomes and advancing the field of animal healthcare. Through dedication, curiosity, and a commitment to excellence, technicians harness the power of pharmacology to make a meaningful impact in the lives of animals and their caretakers. The study of these principles is a dynamic and rewarding pursuit, offering opportunities for growth, discovery, and the chance to make a positive difference in veterinary medicine.

CHAPTER 5
SURGICAL NURSING AND ANESTHESIA

Preoperative Care and Assessment

The journey to a successful surgical outcome begins long before the first incision is made. Preoperative care and assessment are crucial phases in surgical nursing and anesthesia, setting the foundation for patient safety and optimal recovery. Veterinary technicians play a pivotal role in this process, ensuring that each patient is thoroughly evaluated and prepared for the challenges of surgery.

A comprehensive preoperative assessment involves gathering detailed patient history and conducting a thorough physical examination. This step is vital for identifying any underlying conditions or risk factors that could complicate anesthesia or surgery. Veterinary technicians should begin by reviewing the animal's medical records, noting any past surgeries, chronic illnesses, or adverse reactions to medications. This history provides insights into potential anesthetic risks and informs the development of a tailored perioperative plan.

The physical examination allows technicians to assess the animal's overall health and identify any abnormalities that may require further investigation. Key aspects of the examination include evaluating the cardiovascular and respiratory systems, checking for signs of infection or inflammation, and ensuring that the animal's hydration and nutritional status are adequate. Special attention should be paid to any signs of pain or distress, as these can indicate underlying conditions that may need to be addressed before surgery.

Laboratory testing is often an integral part of the preoperative assessment, providing valuable information about the patient's physiological status. Common tests include complete blood counts (CBC), biochemistry panels, and coagulation profiles. CBCs help evaluate the animal's immune function and red blood cell levels, while biochemistry panels assess organ function and electrolyte balance. Coagulation profiles are essential for detecting any clotting disorders that could increase surgical bleeding risk. Veterinary technicians are responsible for collecting and processing these samples, ensuring accurate and timely results.

Pre-anesthetic evaluation also involves assessing the patient's anesthetic risk using standardized classification systems such as the American Society of Anesthesiologists (ASA) physical status classification. This system categorizes patients based on their overall health, from ASA I (healthy) to ASA V (moribund). Understanding the patient's ASA status helps the veterinary team anticipate potential complications and adjust the anesthetic protocol accordingly.

Patient preparation extends beyond physical assessment to include psychological and environmental considerations. Reducing stress and anxiety is crucial for minimizing the physiological impact of surgery and anesthesia. Veterinary technicians can help by maintaining a calm and quiet environment, using pheromone diffusers or calming music, and providing gentle handling and reassurance. Encouraging clients to bring familiar objects from home, such as a blanket or toy, can also provide comfort to the animal.

Fasting protocols are an essential component of preoperative care, reducing the risk of aspiration pneumonia during anesthesia. Veterinary technicians should provide clients with clear instructions on when to withhold food and water before surgery, typically 8-12 hours for food and 2-4 hours for water. Compliance with these guidelines is crucial for patient safety, and technicians should confirm fasting status upon admission.

Medication management is another critical aspect of preoperative preparation. Veterinary technicians must review the patient's current medications and determine which should be continued or withheld before surgery. Some medications, such as anticoagulants or non-steroidal anti-inflammatory drugs (NSAIDs), may need to be paused to reduce bleeding risk. Conversely, medications for chronic conditions, such as heart disease or diabetes, may need to be administered to maintain stability. Technicians should consult with the veterinarian to develop an appropriate medication plan and communicate any changes to the client.

Informed consent is a fundamental ethical and legal requirement in preoperative care. Veterinary technicians play a key role in facilitating this process by providing clients with clear and accurate information about the proposed procedure, potential risks, and expected outcomes. Ensuring that clients understand this information and have the opportunity to ask questions is essential for obtaining valid consent. Documenting the informed consent discussion in the patient's medical record is crucial for both ethical and legal accountability.

Understanding the principles of preoperative care and assessment empowers veterinary technicians to make informed decisions, improving patient outcomes and advancing the field of animal healthcare. Through dedication, curiosity, and a commitment to excellence, technicians harness the power of surgical nursing and anesthesia to make a meaningful impact in the lives of animals and their caretakers. The study of these principles is a dynamic and rewarding pursuit, offering opportunities for growth, discovery, and the chance to make a positive difference in veterinary medicine.

Surgical Instruments and Techniques

Mastering the art of surgical instruments and techniques is essential for veterinary technicians, as they assist in procedures ranging from routine spaying and neutering to complex orthopedic surgeries. A thorough understanding of the tools and methods employed in veterinary surgery not only ensures the smooth execution of procedures but also upholds patient safety and enhances outcomes.

Surgical instruments are the extension of a surgeon's hands, and each has a specific purpose. Scalpels, for example, are indispensable for making precise incisions. These come in various blade sizes and shapes, with the No. 10 blade being a common choice for general surgery due to its versatility. Mastery in handling a scalpel involves a steady hand and an understanding of the angle and pressure needed to achieve clean, controlled cuts.

Forceps, another essential instrument, are used for grasping, holding, or manipulating tissues. Adson forceps, with their fine tips and secure grip, are particularly useful for delicate tissue handling, while Kelly forceps are more robust, ideal for clamping larger tissue or vessels. The choice of forceps can significantly impact the precision of the surgical procedure and the minimization of tissue trauma.

Scissors, available in various designs, serve multiple purposes in surgery. Mayo scissors, with their sturdy construction, are ideal for cutting dense tissue, whereas Metzenbaum scissors, with their longer handles and finer blades, are suited for delicate dissection. Learning the nuances of each type of scissors enables technicians to assist effectively in maintaining the surgical field and facilitating the surgeon's work.

Hemostats are crucial for controlling bleeding during surgery. These clamp onto blood vessels, providing hemostasis until the vessel can be ligated or cauterized. Technicians must be adept at passing hemostats quickly and correctly, as timely intervention is critical in preventing excessive blood loss and ensuring a clear surgical field.

Retractors are designed to hold back tissue and organs, granting the surgeon better visibility and access to the surgical site. Instruments such as Gelpi retractors are self-retaining, freeing the technician's hands, while others like Senn retractors require manual assistance. Proficiency in using retractors involves understanding the appropriate application to prevent tissue damage and maintain optimal exposure.

Sutures and needles are the final components of surgical closure, securing the wound and promoting healing. Various suture materials, from absorbable to non-absorbable, and needle types, such as cutting or tapered, are chosen based on the tissue involved and the desired healing outcome. Technicians must be familiar with suture patterns, such as simple interrupted or continuous, to assist in accurate and efficient wound closure.

Beyond instruments, surgical techniques form the backbone of veterinary surgery. Aseptic technique is paramount in preventing infection, involving meticulous hand scrubbing, donning of sterile gowns and gloves, and maintaining a sterile field. Veterinary technicians play a crucial role in setting up the surgical suite, ensuring that all instruments and materials are sterilized and ready for use.

Positioning the patient is another critical aspect, as it affects access to the surgical site and the patient's physiologic stability. Proper padding and securing of the patient prevent pressure sores and nerve damage, while careful attention to alignment ensures that anesthesia is administered effectively and the surgery proceeds smoothly.

Anesthesia monitoring is integral to surgical success, ensuring that the patient remains stable throughout the procedure. Veterinary technicians are responsible for monitoring vital signs, such as heart rate, respiratory rate, and blood pressure, using both manual techniques and electronic monitors. Recognizing changes in these parameters allows for prompt intervention, whether it involves adjusting anesthetic depth or addressing emergent complications.

Assisting with tissue handling and manipulation requires a delicate touch and keen awareness. Whether suctioning fluids to maintain a clear field or using retractors to hold tissues aside, technicians must anticipate the surgeon's needs and respond swiftly. This collaboration is key to minimizing tissue trauma and optimizing surgical efficiency.

Surgical technique also involves understanding the principles of wound healing and tissue repair. Veterinary technicians must be knowledgeable about the stages of healing and the factors that can impede or promote recovery. This understanding guides postoperative care and client education, ensuring that patients receive the support they need to heal effectively.

Postoperative care is an extension of surgical technique, requiring vigilance in monitoring the patient's recovery and managing pain. Technicians are instrumental in assessing pain levels, administering analgesics, and providing supportive care, such as fluid therapy and nutrition. Educating clients about wound care, activity restrictions, and signs of complications is a crucial component of postoperative management.

Understanding surgical instruments and techniques empowers veterinary technicians to make informed decisions, improving patient outcomes and advancing the field of animal healthcare. Through dedication, curiosity, and a commitment to excellence, technicians harness the power of surgical nursing and anesthesia to make a meaningful impact in the lives of animals and their caretakers. The study of these principles is a dynamic and rewarding pursuit, offering opportunities for growth, discovery, and the chance to make a positive difference in veterinary medicine.

Anesthesia Types and Administration

The realm of anesthesia is integral to surgical nursing, encompassing a spectrum of types and administration techniques that ensure the safety and comfort of animal patients during procedures. Veterinary technicians, equipped with a deep understanding of anesthesia, contribute significantly to the veterinary team's ability to tailor anesthetic plans to each patient's unique needs.

Anesthesia serves the fundamental purpose of rendering a patient insensible to pain, allowing surgical procedures to be performed without distress. The types of anesthesia are broadly categorized into general, local, and regional, each with specific applications and considerations.

General anesthesia involves the induction of unconsciousness, often accompanied by muscle relaxation and analgesia. It is typically achieved through a combination of injectable and inhalant agents. Injectable anesthetics, such as propofol or ketamine, provide rapid induction and are often used to transition patients to inhalant agents like isoflurane or sevoflurane. These inhalants are administered via an endotracheal tube, allowing precise control over anesthetic depth and ensuring a swift recovery. Veterinary technicians play a crucial role in monitoring the patient during general anesthesia, continually assessing vital signs such as heart rate, respiratory rate, and body temperature.

Local anesthesia targets specific areas of the body, providing pain relief without affecting consciousness. Agents such as lidocaine or bupivacaine are injected directly into the tissue surrounding a surgical site, blocking nerve transmission and thus sensation. This type of anesthesia is often used for minor procedures, such as wound repair or dental extractions. Veterinary technicians must be skilled in the precise administration of local anesthetics, ensuring adequate coverage and minimizing the risk of complications such as tissue irritation or systemic toxicity.

Regional anesthesia encompasses techniques that block sensation to larger areas of the body, often by targeting specific nerve plexuses or spinal nerve roots. Epidural anesthesia is a common regional technique in veterinary medicine, providing profound analgesia for procedures involving the hindquarters or pelvis.

Administered into the epidural space, agents such as lidocaine or morphine achieve long-lasting pain relief while allowing the patient to remain conscious. Mastery of regional techniques requires a thorough understanding of anatomy and careful attention to dosing and administration protocols.

Balanced anesthesia, or multimodal anesthesia, is a strategy that combines different types of anesthetic agents to achieve optimal pain control and minimize side effects. By using lower doses of multiple drugs, this approach reduces the reliance on any single agent, thereby decreasing the risk of adverse effects such as cardiovascular depression or prolonged recovery. Veterinary technicians play a pivotal role in implementing balanced anesthesia, assisting in the selection and adjustment of agents based on the patient's response and the specific demands of the procedure.

Pre-anesthetic assessment and preparation are critical components of effective anesthesia administration. A thorough evaluation of the patient's health status, including a review of medical history and laboratory tests, informs the choice of anesthetic agents and protocols. Factors such as age, breed, and underlying medical conditions must be considered, as they can significantly influence anesthetic risk and drug metabolism. Veterinary technicians are responsible for gathering this information and communicating it to the veterinary team, ensuring that the anesthetic plan is both safe and effective.

Premedication, administered prior to induction, aids in calming the patient and reducing the required doses of anesthetic agents. Common premedications include sedatives such as acepromazine or benzodiazepines, and analgesics like opioids. These agents not only facilitate smoother induction but also enhance perioperative analgesia, contributing to a more stable anesthetic course and improved recovery. Veterinary technicians must be adept at calculating and administering premedications, monitoring the patient for any adverse reactions.

Induction of anesthesia marks the transition from consciousness to unconsciousness, achieved through the administration of rapid-acting agents. The choice of induction agent depends on the patient's health status and the anticipated duration and complexity of the procedure. Techniques for induction vary, from intravenous boluses to inhalant mask induction, each with specific advantages and challenges. Veterinary technicians are instrumental in executing induction protocols, ensuring that the patient transitions smoothly and safely into the anesthetized state.

Maintenance of anesthesia involves sustaining the desired anesthetic depth throughout the procedure, requiring continuous monitoring and adjustment of anesthetic agents. Inhalant anesthetics, delivered via precision vaporizers, allow fine-tuning of anesthetic levels based on the patient's physiological response. Monitoring equipment, such as pulse oximeters, capnographs, and ECGs, provide real-time data on the patient's status, enabling timely interventions to prevent complications. Veterinary technicians must be vigilant in interpreting these data and adjusting anesthetic delivery as needed.

Recovery from anesthesia is a critical phase, requiring careful observation and support as the patient regains consciousness. Veterinary technicians must monitor vital signs closely, ensuring a smooth transition and addressing any emergent issues such as hypothermia or pain. Providing a warm, quiet environment and administering postoperative analgesics are essential for promoting recovery and minimizing discomfort. Client education is also a key component of this phase, as technicians provide guidance on postoperative care and alert clients to potential signs of complications.

Understanding anesthesia types and administration empowers veterinary technicians to make informed decisions, improving patient outcomes and advancing the field of animal healthcare. Through dedication, curiosity, and a commitment to excellence, technicians harness the power of surgical nursing and anesthesia to make a meaningful impact in the lives of animals and their caretakers. The study of these principles is a dynamic and rewarding pursuit, offering opportunities for growth, discovery, and the chance to make a positive difference in veterinary medicine.

Monitoring and Postoperative Care

The critical phases of monitoring and postoperative care are essential to the success of any surgical procedure, as they ensure patient stability and promote recovery. Veterinary technicians play a vital role in these stages, diligently observing and supporting the animal as it transitions from surgery to convalescence.

Monitoring begins as soon as anesthesia is induced and continues until the patient is fully recovered. This requires a keen eye and a thorough understanding of the animal's physiological responses to anesthesia. Key parameters to monitor include heart rate, respiratory rate, blood pressure, body temperature, and oxygen saturation. Each of these parameters provides vital information about the patient's cardiovascular and respiratory systems, which are directly impacted by anesthetic agents.

Heart rate and rhythm are monitored using both manual palpation and electronic devices such as ECGs. Any deviations from normal can indicate anesthetic depth issues or cardiovascular distress. Veterinary technicians must be adept at interpreting these signals and alerting the veterinary team to potential complications.

Respiratory rate and effort are equally important, as they reflect the patient's ability to ventilate effectively under anesthesia. Capnography, which measures the concentration of carbon dioxide in exhaled air, provides real-time data on respiratory function. Anomalies in capnograph readings can suggest hypoventilation, airway obstructions, or equipment malfunctions, necessitating immediate corrective actions.

Blood pressure monitoring is critical for assessing perfusion and organ function. Both invasive and non-invasive methods are used, with oscillometric devices and Doppler ultrasound being common non-invasive tools. Hypotension, a frequent anesthetic complication, can lead to inadequate blood flow to vital organs and necessitates prompt intervention to prevent organ damage.

Body temperature regulation is a challenge during anesthesia, as anesthetic agents often disrupt thermoregulatory mechanisms. Hypothermia is common, particularly in small animals, and can prolong recovery and increase the risk of complications. Veterinary technicians must employ warming techniques, such as heated blankets or warmed IV fluids, to maintain normothermia throughout the procedure.

Oxygen saturation, measured via pulse oximetry, provides insight into the patient's oxygenation status. Low saturation levels can indicate hypoxemia, requiring adjustments in ventilation or oxygen delivery. Veterinary technicians must be vigilant in monitoring and interpreting these readings, ensuring that oxygenation remains within safe limits.

The transition from anesthesia to recovery marks the beginning of postoperative care, a phase that demands careful observation and support. As the patient regains consciousness, technicians must monitor for signs of pain, nausea, and disorientation. The use of analgesics and antiemetics is often necessary to manage these symptoms and promote comfort.

Pain management is a cornerstone of postoperative care, as unrelieved pain can impede healing and lead to complications. A multimodal approach, incorporating NSAIDs, opioids, and local anesthetics, provides comprehensive analgesia. Veterinary technicians are responsible for assessing pain levels using standardized pain scales and ensuring timely administration of analgesics.

Wound care is another critical aspect of postoperative management. Veterinary technicians must monitor surgical sites for signs of infection, dehiscence, or excessive bleeding. Proper wound cleaning and dressing changes are essential to prevent complications and promote healing. Educating clients on wound care and activity restrictions is also crucial for successful recovery.

Nutrition and hydration support the healing process, and technicians must ensure that patients receive adequate food and water intake. For patients unable or unwilling to eat voluntarily, assisted feeding techniques, such as syringe feeding or feeding tubes, may be necessary. Monitoring fluid balance and providing IV fluids as needed helps maintain hydration and electrolyte balance.

Understanding monitoring and postoperative care empowers veterinary technicians to make informed decisions, improving patient outcomes and advancing the field of animal healthcare. Through dedication, curiosity, and a commitment to excellence, technicians harness the power of surgical nursing and anesthesia to make a meaningful impact in the lives of animals and their caretakers. The study of these principles is a dynamic and rewarding pursuit, offering opportunities for growth, discovery, and the chance to make a positive difference in veterinary medicine.

Pain Management in Veterinary Practice

Pain management in veterinary practice is a multifaceted discipline that extends beyond mere alleviation of discomfort. It requires a nuanced understanding of animal physiology, pharmacology, and the emotional well-being of patients. Effective pain management not only improves the quality of life for animal patients but also plays a crucial role in their recovery and overall health.

The first step in pain management is accurate assessment. Unlike humans, animals cannot verbally express their pain, necessitating reliance on behavioral and physiological indicators. Veterinary technicians must be adept at interpreting subtle signs such as changes in posture, vocalization, grooming habits, and appetite. Physiological indicators like increased heart rate, respiratory rate, and elevated cortisol levels can also signal pain. Utilizing standardized pain assessment scales, such as the Glasgow Composite Measure Pain Scale for dogs or the Colorado State University Feline Acute Pain Scale, facilitates objective evaluation.

Once pain is identified, a comprehensive and individualized treatment plan is essential. This often involves a multimodal approach, combining pharmacological and non-pharmacological interventions to address different pain pathways. Pharmacological management typically includes analgesics like non-steroidal anti-inflammatory drugs (NSAIDs), opioids, and local anesthetics. Each class of drug has distinct mechanisms of action and potential side effects, necessitating careful selection and dosing.

NSAIDs, such as carprofen or meloxicam, are commonly used for managing mild to moderate pain, particularly in conditions involving inflammation like arthritis. Veterinary technicians must be vigilant about potential side effects, such as gastrointestinal upset or renal dysfunction, and ensure that these drugs are used safely, particularly in patients with pre-existing conditions.

Opioids, including morphine, buprenorphine, and fentanyl, provide potent analgesia for moderate to severe pain. These drugs act centrally to alter pain perception but come with the risk of side effects like sedation, respiratory depression, and gastrointestinal disturbance. Veterinary technicians play a critical role in monitoring patients for these effects and adjusting treatment protocols as needed.

Local anesthetics, such as lidocaine or bupivacaine, are invaluable in both surgical and non-surgical contexts. Administered via local infiltration, nerve blocks, or epidurals, they provide targeted pain relief with minimal systemic effects. Technicians must be proficient in the techniques of administration and understand the pharmacokinetics to avoid toxicity.

Adjunctive therapies, such as gabapentin for neuropathic pain or amantadine as an NMDA antagonist, can enhance analgesic effects when used in combination with other drugs. Veterinary technicians should be familiar with these options, understanding their indications and potential interactions with other medications.

Non-pharmacological interventions are an integral part of comprehensive pain management. Techniques such as physical rehabilitation, acupuncture, laser therapy, and massage can significantly enhance patient comfort and mobility. Veterinary technicians, often at the forefront of administering these therapies, should be trained in their application and aware of their benefits and limitations.

Rehabilitation exercises, tailored to the individual patient's needs, help restore function and alleviate pain through improved strength and flexibility. Technicians must work closely with veterinarians and physical therapists to develop and implement effective rehab plans.

Acupuncture, rooted in traditional Chinese medicine, has gained recognition for its efficacy in pain management. By stimulating specific points on the body, acupuncture can modulate pain pathways and promote healing. Technicians involved in acupuncture must be well-versed in anatomical landmarks and techniques to ensure safe and effective treatment.

Laser therapy, which utilizes specific wavelengths of light to penetrate tissues, can reduce inflammation and pain while promoting tissue repair. Veterinary technicians trained in laser therapy should understand the principles of photobiomodulation and adhere to safety protocols to protect both themselves and the patients.

Massage therapy, an ancient practice, can help alleviate pain by improving circulation, reducing muscle tension, and promoting relaxation. Technicians skilled in massage techniques can provide significant relief to patients, particularly those with chronic pain conditions.

Understanding pain management empowers veterinary technicians to make informed decisions, improving patient outcomes and advancing the field of animal healthcare. Through dedication, curiosity, and a commitment to excellence, technicians harness the power of surgical nursing and anesthesia to make a meaningful impact in the lives of animals and their caretakers. The study of these principles is a dynamic and rewarding pursuit, offering opportunities for growth, discovery, and the chance to make a positive difference in veterinary medicine.

CHAPTER 6
DIAGNOSTIC IMAGING TECHNIQUES

Basics of Radiography

Radiography stands as a cornerstone of diagnostic imaging, offering invaluable insights into the internal structures of animals with remarkable precision. Understanding the basics of radiography is essential for veterinary technicians, who play a crucial role in capturing high-quality images that aid in the diagnosis and treatment of various conditions.

At its core, radiography involves the use of X-rays, a form of electromagnetic radiation, to create images of the body's internal structures. When X-rays pass through the body, they are absorbed at different rates by different tissues. Dense structures like bone absorb more X-rays and appear white on the radiograph, while softer tissues like muscles and organs absorb less and appear in shades of gray. Air-filled spaces, such as the lungs, allow most X-rays to pass through and appear black.

The radiographic process begins with positioning the patient correctly. Proper positioning is paramount to obtaining diagnostic-quality images, as even slight misalignment can obscure critical details or lead to misinterpretation. Veterinary technicians must be well-versed in standard positioning techniques for various anatomical regions, such as lateral and dorsoventral views for thoracic imaging or craniocaudal and mediolateral views for extremities.

Ensuring patient safety during radiography is of utmost importance. This involves minimizing exposure to ionizing radiation through the use of appropriate shielding and adhering to the ALARA (As Low As Reasonably Achievable) principle. Lead aprons, gloves, and thyroid shields are essential protective gear for technicians, while lead barriers or sedation may be necessary to keep the animal still and reduce repeated exposures.

The quality of a radiograph depends on several factors, including exposure settings, which are determined by the kilovoltage (kV) and milliamperage (mA). Kilovoltage affects the penetration power of the X-rays, with higher kV settings used for thicker or denser areas. Milliamperage influences the number of X-rays produced, affecting the overall brightness of the image. Veterinary technicians must skillfully adjust these settings based on the size and density of the patient and the anatomical area being imaged to achieve optimal contrast and detail.

Film-screen systems and digital radiography are the two primary methods of capturing radiographic images. Traditional film-screen systems use a cassette containing a film and an intensifying screen, which converts X-rays into visible light, exposing the film and creating an image. This method requires careful handling and processing of the film in a darkroom to avoid artifacts and ensure image quality.

Digital radiography, on the other hand, captures images using digital detectors, either in direct or computed systems. Direct digital radiography (DR) employs flat-panel detectors that produce images instantaneously, streamlining the imaging process and allowing for immediate evaluation. Computed radiography (CR) uses photostimulable phosphor plates that require scanning to produce a digital image. Both digital methods offer advantages over film, including greater efficiency, reduced exposure times, and the ability to enhance and manipulate images for better diagnostic interpretation.

Radiographic contrast agents can be used to enhance visualization of certain structures or systems. These agents, administered orally, intravenously, or via other routes, highlight areas such as the gastrointestinal tract, urinary system, or vascular structures. Understanding the indications, contraindications, and potential side effects of contrast agents is essential for veterinary technicians, who may be involved in their administration and monitoring for adverse reactions.

Interpreting radiographs requires a methodical approach, focusing on the identification of normal anatomical landmarks and any deviations that may indicate pathology. Veterinary technicians support veterinarians by providing high-quality images and assisting in the initial evaluation of radiographs. Familiarity with common radiographic signs, such as lesions, fractures, or abnormal densities, enhances a technician's ability to contribute to the diagnostic process.

Radiographic artifacts, which can arise from numerous sources, may obscure or mimic pathology, complicating interpretation. Common artifacts include motion blur, grid lines, or foreign objects on the patient or cassette. Veterinary technicians must be adept at recognizing and troubleshooting these artifacts, ensuring that they do not compromise the diagnostic value of the images.

Radiography is not solely about technical proficiency; it also involves effective communication with clients. Veterinary technicians often serve as the first point of contact for pet owners, explaining the purpose and process of radiographic examinations and addressing any concerns. Providing clear and compassionate communication helps alleviate anxiety and fosters trust between the veterinary team and clients.

Understanding the basics of radiography empowers veterinary technicians to make informed decisions, improving patient outcomes and advancing the field of animal healthcare. Through dedication, curiosity, and a commitment to excellence, technicians harness the power of diagnostic imaging to make a meaningful impact in the lives of animals and their caretakers. The study of these principles is a dynamic and rewarding pursuit, offering opportunities for growth, discovery, and the chance to make a positive difference in veterinary medicine.

Ultrasound Utilization

Ultrasound utilization in veterinary practice has revolutionized the way internal structures and organs are examined, offering a non-invasive, safe, and dynamic method of imaging that provides real-time insights. The use of high-frequency sound waves to create images allows for detailed visualization of soft tissues, making it an invaluable tool in diagnosing a variety of conditions.

The mechanics of ultrasound imaging involve a transducer, which emits sound waves that penetrate the body and reflect off tissues at varying speeds. These echoes are captured and converted into images, which are displayed on a monitor. The ability to adjust the frequency of sound waves allows for the examination of structures at different depths, with higher frequencies offering better resolution for superficial tissues and lower frequencies penetrating deeper.

Ultrasound's versatility makes it suitable for a wide range of applications. Abdominal ultrasounds are among the most common, used to assess organs such as the liver, spleen, kidneys, and bladder. The dynamic nature of ultrasound allows veterinarians to observe organ movement and blood flow, providing valuable information about function and pathology. For example, detecting free fluid in the abdomen or identifying masses can guide further diagnostics or interventions.

Cardiac ultrasound, or echocardiography, is another critical application, providing detailed images of the heart's structure and function. It allows for the assessment of cardiac chambers, valves, and blood flow, aiding in the diagnosis of conditions such as cardiomyopathy, valvular disease, and congenital defects. The ability to visualize the heart in real-time helps veterinarians make informed decisions regarding treatment and management.

Reproductive ultrasound is widely used in breeding programs, allowing for the monitoring of pregnancy and assessment of fetal development. It enables the detection of early pregnancy, evaluation of fetal viability, and identification of potential complications. This application is particularly valuable in large animal practice, where early detection of pregnancy can significantly impact breeding management.

Musculoskeletal ultrasound provides insights into injuries and conditions affecting muscles, tendons, and joints. It is particularly useful for diagnosing tendon injuries in equine patients, allowing for precise evaluation of the extent and nature of the damage. This information is essential for developing effective rehabilitation and treatment plans.

When performing an ultrasound examination, proper patient preparation and positioning are crucial for obtaining clear and diagnostic images. The area to be imaged should be shaved and cleaned to eliminate air and debris that can interfere with sound wave transmission. Applying an acoustic coupling gel further enhances wave transmission, ensuring optimal contact between the transducer and skin.

Veterinary technicians play a critical role in the ultrasound process, assisting with patient handling and positioning, as well as operating the ultrasound machine. Familiarity with the machine's controls and settings is essential, as adjustments in gain, depth, and frequency can significantly affect image quality. Technicians must be skilled in recognizing normal anatomical structures and identifying potential abnormalities, providing valuable assistance to veterinarians in interpreting findings.

The interpretation of ultrasound images requires a thorough understanding of anatomy and pathology. Recognizing the echogenicity, or brightness, of tissues is key to identifying normal and abnormal structures. For instance, fluid-filled structures such as cysts or abscesses appear anechoic, or black, due to the lack of internal echoes, while solid tissues like liver or spleen exhibit varying shades of gray. Understanding these patterns aids in distinguishing between different types of lesions and conditions.

While ultrasound is an invaluable diagnostic tool, it has limitations. Sound waves do not penetrate well through bone or air, making it challenging to image structures obscured by these substances. This limitation necessitates the use of complementary imaging modalities, such as radiography or CT, to obtain a complete diagnostic picture.

Understanding ultrasound utilization empowers veterinary technicians to make informed decisions, improving patient outcomes and advancing the field of animal healthcare. Through dedication, curiosity, and a commitment to excellence, technicians harness the power of diagnostic imaging to make a meaningful impact in the lives of animals and their caretakers. The study of these principles is a dynamic and rewarding pursuit, offering opportunities for growth, discovery, and the chance to make a positive difference in veterinary medicine.

Advanced Imaging: CT and MRI

Advanced imaging techniques, such as computed tomography (CT) and magnetic resonance imaging (MRI), have transformed the landscape of veterinary diagnostics, providing unparalleled insights into the anatomy and pathology of animal patients. These modalities offer enhanced visualization and detail, making them indispensable tools for diagnosing complex conditions that may not be apparent with conventional imaging methods.

Computed tomography utilizes X-rays and computer processing to create cross-sectional images of the body, offering a detailed view of both soft tissues and bony structures. The process involves the patient being placed within a circular scanner, where a rotating X-ray beam captures multiple images from different angles. These images are then reconstructed by a computer into a three-dimensional representation, allowing clinicians to examine the body slice by slice.

CT is particularly valuable in assessing complex fractures, evaluating the extent of neoplasms, and visualizing intricate structures such as the skull and spine. Its ability to differentiate between tissues of similar density, such as muscle and fat, provides critical information for surgical planning and treatment decisions. Additionally, CT angiography, a technique that involves the injection of contrast material, enables detailed examination of blood vessels, aiding in the diagnosis of vascular abnormalities.

Magnetic resonance imaging, on the other hand, employs a powerful magnetic field and radiofrequency pulses to generate images. Unlike CT, MRI does not use ionizing radiation, making it a safer option for repeated imaging. The technology excels in visualizing soft tissues, providing exceptional detail of the brain, spinal cord, muscles, and ligaments. The process involves placing the patient within a magnetic coil, where the interaction between the magnetic field and the body's hydrogen atoms produces signals that are converted into images by a computer.

MRI is the gold standard for assessing neurological conditions, such as intervertebral disc disease, brain tumors, and spinal cord lesions. Its superior contrast resolution allows for the differentiation of subtle tissue changes, making it invaluable for diagnosing conditions that affect the central nervous system. MRI is also highly effective in evaluating soft tissue injuries, such as ligament tears or muscle strains, providing detailed information that guides therapeutic interventions.

The preparation and handling of patients undergoing CT or MRI require meticulous attention to detail. Anesthesia is typically necessary to ensure the patient remains still during the procedure, as movement can compromise image quality. Veterinary technicians play a crucial role in anesthetic management, monitoring vital signs and adjusting anesthesia levels as needed to maintain patient stability. Additionally, technicians are responsible for positioning the patient correctly within the scanner, using positioning aids to achieve optimal alignment and reduce the risk of artifacts.

Understanding the indications and limitations of each modality is essential for selecting the appropriate imaging technique. While CT provides rapid imaging and excellent detail of bone and air-filled structures, MRI offers superior soft tissue contrast and is less affected by artifacts from metal implants. The choice between CT and MRI often depends on the clinical question, patient condition, and availability of equipment.

Interpreting CT and MRI images requires a high level of expertise and familiarity with cross-sectional anatomy. Radiologists and veterinary specialists collaborate to analyze the images, identifying abnormalities and correlating findings with clinical signs. Veterinary technicians support this process by preparing high-quality images and assisting with post-processing tasks, such as adjusting image contrast or reconstructing three-dimensional views.

The integration of advanced imaging into veterinary practice has expanded diagnostic capabilities, enabling early detection and accurate characterization of diseases. However, the cost and complexity of these modalities necessitate judicious use, balancing the benefits of advanced imaging with the financial and logistical considerations for pet owners.

Embracing advanced imaging modalities empowers veterinary professionals to make informed decisions, improving diagnostic accuracy and patient outcomes. Through dedication, curiosity, and a commitment to excellence, veterinary technicians harness the power of CT and MRI to make a meaningful impact in the lives of animals and their caretakers. The study and application of these technologies offer opportunities for growth, discovery, and the chance to make a positive difference in veterinary medicine, ensuring that animal patients receive the highest standard of care in an ever-evolving field.

Interpretation of Diagnostic Images

Interpreting diagnostic images is both an art and a science, requiring a blend of technical knowledge, keen observation, and clinical insight. The process of discerning meaningful information from radiographs, ultrasounds, CT scans, and MRIs is fundamental to veterinary diagnostics, guiding decisions that directly impact patient care.

The journey of interpretation begins with understanding the anatomy and physiology of the species being examined. Each animal presents unique anatomical features that must be recognized and understood in the context of the image. Whether it's the intricate bone structures of a canine skull or the delicate soft tissues of a feline abdomen, familiarity with normal anatomy sets the stage for identifying deviations indicative of pathology.

Radiographs, the most traditional form of diagnostic imaging, require a systematic approach for interpretation. Begin by assessing image quality—ensuring proper exposure, positioning, and absence of artifacts. Once image integrity is confirmed, proceed with evaluating the anatomical structures. For skeletal radiographs, scrutinize bone alignment, density, and integrity, looking for signs of fractures, lytic lesions, or abnormal growth patterns. In thoracic radiographs, focus on the heart's silhouette, lung fields, and pleural space, noting any signs of mass effect, fluid accumulation, or air trapping.

Ultrasound interpretation hinges on recognizing the echogenicity and architecture of tissues. Each organ presents a characteristic appearance; for instance, the liver appears as a homogenous medium echogenic structure, while the gall bladder should be anechoic. Deviations from these norms—such as hyperechoic masses, irregular borders, or fluid accumulation—warrant further investigation. The dynamic nature of ultrasound allows for real-time assessment of organ function, such as observing peristalsis in the gastrointestinal tract or cardiac motion in echocardiography.

CT scans offer cross-sectional views that require a three-dimensional understanding of anatomy. Interpretation involves navigating through slices, correlating findings across multiple planes. Pay attention to contrast differentiation between tissues; areas of increased or decreased attenuation may indicate pathology such as tumors or ischemic events. CT is particularly adept at evaluating complex anatomical regions, like the skull or thorax, where overlapping structures on radiographs can obscure details.

MRI interpretation focuses on the intricate detail of soft tissues, leveraging its superior contrast resolution. When examining an MRI, assess signal intensity patterns within tissues, as variations can reveal pathology. For instance, areas of hyperintensity on T2-weighted images might suggest edema or inflammation. Understanding the sequences used—T1, T2, FLAIR, or DWI—guides interpretation, as each sequence highlights different tissue characteristics.

In all imaging modalities, the presence of artifacts can confound interpretation. Recognizing common artifacts—such as motion blur in radiographs, acoustic shadowing in ultrasound, or metal artifacts in CT and MRI—is crucial. Differentiating these from true pathological findings prevents misdiagnosis and ensures accurate clinical decisions.

Interpretation of diagnostic images is a skill honed over time, blending technical proficiency with clinical acumen. By embracing this multifaceted discipline, veterinary professionals enhance their ability to provide accurate diagnoses and effective treatments, ultimately improving patient outcomes and advancing the field of veterinary medicine. Through dedication, curiosity, and a commitment to excellence, veterinary technicians contribute significantly to the lives of animals and their caretakers, making a positive difference in an ever-evolving field.

Safety Protocols and Best Practices

Ensuring safety while utilizing diagnostic imaging techniques in veterinary practice is paramount to protecting both the patient and the personnel involved. As these modalities often involve exposure to radiation or other potential hazards, strict adherence to safety protocols and best practices is essential. This chapter delves into the comprehensive measures required to maintain a safe environment during imaging procedures, emphasizing the importance of education, equipment, and procedural guidelines.

Understanding the potential risks associated with diagnostic imaging is the first step in implementing effective safety protocols. Radiography, for instance, involves ionizing radiation, which poses a risk of cellular damage with prolonged or excessive exposure. While the levels used in veterinary settings are generally low, cumulative exposure over time can increase the risk of health issues in both humans and animals. Therefore, the principle of ALARA—"As Low As Reasonably Achievable"—is a cornerstone of radiation safety, dictating that every effort should be made to minimize exposure while obtaining the necessary diagnostic information.

Personal protective equipment (PPE) is a critical component in safeguarding veterinary staff during radiographic procedures. Lead aprons, gloves, and thyroid shields are essential for reducing radiation exposure. These protective garments are designed to absorb scatter radiation, preventing it from reaching the body. Regular inspection and maintenance of PPE are crucial, as damaged or worn equipment can compromise protection. Additionally, ensuring that all personnel are trained in the correct use and care of PPE enhances its effectiveness.

Positioning devices and restraint techniques play a vital role in minimizing radiation exposure to both patients and staff. Proper positioning not only ensures high-quality diagnostic images but also reduces the need for repeated exposures. In some cases, chemical restraint or sedation may be necessary to keep the animal still, further reducing the risk of unnecessary radiation exposure caused by movement. Veterinary technicians must be adept at selecting and using appropriate positioning aids, such as sandbags, foam wedges, and troughs, to achieve optimal patient alignment.

The use of dosimeters is another essential safety measure for monitoring radiation exposure among veterinary staff. These devices track cumulative exposure over time, allowing for the identification of any individuals at risk of exceeding safety thresholds. Regular review of dosimeter readings enables timely interventions and adjustments to protocols if necessary, ensuring that exposure remains within safe limits.

Training and education are foundational to implementing and maintaining effective safety protocols. All veterinary personnel should receive comprehensive training in radiation safety, including the principles of ALARA, proper use of PPE, and safe operating procedures for imaging equipment. Continuing education opportunities, such as workshops and seminars, provide ongoing learning and updates on the latest safety standards and technologies.

In addition to radiation safety, other imaging modalities such as ultrasound and MRI have their own specific safety considerations. Ultrasound is generally considered safe, as it uses sound waves rather than radiation. However, proper handling of equipment and awareness of ergonomic practices are important to prevent repetitive strain injuries among technicians. MRI safety is primarily concerned with the strong magnetic fields involved; ensuring that no ferromagnetic objects enter the MRI suite is critical to preventing accidents. Comprehensive screening of both patients and personnel for metal implants or devices is necessary prior to MRI procedures.

In summary, the successful implementation of safety protocols and best practices in diagnostic imaging requires a comprehensive approach that encompasses education, equipment, procedural guidelines, and a culture of continuous improvement. By embracing these principles, veterinary professionals enhance the safety and efficacy of imaging techniques, ultimately benefiting patients and advancing the field of veterinary medicine.

CHAPTER 7
LABORATORY PROCEDURES AND TECHNIQUES

Sample Collection and Handling

The foundation of accurate veterinary diagnostics lies in the meticulous collection and handling of samples. Whether it's blood, urine, feces, or tissue biopsies, the quality of these specimens directly influences the reliability of laboratory results. Mastering the art of sample collection and handling is essential for veterinary technicians, who serve as the critical link between clinical evaluation and laboratory analysis.

Blood collection is one of the most common procedures performed in veterinary practice and demands precision and care. The choice of collection site varies depending on the species and size of the animal. For dogs and cats, the cephalic, jugular, or saphenous veins are typically preferred. In larger animals, such as horses and cattle, the jugular vein is often the site of choice due to its accessibility. Proper restraint and positioning are crucial to minimize stress and ensure a successful venipuncture. The use of correct needle gauge and size helps prevent hemolysis and ensures a sufficient sample volume.

Once collected, blood samples must be handled with care to maintain their integrity. Anticoagulants, such as EDTA or heparin, may be used depending on the tests required. It's vital to use the correct anticoagulant to prevent clotting while preserving the sample's components. For serum analysis, allow the blood to clot naturally before centrifugation to separate the serum from cells. Labeling samples accurately with the patient's details and time of collection prevents mix-ups and ensures traceability throughout the laboratory process.

Urine collection is another critical aspect of veterinary diagnostics, providing insights into renal function and overall health. Methods of collection include free catch, catheterization, and cystocentesis. Free catch is the least invasive but may introduce contaminants, affecting test results. Catheterization allows for more controlled collection but requires aseptic technique to prevent infection. Cystocentesis, though invasive, offers the most sterile sample and is preferred for cultures. Once collected, urine should be analyzed promptly or refrigerated to prevent changes in composition.

Fecal samples are essential for diagnosing gastrointestinal disorders and parasitic infections. Collecting fresh samples is imperative, as prolonged exposure to air can alter the presence of certain parasites or affect the pH and moisture content. Technicians should instruct pet owners on proper collection methods, emphasizing the importance of using clean containers and avoiding contamination with soil or litter.

Tissue biopsies provide valuable information about cellular structure and pathology. The technique used for collection—be it fine-needle aspiration, punch biopsy, or surgical excision—depends on the nature of the lesion and its location. Ensuring aseptic conditions during collection minimizes the risk of infection and preserves tissue integrity. Samples should be placed in appropriate fixatives, such as formalin, to prevent degradation and prepare them for histopathological examination.

Handling and transportation of samples are critical steps in maintaining their viability and ensuring accurate laboratory results. Blood and urine samples should be transported in insulated containers to maintain a stable temperature, while tissue samples require secure packaging to prevent leakage or contamination. Adhering to specific transport guidelines, such as those for infectious substances, ensures compliance with regulatory standards and protects both the sample and personnel.

Veterinary technicians must be adept at recognizing common pitfalls in sample collection and handling that can compromise diagnostic accuracy. Hemolysis in blood samples, for example, can result from excessive force during collection or improper handling and may interfere with certain assays. Contamination of urine samples with skin flora can lead to false-positive culture results, while delayed analysis of fecal samples can obscure the presence of parasites.

By mastering the techniques of sample collection and handling, veterinary technicians contribute significantly to the diagnostic process, ensuring that laboratory results accurately reflect the patient's condition. Their expertise in this area supports the accurate diagnosis and effective treatment of animal patients, ultimately advancing the field of veterinary medicine. Through dedication, precision, and collaboration, technicians play a vital role in the health and well-being of the animals they serve.

Hematology and Blood Chemistry

Hematology and blood chemistry are the cornerstones of veterinary diagnostics, offering a detailed glimpse into the physiological status of an animal. These laboratory procedures provide critical information that aids in diagnosing diseases, monitoring health, and guiding therapeutic decisions. Understanding the principles and techniques of hematology and blood chemistry allows veterinary technicians to play an essential role in ensuring the accuracy and reliability of test results.

Hematology involves the study of blood, focusing on the cellular components that make up this vital fluid. A complete blood count (CBC) is the most common hematology test performed, delivering valuable data about red blood cells (RBCs), white blood cells (WBCs), and platelets. Each component carries distinct physiological roles, and any deviation from normal values can indicate underlying health issues.

Red blood cells are responsible for transporting oxygen from the lungs to tissues and returning carbon dioxide for exhalation. Anemia, characterized by a reduced RBC count or hemoglobin concentration, can result from various causes, including nutritional deficiencies, chronic disease, or acute blood loss. Recognizing the signs of anemia, such as pale mucous membranes or lethargy, and correlating them with CBC results is crucial for identifying the underlying cause and guiding treatment.

White blood cells serve as the primary defense against infection and disease, with different types playing specific roles in the immune response. Neutrophils, lymphocytes, monocytes, eosinophils, and basophils each have unique functions and morphologies. A differential WBC count provides insights into the immune status of the patient, revealing conditions like infection, inflammation, or immune-mediated diseases. For instance, an elevated neutrophil count might suggest a bacterial infection, while increased eosinophils could indicate allergies or parasitic infestations.

Platelets are essential for blood clotting and wound healing. Thrombocytopenia, or low platelet count, can lead to excessive bleeding or bruising, making it vital to identify and address the underlying cause. Conditions such as immune-mediated thrombocytopenia, bone marrow disorders, or certain infections can lead to decreased platelet production or increased destruction.

Blood chemistry analyses evaluate the function of organs and systems, providing a comprehensive overview of the patient's metabolic state. Tests such as liver and kidney panels, electrolyte assessments, and glucose measurements are common components of blood chemistry profiles. Each parameter offers insights into specific physiological processes and potential dysfunctions.

Liver function tests, including alanine aminotransferase (ALT) and alkaline phosphatase (ALP), assess the liver's ability to metabolize and detoxify substances. Elevated enzyme levels may indicate liver disease, bile duct obstruction, or damage from toxins or medications. Identifying the cause of liver dysfunction is crucial for implementing effective treatment strategies and monitoring response to therapy.

Kidney function is evaluated through tests such as blood urea nitrogen (BUN) and creatinine. These parameters reflect the kidneys' ability to filter waste products from the blood. Elevated levels may indicate renal insufficiency or failure, necessitating further investigation and management. Monitoring kidney function is also essential in patients receiving medications that can affect renal health.

Electrolyte imbalances can result in a variety of clinical signs, from muscle weakness to cardiac arrhythmias. Assessing levels of sodium, potassium, chloride, and calcium helps identify disturbances that require correction. Conditions such as dehydration, endocrine disorders, or certain medications can lead to electrolyte imbalances, making regular monitoring essential.

Glucose levels provide insight into carbohydrate metabolism and pancreatic function. Hyperglycemia, or elevated glucose levels, may suggest diabetes mellitus, while hypoglycemia can result from insulin overdose, liver disease, or certain tumors. Accurate measurement and interpretation of glucose levels are critical for managing diabetic patients and preventing complications.

The accuracy of hematology and blood chemistry results relies on proper sample collection, handling, and processing. Ensuring that samples are collected in the correct tubes with appropriate anticoagulants and transported under optimal conditions prevents pre-analytical errors that could affect results. For instance, EDTA tubes are used for CBCs, while serum separator tubes are suitable for chemistry panels.

Veterinary technicians play a pivotal role in performing and interpreting hematology and blood chemistry tests. Familiarity with laboratory equipment, such as automated analyzers and microscopes, is essential for generating accurate results. Technicians must also be skilled in performing manual differential counts and identifying morphological abnormalities in blood smears.

Quality control is a critical aspect of laboratory testing, ensuring the reliability and accuracy of results. Regular calibration and maintenance of equipment, along with adherence to standard operating procedures, are fundamental to achieving consistent results. Participation in proficiency testing programs and external quality assessments further validates the accuracy of laboratory processes.

By mastering the principles and techniques of hematology and blood chemistry, veterinary technicians contribute significantly to the diagnostic process, ensuring that laboratory results accurately reflect the patient's condition. Through precision, dedication, and collaboration, they play a crucial role in the health and well-being of the animals they serve, advancing the field of veterinary medicine and improving patient outcomes.

Microbiology and Parasitology

Navigating the intricate world of microbiology and parasitology is essential for veterinary technicians, as these disciplines uncover the unseen culprits behind many animal diseases. By understanding the complexities of microorganisms and parasites, technicians can aid veterinarians in diagnosing infections, implementing effective treatments, and preventing disease spread.

In microbiology, the focus is on identifying bacteria, fungi, and viruses that can cause illness in animals. The process begins with the collection of appropriate samples, such as swabs, tissue biopsies, or bodily fluids. Ensuring aseptic technique during collection is critical to avoid contamination, which could skew results and lead to misdiagnosis. Once collected, samples are transported to the laboratory under conditions that preserve their integrity, such as refrigeration for bacterial cultures.

Culturing is a primary method for identifying bacterial and fungal pathogens. In the laboratory, technicians inoculate samples onto selective and differential media, which promote the growth of specific organisms while inhibiting others. For example, blood agar is a common medium that supports the growth of many bacteria, allowing for the observation of hemolytic activity. MacConkey agar, on the other hand, differentiates between lactose fermenters and non-fermenters, aiding in the identification of Gram-negative bacteria.

After incubation, colonies are examined for morphological characteristics, such as shape, size, and color. These observations guide further testing, including Gram staining and biochemical assays. Gram staining differentiates bacteria based on cell wall structure, classifying them as Gram-positive or Gram-negative. This distinction is crucial for guiding antibiotic therapy, as it influences drug susceptibility.

Biochemical tests assess the metabolic capabilities of bacteria, providing additional identification clues. Tests such as catalase, oxidase, and urease reactions, along with carbohydrate fermentation profiles, help pinpoint the specific species. Advanced methods like polymerase chain reaction (PCR) can also be employed for rapid and precise identification. PCR amplifies target DNA sequences, allowing for the detection of pathogens that are difficult to culture or identify through traditional methods.

Antimicrobial susceptibility testing is a vital component of microbiology, determining the sensitivity or resistance of bacteria to various antibiotics. Techniques such as the disk diffusion method or broth dilution assays provide valuable information for selecting effective treatments, minimizing the use of broad-spectrum antibiotics, and combating antimicrobial resistance.

Parasitology delves into the study of parasites that affect animals, including protozoa, helminths, and arthropods. Identifying these organisms is crucial for diagnosing parasitic infections and implementing control measures. Fecal examinations are a common parasitology technique, used to detect intestinal parasites such as Giardia, roundworms, and tapeworms. Techniques like flotation and sedimentation concentrate parasite eggs or cysts, enhancing detection under the microscope.

For protozoal infections, direct smears or stained preparations may be necessary to visualize organisms such as coccidia or Tritrichomonas. Blood smears can reveal hemoparasites like Babesia or Anaplasma, providing insights into infections that affect blood cells. Accurate identification of parasites involves recognizing their distinct morphological features, such as size, shape, and internal structures.

Understanding the life cycles of parasites is essential for effective diagnosis and treatment. Many parasites have complex life cycles involving multiple hosts or environmental stages, which can impact transmission and persistence in the environment. For example, the lifecycle of heartworms involves both mosquitoes and definitive hosts, requiring a multifaceted approach to prevention and control.

By mastering the principles and techniques of microbiology and parasitology, veterinary technicians contribute significantly to the diagnostic process, ensuring that laboratory results accurately reflect the patient's condition. Through precision, dedication, and collaboration, they play a crucial role in the health and well-being of the animals they serve, advancing the field of veterinary medicine and improving patient outcomes.

Urinalysis and Cytology

Urinalysis and cytology are indispensable components of veterinary diagnostics, offering insights into a wide range of physiological and pathological conditions. These laboratory procedures provide critical information about the health status of an animal, guiding clinical decisions and therapeutic interventions. Understanding the principles and techniques of urinalysis and cytology is essential for veterinary technicians, who play a vital role in ensuring the accuracy and reliability of test results.

Urinalysis involves the examination of urine to assess renal function and detect systemic diseases. It begins with the collection of a urine sample, where the method of collection—whether free catch, catheterization, or cystocentesis—can impact the quality and interpretation of results. A clean sample is crucial for accurate analysis, minimizing the risk of contamination that could lead to false findings. Once collected, the urine should be analyzed promptly or refrigerated to prevent decomposition of its components.

The urinalysis process comprises several key components: physical examination, chemical analysis, and microscopic examination. The physical examination evaluates the urine's color, clarity, and odor. These characteristics can provide initial clues about potential issues. For instance, dark yellow urine might indicate dehydration, while cloudy urine could suggest the presence of cells or crystals.

Chemical analysis involves the use of reagent strips to assess various parameters, such as pH, specific gravity, protein, glucose, ketones, bilirubin, and blood. Each of these can reveal important information about the animal's health. A high specific gravity, for example, might indicate concentrated urine due to dehydration, while the presence of glucose could suggest diabetes mellitus. Accurate interpretation of chemical test results requires an understanding of the normal ranges and potential implications of deviations.

Microscopic examination of urine sediment is a critical step in urinalysis, revealing the presence of cells, crystals, casts, and microorganisms. Red and white blood cells in the sediment can indicate inflammation, infection, or bleeding within the urinary tract. Crystals, such as struvite or calcium oxalate, may suggest urinary calculi or predisposition to stone formation. Casts, which are cylindrical structures formed in the renal tubules, can provide insights into kidney health, with different types indicating specific renal conditions.

Cytology, the study of cells, extends beyond urinalysis to encompass the examination of samples from various body sites, such as skin lesions, lymph nodes, and body cavities. This technique allows for the identification of cellular changes associated with inflammation, infection, or neoplasia. Accurate sample collection and preparation are crucial for obtaining diagnostic-quality cytological specimens.

Fine-needle aspiration (FNA) is a common technique used to collect cytological samples from masses or lymph nodes. This minimally invasive procedure involves using a small gauge needle to aspirate cells, which are then spread onto a microscope slide for examination. Proper technique is essential to minimize blood contamination and ensure adequate cellular material is obtained. Air-drying slides rapidly and staining them with appropriate dyes, such as Diff-Quik, enhances cellular detail and facilitates interpretation.

The examination of cytological samples under the microscope requires careful attention to cellular morphology and patterns. Inflammatory conditions often present with an abundance of neutrophils or macrophages, while the presence of bacteria or fungi can indicate infectious processes. Neoplastic conditions may be identified by observing abnormal cell shapes, sizes, and arrangements. Differentiating between benign and malignant neoplasms is a critical skill, guided by criteria such as cellular uniformity, nuclear characteristics, and mitotic figures.

Veterinary technicians must be adept at recognizing common artifacts and pitfalls that can affect the interpretation of urinalysis and cytology results. For instance, prolonged exposure of urine sediment to air can cause crystal formation, leading to misdiagnosis. Similarly, improper slide preparation in cytology can result in cell damage or poor staining, obscuring diagnostic features.

Through precision, dedication, and collaboration, veterinary technicians play a crucial role in the health and well-being of the animals they serve, advancing the field of veterinary medicine and improving patient outcomes. By mastering the principles and techniques of urinalysis and cytology, technicians contribute significantly to the diagnostic process, ensuring that laboratory results accurately reflect the patient's ondition.

Quality Control in Veterinary Laboratories

Quality control in veterinary laboratories serves as the backbone of reliable diagnostics, ensuring that test results are accurate, consistent, and trustworthy. The importance of maintaining rigorous quality control measures cannot be overstated, as they directly impact the efficacy of clinical decisions and the health outcomes of animal patients. For veterinary technicians, mastering quality control protocols is essential for delivering dependable laboratory services.

The foundation of quality control lies in understanding the concept of precision and accuracy. Precision refers to the consistency of test results when repeated under the same conditions, while accuracy denotes how close a test result is to the true value. Both elements are critical for producing reliable data, and achieving them requires meticulous attention to detail and adherence to established procedures.

Implementing standard operating procedures (SOPs) is a crucial step in maintaining quality control. SOPs provide a detailed guide for performing laboratory tests, outlining every step from sample collection to result analysis. By following these protocols, technicians can minimize variability and ensure that each test is conducted consistently. Regular training and updates to SOPs are necessary to incorporate new techniques and address any procedural gaps.

Calibration and maintenance of laboratory equipment are integral to quality control. Instruments such as microscopes, analyzers, and centrifuges must be regularly calibrated to ensure their accuracy. This process involves comparing the equipment's output to a known standard and making adjustments as needed. Routine maintenance, such as cleaning and replacing parts, prevents equipment malfunctions that could compromise test results.

Participation in proficiency testing programs is another essential element of quality control. These programs involve analyzing samples provided by external organizations and comparing results with those of other laboratories. This external validation helps identify any discrepancies or areas for improvement, providing an opportunity to enhance laboratory practices. Proficiency testing also fosters confidence in the accuracy of laboratory results, both for the veterinary team and for clients.

Internal quality control measures, such as running control samples alongside patient specimens, offer continuous monitoring of test performance. Control samples are designed to mimic patient samples but have known values, allowing technicians to assess whether the test system is functioning correctly. If control results fall outside the expected range, it may indicate an issue with the test method, reagents, or equipment, prompting further investigation and corrective action.

Documentation plays a pivotal role in quality control, ensuring traceability and accountability throughout the laboratory process. Detailed records of test results, equipment maintenance, calibrations, and proficiency testing outcomes provide a comprehensive overview of laboratory performance. These records are invaluable for identifying trends, addressing recurring issues, and demonstrating compliance with regulatory standards.

By mastering the principles and techniques of quality control, veterinary technicians contribute significantly to the diagnostic process, ensuring that laboratory results accurately reflect the patient's condition. Their expertise in this area supports the accurate diagnosis and effective treatment of animal patients, ultimately advancing the field of veterinary medicine. Through precision, dedication, and collaboration, technicians play a critical role in the health and well-being of the animals they serve, improving patient outcomes and fostering trust with clients.

CHAPTER 8
DENTISTRY AND ORAL HEALTH IN ANIMALS

Anatomy of the Oral Cavity

Understanding the anatomy of the oral cavity in animals is essential for anyone involved in veterinary dentistry and oral health care. This knowledge provides a foundation for diagnosing dental diseases, performing procedures, and offering comprehensive care to animal patients. The oral cavity is a complex system, intricately designed for various functions, including ingestion, vocalization, and, in some species, defense.

The oral cavity begins at the lips and extends to the pharynx. It comprises several key structures: the lips, cheeks, teeth, gums, tongue, hard and soft palates, salivary glands, and the oropharynx. Each component plays a specific role in the functionality and health of the mouth.

The lips, forming the anterior boundary of the oral cavity, are muscular structures that help manipulate food, facilitating the initial stages of mastication and preventing food spillage. They vary significantly between species, influencing the way animals interact with their environment. For instance, horses have highly sensitive and mobile lips to aid in selective foraging, while carnivores like cats and dogs use theirs primarily for holding and manipulating prey.

Cheeks form the lateral walls of the oral cavity and are instrumental in keeping food between the teeth during chewing. They are lined with mucous membranes that provide lubrication and protection, supporting the process of digestion. In rodents, the cheeks are more pronounced, allowing for food storage—a trait that highlights the diversity in oral cavity function across species.

Teeth are perhaps the most prominent and functionally diverse structures within the oral cavity. They are classified into incisors, canines, premolars, and molars, each serving distinct purposes. Incisors are primarily for cutting or nibbling food, canines for tearing and holding, and premolars and molars for grinding. The dental formula varies between species, reflecting dietary adaptations. For example, herbivores like rabbits have continuously growing teeth to compensate for constant wear from fibrous plant material, whereas carnivores possess sharp, pointed teeth suitable for slicing through flesh.

The gums, or gingiva, are the soft tissue that surrounds and supports the teeth. Healthy gums are crucial for overall oral health, providing a barrier against pathogens and contributing to the stability of the teeth. Signs of gingival inflammation, such as redness or swelling, can indicate periodontal disease, necessitating prompt veterinary attention.

The tongue is a muscular organ that plays multiple roles, including food manipulation, taste, and, in some species, thermoregulation. Its surface is covered with papillae, which house taste buds and aid in the mechanical processing of food. The tongue's mobility and dexterity are particularly important in species-specific feeding behaviors, such as the lapping of water by cats and dogs or the prehensile action seen in cows.

The hard palate forms the roof of the mouth and separates the oral and nasal cavities. It is ridged and provides a surface against which the tongue can press food during mastication. Posteriorly, the hard palate transitions to the soft palate, a flexible structure that rises during swallowing to close off the nasopharynx, preventing food from entering the nasal passages.

Salivary glands are scattered throughout the oral cavity, producing saliva that lubricates food, aids in digestion, and maintains oral health. Saliva contains enzymes such as amylase, which begin the breakdown of carbohydrates, and antimicrobial agents that help control oral bacteria. The major salivary glands include the parotid, mandibular, and sublingual glands, each contributing to the production and secretion of saliva.

The oropharynx is the section of the pharynx that lies behind the oral cavity and functions as a passageway for food and air. During swallowing, the epiglottis, a flap of cartilage, covers the trachea to prevent aspiration.

Understanding the anatomy of the oropharynx is vital for recognizing and managing conditions that affect swallowing or breathing.

In addition to these structures, the oral cavity is richly supplied with nerves and blood vessels, essential for sensation and nourishment. The trigeminal nerve provides sensory innervation to the teeth and gums, while the facial nerve contributes to the movement of the lips and cheeks. Blood supply is primarily through branches of the external carotid artery, ensuring that tissues receive the necessary nutrients and oxygen.

In conclusion, the oral cavity is a multifunctional and complex system, integral to an animal's health and survival. Mastery of its anatomy provides the foundation for effective veterinary dental care, enabling professionals to diagnose and treat a wide range of conditions. Through ongoing education and practice, veterinary technicians and other professionals can ensure that they deliver the highest standard of care, ultimately enhancing the quality of life for their animal patients.

Common Dental Diseases

Dental diseases in animals are a significant concern, often impacting their overall health and quality of life. As animals cannot verbally communicate discomfort, it's crucial for veterinary professionals to recognize the signs of dental issues and address them promptly. Understanding common dental diseases allows for early intervention, preventing complications that can affect an animal's systemic health.

Periodontal disease is among the most prevalent dental conditions in both domestic and wild animals, particularly in dogs and cats. It starts with gingivitis, an inflammation of the gums caused by plaque accumulation. Plaque, a sticky biofilm of bacteria, hardens into tartar when not removed, irritating the gums and leading to infection. As the disease progresses, periodontal disease affects the structures supporting the teeth, eventually causing tooth loss if untreated. Symptoms include bad breath, red or swollen gums, and reluctance to chew. Regular dental cleanings and at-home oral care are vital in managing periodontal disease.

Tooth resorption is another common issue, especially in cats, where it affects a significant portion of the feline population. This condition involves the gradual destruction of the tooth structure, often beginning at the root and progressing to the crown. The cause of tooth resorption remains unclear, but it results in painful lesions that can lead to tooth loss. Affected cats may show signs such as drooling, difficulty eating, or pawing at the mouth. Radiographs are essential for diagnosing tooth resorption, as lesions often occur below the gumline.

Fractured teeth are frequently encountered in animals, resulting from trauma such as chewing on hard objects or accidents. Fractures can expose the tooth pulp, leading to pain and potential infection. Depending on the fracture's severity, treatment options range from extraction to root canal therapy. Immediate veterinary attention is crucial to prevent further complications and alleviate discomfort.

Malocclusion, or misalignment of the teeth, is another dental concern, particularly in brachycephalic breeds and rodents. In these cases, improper alignment can cause excessive wear on the teeth, difficulty eating, and oral trauma. In rodents, malocclusion can lead to overgrown incisors, as their teeth continuously grow. Regular dental check-ups and appropriate interventions, such as teeth trimming or orthodontic devices, are necessary to manage malocclusion effectively.

Stomatitis, an inflammation of the oral mucosa, is a painful condition often seen in cats. It may be linked to viral infections, immune-mediated diseases, or dental plaque. Affected animals exhibit symptoms such as drooling, bad breath, and reluctance to eat. Treatment typically involves addressing the underlying cause, managing pain, and maintaining oral hygiene. In severe cases, full-mouth extractions may be considered to alleviate discomfort.

Oral tumors, both benign and malignant, can occur in animals, with older pets being more susceptible. Squamous cell carcinoma is one of the most common malignant tumors in cats, while dogs frequently develop melanomas and fibrosarcomas. These tumors can cause swelling, bleeding, and difficulty eating. Early detection through regular oral examinations is crucial for successful treatment, which may involve surgery, radiation, or chemotherapy.

Feline odontoclastic resorptive lesions (FORLs) are a specific type of tooth resorption seen in cats. These lesions result in the gradual destruction of dental tissue, often causing significant pain. The exact cause of FORLs is still unknown, but they are characterized by the presence of resorptive lesions at the tooth neck or crown. Treatment typically involves extraction of the affected teeth to relieve pain and prevent further progression.

Halitosis, or bad breath, is a common indicator of underlying dental issues. While it may seem benign, persistent halitosis should not be ignored, as it often signals periodontal disease, oral infections, or systemic health problems. Identifying and addressing the root cause of halitosis is essential for improving oral health and overall well-being.

Dental caries, or cavities, are less common in animals than humans but can still occur, particularly in dogs. Cavities result from the demineralization of tooth enamel by bacterial acids, leading to decay. Affected teeth may exhibit dark spots or visible holes and can cause pain or sensitivity. Treatment options include fillings or extractions, depending on the severity of the decay.

In summary, common dental diseases in animals range from periodontal disease and tooth resorption to malocclusions and oral tumors. Each presents unique challenges and requires specific diagnostic and therapeutic strategies. By recognizing the signs of these conditions and promoting preventive care, veterinary professionals can significantly impact the health and comfort of their patients. Through expertise, dedication, and collaboration, they ensure that animals receive the highest standard of dental care, ultimately improving their overall quality of life.

Dental Prophylaxis and Treatments

Maintaining optimal oral health in animals is essential for their overall well-being, and dental prophylaxis plays a pivotal role in this process. Dental prophylaxis refers to preventive measures and treatments aimed at preserving oral health and preventing dental diseases. As veterinary professionals, understanding the techniques and practices involved in dental prophylaxis and treatments is crucial for providing comprehensive care to animal patients.

Dental prophylaxis begins with a thorough oral examination, which serves as the foundation for identifying existing dental issues and assessing the overall health of the oral cavity. During this examination, veterinarians and technicians inspect the teeth, gums, tongue, and other oral structures for signs of disease, such as plaque buildup, gingival inflammation, or tooth fractures. This initial assessment helps determine the appropriate course of action for each patient.

Once the examination is complete, the next step in dental prophylaxis is scaling and polishing. Scaling involves the removal of plaque and tartar from the tooth surfaces and below the gumline. This is achieved using specialized instruments, such as ultrasonic scalers and hand scalers, which effectively dislodge and remove deposits without damaging the tooth enamel. Proper technique is essential to avoid trauma to the gums and to ensure thorough cleaning.

After scaling, polishing the teeth is critical to smooth the enamel surfaces and reduce the likelihood of future plaque accumulation. Polishing is performed with a low-speed handpiece and a prophylaxis paste, which helps remove any remaining microabrasions and leaves the teeth with a smooth, glossy finish. This step not only enhances the appearance of the teeth but also contributes to prolonging the effects of the cleaning.

In some cases, dental radiographs are necessary to gain a complete understanding of the animal's oral health. Radiographs can reveal issues not visible to the naked eye, such as root fractures, resorptive lesions, or bone loss associated with periodontal disease. By identifying these hidden problems, veterinary professionals can develop a more comprehensive treatment plan tailored to the individual needs of the patient.

For animals with diagnosed dental diseases, additional treatments may be required beyond prophylaxis. One common procedure is tooth extraction, which becomes necessary when a tooth is severely compromised by infection, fracture, or resorption. Extractions are performed with care to minimize trauma and discomfort, ensuring that all root fragments are removed to prevent complications.

Root canal therapy offers an alternative to extraction for certain teeth, particularly those that are essential for function or aesthetics. This procedure involves removing the infected pulp from the tooth's interior, cleaning and disinfecting the canal, and filling it with a biocompatible material to restore the tooth's integrity. While more complex than extractions, root canals can save teeth that would otherwise be lost.

For animals with malocclusions or orthodontic issues, orthodontic treatments may be indicated to improve oral function and comfort. These treatments can include the use of braces, appliances, or selective tooth extractions to correct misalignments and create a more balanced occlusion. Veterinary orthodontics is a specialized field, requiring a deep understanding of dental anatomy and biomechanics to achieve successful outcomes.

Periodontal therapy is another important aspect of dental treatments, particularly for animals with advanced periodontal disease. This therapy may involve deep cleaning procedures, such as root planing and gingival curettage, to remove plaque and tartar from below the gumline and promote healing of periodontal tissues. In severe cases, surgical interventions, such as flap surgery, may be necessary to access and clean deep periodontal pockets.

In addition to professional dental cleanings and treatments, at-home oral care is vital for maintaining oral health between veterinary visits. Educating pet owners on the importance of regular tooth brushing, the use of dental chews, and providing a balanced diet can significantly reduce the risk of dental disease. Veterinary technicians play a key role in demonstrating proper brushing techniques and recommending appropriate oral care products tailored to each animal's needs.

Through expertise, dedication, and a commitment to excellence, veterinary professionals play a vital role in maintaining the oral health of animals. By mastering the principles and techniques of dental prophylaxis and treatments, they ensure that animals receive the highest standard of care. This proactive approach not only prevents dental disease but also enhances the overall well-being of animal patients, fostering a healthier and happier life.

Tools and Techniques in Veterinary Dentistry

Veterinary dentistry has evolved considerably over the years, with advancements in tools and techniques significantly improving the quality of care that animals receive. Understanding these tools and techniques is crucial for veterinary professionals who are responsible for ensuring optimal oral health in their patients. The right equipment, combined with skilled techniques, allows for precise diagnostics and effective treatments, ultimately enhancing the well-being of animals.

One of the fundamental tools in veterinary dentistry is the dental scaler. Available in both manual and ultrasonic forms, scalers are essential for removing plaque and tartar from tooth surfaces. Manual scalers require meticulous hand movements to effectively clean the teeth, while ultrasonic scalers use high-frequency vibrations to break up deposits with less physical effort. The choice between the two often depends on the specific needs of the patient and the preference of the practitioner. Ultrasonic scalers are particularly useful in reducing the time required for cleaning, which can be beneficial in minimizing anesthesia time for the patient.

Dental probes and explorers are indispensable for examining the oral cavity. These slender, pointed instruments help identify pockets, cavities, and other abnormalities by providing tactile feedback to the practitioner. Probes are particularly useful for measuring periodontal pocket depth, which is a key indicator of periodontal health. Explorers, with their sharp tips, are used to detect irregularities on the tooth surface, such as caries or fractures. Mastery of these instruments is crucial for accurate diagnostics and treatment planning.

Dental radiography is another critical component of veterinary dentistry. Radiographs provide a detailed view of the teeth, roots, and surrounding bone structures, revealing issues that are not visible during a standard oral examination. Digital radiography has become increasingly popular due to its ability to produce high-quality images quickly, allowing for immediate analysis and decision-making. It also reduces radiation exposure and eliminates the need for chemical processing, making it a more environmentally friendly option.

Extraction forceps and elevators are vital for performing tooth extractions. Elevators are used to loosen the tooth from its socket by severing the periodontal ligament, while forceps are employed to grasp and remove the tooth. The design of these instruments varies based on the size and type of tooth being extracted. Proper technique is essential to minimize trauma to surrounding tissues and ensure complete removal of the tooth and roots. Training and experience are crucial for mastering these procedures and reducing the risk of complications.

Polishing equipment is essential for finishing the cleaning process. After scaling, polishing smooths the tooth surface, reducing the likelihood of plaque re-accumulation. Polishing is performed using a low-speed handpiece with a rubber cup or brush, along with a polishing paste. This step not only enhances the appearance of the teeth but also contributes to long-term oral health by creating an environment less conducive to bacterial growth.

Dental units, which integrate various instruments and functionalities, are central to a well-equipped veterinary dental suite. These units typically include air and water syringes, high and low-speed handpieces, suction devices, and piezoelectric scalers. Having all necessary tools in one unit streamlines procedures, allowing for efficient workflow and reducing the time the patient spends under anesthesia.

For more advanced procedures, such as root canals or orthodontics, specialized instruments are required. Endodontic files and reamers are used in root canal therapy to clean and shape the root canal before filling it with a biocompatible material. Orthodontic tools, including braces and aligners, help correct malocclusions and improve dental function. These specialized instruments require additional training and expertise to ensure successful outcomes.

Anesthesia is a critical component of veterinary dentistry, as most procedures require the patient to be still and pain-free. Understanding anesthesia protocols, monitoring equipment, and recovery techniques is essential for ensuring patient safety and comfort. Anesthesia machines, equipped with vaporizer settings and oxygen delivery systems, are vital for maintaining appropriate anesthesia levels throughout the procedure. Monitoring devices track vital signs, ensuring that any changes in the patient's condition are promptly addressed.

Through dedication, expertise, and a commitment to excellence, veterinary professionals play a vital role in maintaining the oral health of animals. By mastering the tools and techniques of veterinary dentistry, they ensure that animals receive the highest standard of care. This proactive approach not only prevents dental disease but also enhances the overall well-being of animal patients, fostering a healthier and happier life.

Client Education on Oral Health

Educating clients about oral health is a fundamental aspect of veterinary care, ensuring that pet owners understand the importance of maintaining their animals' dental hygiene. By fostering a collaborative relationship between veterinary professionals and clients, the health and well-being of animal companions can be significantly enhanced. Communication is key, and providing clear, accessible information empowers pet owners to take an active role in their animals' oral health.

The journey to effective client education begins with understanding the common misconceptions and gaps in knowledge that many pet owners have about animal oral health. For instance, some may believe that bad breath in pets is normal, while others might underestimate the impact of dental disease on overall health. By addressing these misconceptions, veterinary professionals can lay the groundwork for more informed and proactive pet care.

One effective approach to client education is the use of visual aids and demonstrations. Showing clients images of healthy vs. diseased teeth and gums can be a powerful tool in illustrating the importance of regular dental care. Demonstrations of tooth brushing techniques, using models or even their own pets, can help demystify the process and encourage owners to incorporate it into their routine. Visual aids not only enhance understanding but also leave a lasting impression, making it more likely that clients will adhere to recommended practices.

Regular communication with clients about their pets' oral health status is essential. During check-ups and dental cleanings, veterinary professionals should provide detailed explanations of any findings, such as plaque buildup, gingivitis, or tooth fractures. Offering a clear assessment and discussing potential consequences of neglecting dental care can motivate clients to prioritize oral hygiene. Providing written reports or digital summaries can further reinforce the information shared during consultations.

Customized oral health plans are an invaluable tool in client education. Tailoring advice and recommendations to the specific needs of each pet ensures that clients receive relevant and practical guidance. For instance, a young dog with minimal tartar buildup may benefit from preventive measures such as regular tooth brushing and dental chews, while an older cat with periodontal disease might require more intensive treatments and frequent veterinary visits. Personalizing the approach fosters a sense of partnership and responsibility, encouraging clients to take an active role in their pets' oral care.

Highlighting the benefits of good oral hygiene can also be a compelling motivator for clients. Emphasizing the connection between oral health and overall well-being, such as improved breath, reduced risk of systemic diseases, and increased longevity, can help clients understand the value of investing in dental care. Sharing success stories or case studies of pets whose lives have improved through diligent oral hygiene can inspire clients and reinforce the importance of their efforts.

Veterinary technicians play a crucial role in client education, as they often have more direct contact with clients and can provide practical, hands-on guidance. Their expertise and approachable demeanor make them ideal educators, capable of answering questions and addressing concerns. By building rapport and trust with clients, technicians can effectively communicate the significance of oral health and encourage compliance with recommended practices.

Educational materials, such as brochures, handouts, and online resources, are valuable tools for reinforcing the information shared during consultations. Providing clients with easy-to-understand materials that they can reference at home enhances their ability to care for their pets' oral health. These resources should cover a range of topics, from tooth brushing techniques and dietary recommendations to signs of dental disease and when to seek veterinary care.

Workshops and seminars on pet oral health are another effective way to engage clients and promote education. Hosting events at the clinic or partnering with local pet organizations can provide a platform for sharing knowledge and addressing common concerns. These interactive sessions offer an opportunity for clients to learn from experts, ask questions, and practice techniques in a supportive environment. Additionally, they foster a sense of community among pet owners, who can share experiences and advice with one another.

Through dedication, communication, and a commitment to excellence, veterinary professionals can play a transformative role in improving the oral health of animals. By equipping clients with the knowledge and tools they need, they ensure that pets receive the highest standard of care. This proactive approach not only prevents dental disease but also enhances the overall well-being of animal patients, fostering a healthier and happier life.

CHAPTER 9
UNDERSTANDING ANIMAL BEHAVIOR

Fundamentals of Animal Behavior

Animal behavior is an intricate and fascinating field, encompassing a wide range of actions and interactions influenced by genetics, environment, and experience. Understanding the fundamentals of animal behavior provides insight into how animals communicate, survive, and thrive in their natural habitats and in human care. Grasping these basics is crucial for both professional animal caretakers and pet owners, as it enhances the ability to meet the needs of animals and foster harmonious relationships.

At the core of animal behavior lies the concept of instinct. Instinctive behaviors are innate, hardwired actions that animals perform without prior learning or experience. These behaviors are essential for survival and reproduction, such as a bird building a nest or a spider spinning a web. Instincts are typically triggered by specific stimuli and are often consistent across individuals of a species. Understanding the instinctual drives of an animal can help predict its actions and provide appropriate enrichment or interventions to support its natural tendencies.

Learning is another fundamental aspect of animal behavior, allowing animals to adapt to their environments and experiences. Learning can occur through various mechanisms, including habituation, classical conditioning, operant conditioning, and observational learning. Habituation involves an animal becoming accustomed to a stimulus over time, reducing its response to it. This process is crucial for animals living in dynamic environments, as it prevents them from wasting energy on non-threatening stimuli.

Classical conditioning, famously demonstrated by Pavlov's experiments with dogs, involves associating a neutral stimulus with a significant one, leading to a learned response. For instance, if a dog hears a bell before being fed repeatedly, it may begin to salivate at the sound of the bell alone. This type of learning is prevalent in animal training, where signals or cues are paired with desired behaviors.

Operant conditioning, on the other hand, involves learning through consequences. Animals learn to associate their actions with rewards or punishments, which can increase or decrease the likelihood of a behavior recurring. Positive reinforcement, where a desired behavior is followed by a rewarding stimulus, is a powerful tool for shaping animal behavior. Conversely, negative reinforcement involves the removal of an unpleasant stimulus following a behavior, also increasing the likelihood of that behavior.

Observational learning, or social learning, occurs when animals learn by watching and imitating others. This type of learning is particularly significant in species that live in social groups, as it allows individuals to acquire essential skills without direct experience. For example, young primates often learn foraging techniques by observing their mothers, while wolf pups may learn hunting strategies by watching adult pack members.

Communication is a vital component of animal behavior, facilitating interactions between individuals and groups. Animals use a variety of signals, including visual, auditory, olfactory, and tactile cues, to convey information. Visual signals, such as body postures or color changes, can indicate an animal's intentions or emotional state. Auditory signals, such as bird songs or wolf howls, can serve purposes ranging from attracting mates to warning of danger.

Olfactory communication involves the use of scents or pheromones to convey messages. Many animals, such as dogs and cats, use scent marking to establish territory or signal reproductive status. Tactile communication, involving physical contact, can reinforce social bonds or communicate aggression, as seen in grooming behaviors among primates or the nuzzling of horses.

Social behavior is another important aspect of animal interactions, varying widely among species. Some animals, like lions or elephants, live in complex social structures with clear hierarchies and cooperative behaviors. These social groups provide benefits such as increased protection from predators and assistance in raising offspring. Understanding the social dynamics of animals can aid in their care and management, particularly in captive settings.

Conversely, some species are solitary, interacting with others primarily for mating purposes. These animals may exhibit territorial behaviors to defend their space and resources. Recognizing the social preferences of a species is crucial for providing appropriate living conditions and minimizing stress.

Reproductive behavior encompasses the actions and strategies animals use to attract mates, reproduce, and care for their offspring. Courtship displays, mating rituals, and parental care vary significantly across species and are often influenced by environmental factors. For instance, birds may engage in elaborate dances or song displays to attract partners, while some fish species may build nests or care for eggs. Understanding these behaviors can inform breeding programs and improve reproductive success in captive populations.

Aggression and territoriality are also key elements of animal behavior, often driven by the need to secure resources or establish dominance. Aggressive behaviors can manifest as physical confrontations, vocalizations, or displays intended to intimidate rivals. Territorial behaviors involve the defense of a specific area, often through scent marking or visual displays. Recognizing the underlying motivations for aggression or territoriality can aid in managing conflicts and ensuring the well-being of animals in group settings.

By understanding the fundamentals of animal behavior, caregivers and professionals can create environments that meet the physical and psychological needs of animals. This knowledge enhances the ability to interpret and respond to animal actions, fostering positive interactions and improving care standards. As our understanding of animal behavior continues to grow, it opens new avenues for conservation, welfare, and the deepening of our connection with the animal world.

Behavioral Disorders and Treatments

Behavioral disorders in animals can present significant challenges for both the animals themselves and their caregivers. These disorders often manifest as deviations from normal behavior, causing distress or harm to the animal or those around it. Understanding these disorders and their treatments is essential for improving the quality of life for affected animals and fostering better relationships between them and their human companions.

One of the most common behavioral disorders in animals is separation anxiety, particularly prevalent in dogs. This condition arises when an animal becomes excessively anxious or distressed in the absence of its owner or primary attachment figure. Symptoms can include destructive behaviors, vocalization, and attempts to escape. To address separation anxiety, a comprehensive treatment plan often combines behavior modification techniques with environmental management. Gradual desensitization to the owner's departure, along with positive reinforcement for calm behavior, can help alleviate anxiety. In some cases, anti-anxiety medications prescribed by a veterinarian may be necessary to support the behavior modification process.

Aggression is another significant behavioral issue that can occur in various forms, such as fear-based aggression, territorial aggression, or redirected aggression. Identifying the underlying cause of aggression is crucial for effective treatment. Behavior modification techniques, such as counter-conditioning and desensitization, can help change the animal's emotional response to triggers. Additionally, providing a structured environment with clear boundaries and consistent training can reduce aggressive tendencies. Professional guidance from a behaviorist or veterinarian is often necessary to develop a safe and effective treatment plan.

Compulsive behaviors, similar to obsessive-compulsive disorders in humans, can also affect animals. These behaviors may manifest as repetitive actions, such as excessive licking, tail chasing, or pacing. Compulsions often arise from stress, anxiety, or a lack of mental stimulation. Addressing compulsive behaviors involves identifying and mitigating stressors, providing ample mental and physical enrichment, and establishing a consistent routine. In some cases, medications that alter brain chemistry may be prescribed to help manage the condition.

Fear and phobias are common behavioral issues that can significantly impact an animal's quality of life. These may include fear of loud noises, unfamiliar people, or specific objects. Gradual exposure to the fear-inducing stimulus, paired with positive reinforcement, can help animals build confidence and reduce fear responses. Creating a safe and secure environment, along with providing hiding places or safe zones, can further support the animal's well-being. Professional intervention may be required for severe phobias to ensure the safety and comfort of the animal.

House soiling is a behavioral issue that can be particularly frustrating for pet owners. This behavior may result from medical issues, anxiety, or improper house-training. A thorough veterinary examination is essential to rule out any underlying medical conditions. If the issue is behavioral, re-establishing a consistent house-training routine, along with positive reinforcement, can often resolve the problem. Identifying and addressing any anxiety-inducing factors is also crucial for preventing recurrence.

Destructive behavior, such as chewing or digging, can result from boredom, anxiety, or lack of proper outlets for natural behaviors. Providing appropriate toys, activities, and enrichment can redirect these behaviors into more acceptable channels. Ensuring that the animal receives adequate exercise and mental stimulation is essential for preventing destructive tendencies. Training and supervision are also critical components of managing and modifying these behaviors.

In multi-animal households, inter-animal aggression or hierarchy disputes can arise, leading to tension and conflict. Understanding the social dynamics and body language of the animals involved is essential for managing these situations. Providing separate spaces, resources, and supervised interactions can help mitigate aggression. In some cases, a gradual introduction or reintroduction process may be necessary to establish harmony within the group.

Professional intervention is often beneficial for diagnosing and treating complex behavioral disorders. Veterinary behaviorists or certified animal behaviorists can provide expert assessments and develop tailored treatment plans. These professionals have the training and experience to address the nuances of animal behavior and implement evidence-based interventions.

By understanding and addressing behavioral disorders in animals, caregivers can improve the lives of their animal companions and enhance the bond they share. Through compassion, patience, and informed intervention, it is possible to guide animals toward healthier and more harmonious behavior. This approach not only benefits the individual animal but also contributes to a more positive and understanding relationship between humans and the animal world.

Techniques for Behavior Modification

Behavior modification techniques in animals are designed to change undesirable behaviors into more acceptable ones, enhancing the relationship between animals and their caregivers. These techniques rely on understanding the underlying motivations and triggers for behaviors, allowing for targeted and effective interventions. By employing strategic methods, caregivers can guide animals toward positive behavior while fostering trust and cooperation.

A fundamental principle of behavior modification is reinforcement, which involves increasing the likelihood of a behavior through positive or negative reinforcement. Positive reinforcement is a widely used technique that involves rewarding desirable behavior with something the animal finds pleasurable, such as treats, praise, or playtime. The key to successful positive reinforcement is timing and consistency. The reward should be given immediately following the desired behavior to strengthen the association, and it should be applied consistently to establish a clear link between the behavior and the reward.

Negative reinforcement involves removing an unpleasant stimulus when the desired behavior occurs, thereby increasing the likelihood of that behavior being repeated. For example, applying gentle pressure on a dog's back to encourage it to sit, then releasing the pressure when the dog complies, can reinforce the sitting behavior. While effective in some cases, negative reinforcement should be used cautiously to avoid causing stress or anxiety in the animal.

In contrast, punishment seeks to decrease the likelihood of undesirable behavior by introducing an aversive consequence. However, punishment can lead to fear, anxiety, and aggression, potentially damaging the trust between the animal and its caregiver. Therefore, punishment is generally discouraged in favor of positive reinforcement strategies, which encourage learning and cooperation without negative side effects.

Shaping is a technique that involves reinforcing successive approximations of a desired behavior. This method is particularly useful for teaching complex behaviors that the animal may not naturally exhibit. By rewarding small steps toward the final goal, caregivers can gradually shape the animal's behavior. For instance, if training a dog to fetch, the initial reward might be given for simply looking at or touching the toy. As the dog progresses, rewards are given for picking up the toy, carrying it, and finally delivering it to the caregiver.

Desensitization and counter-conditioning are techniques used to address fear-based behaviors or phobias. Desensitization involves exposing the animal to a fear-inducing stimulus at a low and non-threatening level, gradually increasing the intensity as the animal becomes more comfortable. Counter-conditioning pairs the fear-inducing stimulus with a positive experience, such as treats or play, to change the animal's emotional response. Together, these techniques can help animals overcome fears and develop positive associations with previously distressing stimuli.

Clicker training is a popular method that utilizes a small device that makes a distinct clicking sound to mark desired behavior. The clicker serves as a precise signal that the behavior is correct and will be followed by a reward. This technique is effective because it provides clear and immediate feedback, helping animals learn new behaviors quickly. Clicker training can be used for various tasks, from basic obedience commands to advanced tricks and tasks.

Modeling, or social learning, involves teaching an animal a behavior by having it observe another animal or human performing the behavior. This technique leverages the natural tendency of animals to learn through observation and imitation. For example, a dog may learn to navigate an agility course by watching another dog successfully complete it. Modeling can be particularly effective in social species, where individuals are accustomed to learning from group members.

Setting clear and achievable goals is important in behavior modification. Caregivers should identify specific behaviors they wish to encourage or discourage and develop a structured plan for addressing them. Breaking down complex behaviors into smaller, manageable steps can facilitate learning and prevent frustration for both the animal and the caregiver. Regular monitoring and adjustment of the training plan ensure that it remains effective and responsive to the animal's progress.

By using these techniques, caregivers can foster positive behavior changes in animals, promoting a harmonious and enriching relationship. The success of behavior modification rests on a foundation of understanding, trust, and communication, ensuring that animals are not only well-behaved but also happy and secure in their environments. Through dedication and informed methods, caregivers can guide animals toward a more balanced and fulfilling life.

Human-Animal Bond and Its Implications

The human-animal bond is a profound and multifaceted connection, rooted in centuries of shared history and mutual reliance. This relationship holds significant implications for both humans and animals, affecting their well-being, behavior, and social interactions. Understanding the dynamics of this bond can enhance the care and companionship we provide to animals, as well as improve human health and happiness.

Animals have long been companions to humans, providing not just physical labor but also emotional support and companionship. This bond is evident in the way animals are integrated into human families, often considered members with their own personalities and roles. The emotional attachment between humans and animals can lead to improved mental health and reduced feelings of loneliness, as numerous studies have shown the positive effects of pets on human well-being. For instance, spending time with animals can lower stress levels, decrease blood pressure, and increase feelings of happiness and relaxation.

From the animal's perspective, the bond with humans can influence behavior and social dynamics. Animals that are closely bonded with their human caregivers often exhibit behaviors that reflect trust and affection, such as seeking physical contact, following their owners, and responding to vocal cues. This bond can enhance an animal's sense of security and reduce anxiety, contributing to a more stable and content demeanor.

The human-animal bond is not limited to domestic pets; it extends to working animals, therapy animals, and service animals. Each of these relationships involves a unique dynamic, where animals contribute to human tasks or well-being while receiving care and attention in return. Working animals, such as guide dogs or police horses, form partnerships with humans that rely on mutual trust and communication. These animals must be attuned to human signals and cues, while humans must understand and respect the animal's capabilities and limits.

Therapy and service animals offer another dimension to the human-animal bond, providing support to individuals with physical, emotional, or psychological needs. These animals are trained to perform specific tasks, such as guiding individuals with vision impairments, detecting seizures, or offering comfort to those with mental health challenges. The bond between therapy animals and their handlers is often deeply personal, built on a foundation of empathy and understanding that transcends verbal communication.

The implications of the human-animal bond extend to the field of animal-assisted therapies, where animals are integrated into therapeutic settings to support human health and healing. These programs can involve various species, from dogs and cats to horses and dolphins, each offering unique benefits. Animal-assisted therapy has been shown to improve social interactions, increase motivation for rehabilitation exercises, and provide comfort in clinical settings. The presence of animals can create a more relaxed and supportive environment, encouraging patients to engage more fully in their treatment.

In the context of animal welfare, the human-animal bond plays a critical role in shaping attitudes toward the care and treatment of animals. A strong bond can lead to increased awareness and advocacy for animal welfare issues, as individuals who feel connected to animals are more likely to support ethical and humane practices. This bond motivates caregivers to provide high-quality care, ensuring that animals' physical and emotional needs are met. Conversely, neglect or misunderstanding of this bond can result in inadequate care or mistreatment, highlighting the importance of education and awareness in fostering positive relationships between humans and animals.

The human-animal bond also influences conservation efforts, as people who feel connected to animals are often more invested in protecting wildlife and natural habitats. Conservation programs that involve community engagement and education can strengthen this bond, fostering a sense of stewardship and responsibility for the natural world. By cultivating empathy and understanding toward animals, conservationists can inspire action and support for initiatives aimed at preserving biodiversity and ecosystems.

In research settings, the human-animal bond can impact the ethical considerations and treatment of animals used in scientific studies. Researchers who recognize the significance of this bond are more likely to prioritize humane treatment and seek alternatives to animal testing when possible. This awareness can lead to advancements in research methodologies that reduce the need for animal subjects while still achieving scientific objectives.

The human-animal bond is a dynamic and evolving relationship, influenced by cultural, social, and individual factors. Cultural attitudes toward animals can shape the nature of this bond, affecting how animals are perceived and treated in different societies. Social norms and values also play a role, influencing the acceptance and integration of animals into various aspects of human life.

At the individual level, personal experiences and beliefs shape the bond between humans and animals. Factors such as childhood experiences with pets, exposure to nature, and personal values can influence how individuals relate to animals and the significance they place on these relationships. The bond is often strengthened through shared experiences and interactions, such as play, training, and caregiving, which foster mutual understanding and connection.

To nurture and enhance the human-animal bond, caregivers and professionals can focus on building trust, communication, and empathy. Providing consistent care, positive reinforcement, and opportunities for enrichment can strengthen the bond and improve the quality of life for both humans and animals. Education and awareness are also crucial, helping individuals understand the needs and behaviors of animals, as well as the benefits of a strong bond.

By recognizing and valuing the human-animal bond, we can create environments and relationships that promote the well-being of all involved. This bond has the power to inspire compassion, drive social change, and enhance the lives of humans and animals alike. As we continue to explore and deepen our understanding of this connection, we uncover new opportunities for growth, healing, and collaboration, ultimately enriching the tapestry of life that we share with the animal kingdom.

Case Studies in Veterinary Behavior

Veterinary behavior is an intricate field that combines the principles of veterinary medicine with the study of animal behavior. Through the examination of case studies, we gain valuable insights into the complexities of diagnosing and treating behavioral issues in animals. These real-world examples illustrate the diverse challenges faced by veterinary behaviorists and shed light on the strategies employed to address them effectively.

Consider the case of Max, a three-year-old Labrador Retriever who developed severe separation anxiety. Max's owners reported that he would become highly anxious whenever they prepared to leave the house, exhibiting behaviors such as excessive barking, destructive chewing, and attempts to escape. The veterinary behaviorist began by conducting a comprehensive assessment, which included a thorough history of Max's behavior, his environment, and any previous training. This assessment revealed that Max's anxiety was exacerbated by a lack of consistent routine and insufficient mental stimulation.

The treatment plan for Max involved a multi-faceted approach. First, the behaviorist recommended establishing a consistent daily routine to help Max anticipate and adjust to his owners' departures. Additionally, enrichment activities, such as puzzle toys and interactive play sessions, were introduced to provide mental stimulation and alleviate boredom. Desensitization techniques were employed, gradually acclimating Max to short periods of separation, paired with positive reinforcement for calm behavior. In this case, the use of anti-anxiety medication was considered, but behavioral interventions proved sufficient in alleviating Max's anxiety over time.

Another case involved Luna, a five-year-old domestic shorthair cat who exhibited inexplicable aggression towards her owners. The aggression appeared unprovoked, with Luna lashing out during routine interactions such as petting or grooming. The veterinary behaviorist approached the situation by first ruling out any underlying medical conditions that could contribute to Luna's behavior. A physical examination and blood tests were conducted to ensure there were no underlying health issues.

Once medical causes were ruled out, the focus shifted to identifying potential environmental triggers. It was discovered that Luna's aggression was often preceded by overstimulation during petting sessions. The behaviorist introduced a strategy of observing Luna's body language closely to identify subtle signs of discomfort or agitation. By limiting petting sessions to shorter durations and providing Luna with opportunities to initiate contact, her aggression decreased significantly. Additionally, the introduction of vertical spaces and hiding spots within the home environment helped Luna feel more secure and in control of her surroundings.

In the case of Bella, a two-year-old German Shepherd with a history of relentless barking and lunging at other dogs during walks, the veterinary behaviorist faced a challenge rooted in fear-based reactivity. Bella's owners were at a loss, feeling embarrassed and overwhelmed by her behavior. The behaviorist conducted an assessment that revealed Bella's reactions were primarily driven by fear and anxiety when encountering unfamiliar dogs.

The treatment plan for Bella involved a combination of behavior modification techniques and environmental management. Counter-conditioning and desensitization were employed to change Bella's emotional response to other dogs. This involved gradually exposing her to controlled scenarios where she could observe other dogs from a distance without reacting, paired with high-value rewards for calm behavior. As Bella became more comfortable, the distance was gradually decreased. Additionally, her owners were encouraged to practice relaxation exercises with Bella, teaching her to focus on them rather than external stimuli.

A case involving a rabbit named Thumper highlighted the importance of understanding species-specific behaviors. Thumper, a one-year-old Holland Lop, exhibited persistent digging and destructive chewing habits. His owners were concerned about the damage to their home and sought guidance from a veterinary behaviorist. The behaviorist recognized that Thumper's actions were rooted in natural burrowing instincts and a lack of appropriate outlets for these behaviors.

To address Thumper's behavior, the behaviorist recommended creating a more enriched environment that catered to his natural instincts. This included providing digging boxes filled with hay and safe chew toys to redirect his behaviors. Additionally, Thumper's owners were encouraged to offer supervised outdoor playtime in a secure area, allowing him to engage in natural behaviors in a controlled environment. With these adjustments, Thumper's destructive habits diminished, and his overall well-being improved.

The case of Charlie, a ten-year-old African Grey Parrot, demonstrated the complexities of feather-plucking behavior in birds. Charlie began plucking his feathers, leading to bald patches and skin irritation. The veterinary behaviorist conducted a thorough evaluation, considering factors such as diet, environment, and potential stressors. It was determined that Charlie's feather-plucking was linked to stress caused by changes in his routine and environment.

The behaviorist implemented a comprehensive plan to address Charlie's behavior. This involved creating a stable and predictable daily routine, enhancing his environment with foraging opportunities and interactive toys, and incorporating regular social interaction with his owners. By identifying and addressing the sources of stress, Charlie's feather-plucking behavior gradually decreased, and his plumage began to recover.

These case studies underscore the importance of a holistic and individualized approach to veterinary behavior. Successful interventions often involve a combination of behavior modification techniques, environmental enrichment, and, when necessary, pharmacological support. Collaboration between veterinary behaviorists, pet owners, and other professionals is essential for accurately diagnosing and addressing behavioral issues.

Through these case studies, it becomes evident that veterinary behavior is a field that requires not only scientific knowledge but also empathy and creativity. The ability to interpret an animal's behavior and develop innovative solutions is essential for fostering harmonious relationships between humans and animals. As we continue to learn from these experiences, we gain valuable insights into the intricate tapestry of animal behavior and the ways in which we can support and enhance the lives of our animal companions.

CHAPTER 10
PRACTICE MANAGEMENT FOR VETERINARY TECHNICIANS

Fundamentals of Practice Management

Practice management is an essential component of veterinary medicine, ensuring that clinics and hospitals operate smoothly and efficiently while delivering high-quality care to animals. For veterinary technicians, understanding the fundamentals of practice management is crucial, as it empowers them to contribute effectively to the administrative and operational aspects of the practice. This chapter delves into the key elements of practice management, highlighting the roles and responsibilities of veterinary technicians in this dynamic environment.

At the core of practice management is the efficient organization of daily operations. This involves scheduling appointments, managing patient records, and coordinating the flow of patients through the clinic. Veterinary technicians play a pivotal role in maintaining the schedule, ensuring that appointments are booked appropriately to maximize the use of resources while minimizing wait times for clients. By efficiently managing the schedule, technicians help maintain a steady workflow and prevent bottlenecks that can disrupt the clinic's operations.

Patient record management is another critical aspect of practice management. Accurate and up-to-date records are essential for providing effective care, as they contain vital information about the animal's medical history, treatments, and ongoing health needs. Veterinary technicians are often responsible for maintaining these records, ensuring that they are organized, accessible, and secure. This involves entering data into electronic medical record systems, updating information as needed, and ensuring compliance with legal and ethical standards for record-keeping.

Inventory management is a fundamental task within practice management, as it ensures that the clinic has the necessary supplies and medications to provide care. Veterinary technicians are often tasked with monitoring inventory levels, ordering supplies, and managing stock to prevent shortages or overstocking. Effective inventory management requires attention to detail and an understanding of the specific needs of the practice, as well as the ability to anticipate future demands based on patient volume and seasonal trends.

Financial management is another key element of practice management, encompassing budgeting, billing, and financial reporting. While veterinarians often oversee the financial aspects of a practice, veterinary technicians may be involved in tasks such as processing payments, preparing invoices, and assisting with financial record-keeping. Understanding the financial operations of a practice enables technicians to contribute to cost-effective decision-making and ensure that the clinic remains financially sustainable.

Client communication and service are integral to the success of any veterinary practice. Veterinary technicians often serve as the first point of contact for clients, whether in person, over the phone, or through digital communication. Providing excellent client service involves clear communication, empathy, and responsiveness to client needs and concerns. Technicians must be adept at explaining medical procedures, discussing treatment options, and providing follow-up care instructions, all while ensuring that clients feel heard and valued.

Team collaboration is essential in practice management, as veterinary clinics rely on the coordinated efforts of veterinarians, technicians, and support staff to deliver comprehensive care. Veterinary technicians play a key role in fostering a collaborative work environment by facilitating communication, sharing information, and supporting team members in their roles. This collaboration extends to working closely with veterinarians during medical procedures, assisting with diagnostic tests, and ensuring that the clinic operates efficiently and safely.

Compliance with regulatory and legal requirements is a crucial aspect of practice management. Veterinary technicians must be familiar with the laws and regulations governing veterinary medicine, including those related to controlled substances, animal welfare, and professional conduct. Ensuring compliance involves adhering to established protocols, maintaining accurate records, and participating in continuing education to stay informed about changes in regulations and best practices.

Continuing education and professional development are vital for veterinary technicians involved in practice management. Staying current with industry trends, technological advancements, and evolving standards of care ensures that technicians can contribute effectively to the practice's success. This may involve attending workshops, conferences, and training sessions, as well as pursuing certifications in areas such as practice management or specialized veterinary care.

Technology plays an increasingly important role in practice management, streamlining operations and enhancing the quality of care. Veterinary technicians must be proficient in using practice management software, electronic medical records, and diagnostic equipment. Familiarity with these technologies not only improves efficiency but also enables technicians to provide accurate and timely information to clients and team members.

Crisis management and problem-solving are essential skills for veterinary technicians involved in practice management. Clinics may face unexpected challenges, such as equipment failures, staffing shortages, or emergency cases. Technicians must be prepared to respond quickly and effectively, using critical thinking and resourcefulness to address issues and minimize disruptions to patient care. Developing contingency plans and maintaining open communication with team members can help manage crises and ensure continuity of operations.

In summary, veterinary technicians play a crucial role in the practice management of veterinary clinics and hospitals. Through effective organization, communication, and collaboration, they ensure that the practice operates smoothly and efficiently, delivering high-quality care to animals. By embracing their responsibilities and continually developing their skills, veterinary technicians contribute to the success and sustainability of the practice, ultimately enhancing the well-being of both animals and their human companions.

Client Communication and Customer Service

Client communication and customer service form the backbone of any successful veterinary practice, playing a crucial role in fostering trust and satisfaction among pet owners. For veterinary technicians, mastering these skills is essential, as they are often the primary point of contact for clients and serve as the bridge between veterinarians and pet owners. Understanding the nuances of effective communication and delivering exceptional customer service can significantly enhance client relationships and ensure the smooth operation of the practice.

The first impression is a lasting one, and veterinary technicians are often responsible for setting the tone from the moment a client enters the clinic or calls to schedule an appointment. Greeting clients warmly and professionally, whether in person or over the phone, establishes a positive atmosphere and reassures clients that their concerns will be addressed with care and competence. Using a friendly tone, maintaining eye contact, and offering a genuine smile can help put clients at ease and create a welcoming environment.

Active listening is a fundamental component of effective client communication. Veterinary technicians must be attentive and empathetic, taking the time to fully understand the client's concerns, questions, and needs. This involves not only hearing the words being spoken but also paying attention to non-verbal cues, such as body language and facial expressions, which can provide additional context and insight. By demonstrating genuine interest and empathy, technicians can build rapport with clients and foster a sense of trust and collaboration.

Clear and concise communication is essential when conveying information to clients, particularly when discussing medical procedures, treatment plans, or follow-up care instructions. Veterinary technicians should aim to use language that is easily understood by individuals without a medical background, avoiding jargon and technical terms that may confuse or overwhelm clients. When explaining complex information, breaking it down into simple, manageable steps and using visual aids or written handouts can enhance understanding and retention.

Providing accurate and timely information is key to effective client communication. Veterinary technicians must be knowledgeable about the practice's policies, services, and procedures, as well as the specific needs and conditions of each patient. When clients have questions or concerns, technicians should respond promptly and accurately, seeking clarification from the veterinarian when necessary. By ensuring that clients receive consistent and reliable information, technicians can enhance their confidence in the care provided and prevent misunderstandings or miscommunications.

Empathy and compassion are integral to customer service in a veterinary setting, as clients often seek care for their beloved pets during times of stress or uncertainty. Veterinary technicians must approach each interaction with sensitivity and understanding, acknowledging the emotional bond between clients and their animals. Offering reassurance, support, and a listening ear can help alleviate clients' concerns and demonstrate the practice's commitment to compassionate care.

Managing difficult or emotional situations is a critical skill for veterinary technicians, as they may encounter clients who are upset, frustrated, or grieving. In such cases, it is important to remain calm and composed, allowing clients to express their emotions without judgment or interruption. By validating their feelings and offering solutions or alternatives, technicians can help de-escalate tense situations and work toward a resolution that meets the client's needs.

Client education is a valuable aspect of customer service, empowering pet owners to make informed decisions about their animals' health and well-being. Veterinary technicians can play a key role in educating clients about preventive care, nutrition, behavior, and common health issues. By providing resources, answering questions, and encouraging an open dialogue, technicians can enhance clients' understanding and involvement in their pets' care, ultimately leading to better health outcomes.

Follow-up communication is an important aspect of client service, reinforcing the practice's commitment to patient care and client satisfaction. Veterinary technicians may be responsible for conducting follow-up calls or sending reminders for appointments, vaccinations, or rechecks. These touchpoints provide an opportunity to address any ongoing concerns, answer questions, and ensure that clients feel supported throughout their pets' care journey.

Digital communication tools, such as email, text messaging, and social media, offer additional avenues for client engagement and service. Veterinary technicians should be familiar with the practice's digital communication policies and procedures, ensuring that they respond to inquiries and messages in a timely and professional manner. Utilizing these tools effectively can enhance convenience and accessibility for clients, while also streamlining communication and record-keeping for the practice.

Feedback and continuous improvement are essential components of customer service, as they allow the practice to identify areas for growth and enhancement. Veterinary technicians can encourage clients to provide feedback on their experiences, whether through informal conversations, surveys, or online reviews. By actively seeking and responding to feedback, the practice can demonstrate its commitment to excellence and adaptability, fostering long-term client loyalty and satisfaction.

Building lasting relationships with clients is a key objective of client communication and customer service. Veterinary technicians can achieve this by consistently delivering high-quality service, demonstrating reliability, and showing genuine care for clients and their pets. By cultivating strong connections with clients, technicians contribute to a positive practice reputation and a supportive community of pet owners who trust and value the care provided.

In conclusion, effective client communication and exceptional customer service are essential skills for veterinary technicians, contributing to the overall success and reputation of the practice. By mastering these skills, technicians can enhance client satisfaction, build trust and loyalty, and ensure the delivery of compassionate, high-quality care to animals and their owners. Through ongoing education, empathy, and dedication, veterinary technicians play a vital role in fostering positive relationships and creating a welcoming and supportive environment for clients and patients alike.

Inventory and Financial Management

Inventory and financial management are critical components of practice management in veterinary settings, serving as the backbone for maintaining operational efficiency and sustainability. For veterinary technicians, mastering these areas not only enhances the smooth functioning of the clinic but also contributes to overall financial health. This chapter delves into the fundamentals of managing inventory and finances, providing practical strategies and insights for veterinary technicians to implement effectively.

Inventory management begins with understanding the needs of the practice and establishing a system that ensures the availability of necessary supplies and medications. Veterinary technicians play a key role in this process, as they are often responsible for tracking inventory levels, placing orders, and organizing stock. An effective inventory management system involves several key steps, starting with accurate record-keeping. Technicians must meticulously document inventory levels, usage rates, and expiration dates to prevent shortages or overstocking.

Regular inventory audits are essential to maintaining an accurate and up-to-date inventory system. By conducting routine checks, technicians can identify discrepancies, expired items, or inefficiencies in inventory turnover. This proactive approach allows for timely adjustments, reducing waste and ensuring that the clinic is equipped to meet patient needs. Implementing a digital inventory management system can streamline this process, providing real-time data and alerts for low-stock items or upcoming expiration dates.

The selection of suppliers and negotiation of contracts are also important aspects of inventory management. Building strong relationships with reliable suppliers ensures consistent access to high-quality products at competitive prices. Veterinary technicians may be involved in evaluating supplier performance, comparing pricing, and negotiating terms to achieve the best value for the practice. By fostering positive supplier relationships, technicians can contribute to cost savings and ensure the availability of critical supplies.

Effective inventory management also requires strategic planning based on anticipated demand and seasonal trends. Veterinary technicians should consider factors such as patient volume, common procedures, and historical usage patterns when forecasting inventory needs. This foresight enables the practice to maintain optimal stock levels, reduce the risk of shortages, and minimize the financial impact of excess inventory.

Financial management in a veterinary practice encompasses budgeting, billing, and financial reporting, each of which plays a vital role in the practice's sustainability. Veterinary technicians can support financial management by assisting with billing processes, preparing invoices, and ensuring accurate financial record-keeping. This involvement requires attention to detail and a solid understanding of the practice's pricing structure, services, and payment policies.

Accurate billing and invoicing are essential for maintaining cash flow and ensuring that the practice receives timely payment for services rendered. Veterinary technicians must ensure that invoices are clear, detailed, and correctly reflect the services provided. This transparency helps prevent disputes and fosters trust with clients. Additionally, technicians may assist in managing accounts receivable by following up on outstanding payments and implementing payment plans if needed.

Budgeting is a critical component of financial management, guiding the allocation of resources and setting financial goals for the practice. While veterinarians often oversee the budgeting process, veterinary technicians can contribute by providing insights into operational needs and identifying areas for cost savings. By understanding the practice's financial priorities, technicians can make informed decisions that align with the clinic's goals and objectives.

Financial reporting provides a snapshot of the practice's financial health, enabling informed decision-making and strategic planning. Veterinary technicians may assist in generating financial reports, analyzing data, and identifying trends that impact the practice's profitability. This analysis can reveal opportunities for growth, areas for improvement, and potential risks, allowing the practice to adapt and thrive in a competitive environment.

Cost control is an important aspect of financial management, as it directly impacts the practice's bottom line. Veterinary technicians can support cost control efforts by identifying and implementing efficiency improvements, such as reducing waste, optimizing inventory turnover, and minimizing unnecessary expenses. By actively seeking ways to enhance operational efficiency, technicians can contribute to the practice's overall financial success.

Client communication also plays a role in financial management, particularly when discussing treatment costs, payment options, and financial policies. Veterinary technicians must be prepared to address client inquiries and concerns with transparency and empathy, ensuring that clients understand the value of the services provided and the options available for managing costs. By fostering open and honest communication, technicians can enhance client satisfaction and promote financial transparency.

In summary, inventory and financial management are integral to the success of a veterinary practice, requiring a strategic and proactive approach. Veterinary technicians play a vital role in these areas, ensuring that the practice operates efficiently, maintains financial stability, and delivers high-quality care to patients. By embracing their responsibilities and continually developing their skills, technicians contribute to the practice's sustainability and growth, ultimately enhancing the well-being of both animals and their human companions.

Legalities in Veterinary Practice

Navigating the legal landscape of veterinary practice is a crucial responsibility for veterinary technicians, who must ensure compliance with a myriad of regulations and standards that govern the profession. Understanding these legalities is not only fundamental to maintaining the practice's integrity but also vital for safeguarding the welfare of both patients and clients. This chapter delves into the legal aspects pertinent to veterinary practice, focusing on the role of veterinary technicians in upholding these standards and navigating potential challenges.

At the heart of legal compliance in veterinary practice is the adherence to state and federal regulations that dictate the scope of practice for veterinary professionals. Each state has its own veterinary practice act, which outlines the legal framework within which veterinarians and veterinary technicians operate. These acts delineate the roles, responsibilities, and limitations of each position, ensuring that professionals provide care within the bounds of their licensure. Veterinary technicians must be well-versed in their state's practice act, recognizing what tasks they are authorized to perform and when veterinarian supervision is required.

Licensure and certification are fundamental legal requirements for veterinary technicians, serving as proof of their qualifications and competence. Maintaining an active license often entails fulfilling continuing education requirements and adhering to ethical standards. Veterinary technicians must be diligent in renewing their licenses on time and documenting their educational activities to demonstrate compliance. This commitment to ongoing learning not only ensures legal compliance but also enhances the quality of care provided to patients.

Confidentiality and privacy are paramount in veterinary practice, with legal obligations mirroring those found in human healthcare settings. Veterinary technicians are entrusted with sensitive information about patients and clients, necessitating strict adherence to confidentiality protocols. This includes safeguarding medical records, refraining from discussing patient details with unauthorized individuals, and ensuring that all communications are conducted with discretion. By maintaining confidentiality, technicians uphold the trust placed in them by clients and protect the practice from potential legal repercussions.

Controlled substances management is a critical area of legal compliance, as veterinary practices often handle medications that are subject to stringent regulations. Veterinary technicians may be involved in the handling, dispensing, and record-keeping of controlled substances, necessitating a thorough understanding of relevant laws and protocols. This includes maintaining accurate logs, securing medications, and monitoring inventory to prevent theft or misuse. Compliance with controlled substances regulations is essential to avoid legal penalties and ensure the responsible use of medications.

Animal welfare laws represent another significant aspect of legal compliance, reflecting society's commitment to the humane treatment of animals. Veterinary technicians must be familiar with these laws, which encompass issues such as animal cruelty, neglect, and proper care standards. This knowledge empowers technicians to recognize and report suspected cases of animal abuse, thereby playing an active role in protecting vulnerable animals and upholding the practice's ethical standards.

Informed consent is a legal and ethical obligation in veterinary practice, requiring that clients are fully apprised of the risks, benefits, and alternatives to proposed treatments or procedures. Veterinary technicians may assist in the informed consent process by providing clients with clear, accurate information and answering their questions. Ensuring that clients understand and agree to the proposed care plan is essential for protecting the practice from liability and fostering transparent communication.

Documentation and record-keeping are integral to legal compliance, providing a detailed account of patient care and interactions with clients. Veterinary technicians must ensure that medical records are accurate, complete, and up-to-date, capturing all relevant information about diagnoses, treatments, and client communications. This meticulous documentation serves as a legal record of the care provided and can be critical in defending the practice against potential legal challenges.

Animal ownership disputes can present legal challenges in veterinary practice, particularly when multiple parties claim ownership of a pet. Veterinary technicians may be called upon to verify ownership documentation, such as microchip registrations or adoption papers, to resolve these disputes. Understanding the legal aspects of animal ownership helps technicians navigate these situations with sensitivity and adherence to legal protocols.

Professional liability and malpractice are concerns for all veterinary professionals, underscoring the importance of adhering to established standards of care. Veterinary technicians must be aware of the potential for malpractice claims and take proactive steps to minimize risk, such as following protocols, maintaining clear communication with clients, and documenting all aspects of patient care. By demonstrating competence and professionalism, technicians contribute to the practice's reputation and reduce the likelihood of legal disputes.

In summary, legal compliance is a cornerstone of veterinary practice, requiring veterinary technicians to navigate a complex array of regulations and standards. By understanding and adhering to these legalities, technicians play a critical role in maintaining the practice's integrity, protecting patient welfare, and ensuring the delivery of high-quality care. Through diligence, collaboration, and a commitment to professional development, veterinary technicians contribute to a legal and ethical practice environment that benefits both animals and their human companions.

Strategies for Effective Team Collaboration

Effective team collaboration is a cornerstone of successful veterinary practice management, fostering an environment where veterinary technicians, veterinarians, and support staff work cohesively to deliver high-quality patient care. In the bustling environment of a veterinary clinic, the ability to collaborate efficiently and harmoniously is not only beneficial but essential for achieving common goals and ensuring smooth operations. This chapter delves into strategies for veterinary technicians to enhance team collaboration, emphasizing communication, mutual respect, and shared responsibilities.

Open and transparent communication is the foundation of any collaborative effort. In a veterinary setting, clear communication ensures that all team members are informed about patient needs, treatment plans, and any changes in the schedule. Veterinary technicians can facilitate effective communication by actively listening to their colleagues, asking clarifying questions, and providing feedback in a constructive manner. Regular team meetings and briefings can be instrumental in keeping everyone on the same page, allowing team members to share updates, discuss challenges, and brainstorm solutions together.

Understanding the roles and responsibilities of each team member is crucial for fostering collaboration. Veterinary technicians should be aware of the specific duties of veterinarians, receptionists, and other support staff, recognizing how their roles interconnect to support patient care. This understanding helps prevent overlap or gaps in responsibilities, ensuring that tasks are completed efficiently and that team members can rely on each other's expertise. By respecting each other's roles, veterinary technicians contribute to a culture of mutual trust and accountability.

Conflict resolution skills are essential for maintaining a harmonious team dynamic, as disagreements or misunderstandings can arise in any workplace. Veterinary technicians should approach conflicts with a solution-oriented mindset, seeking to understand the perspectives of all parties involved and working towards a compromise that benefits the team and the patients. Techniques such as active listening, empathy, and open dialogue can help de-escalate tensions and foster a collaborative atmosphere where team members feel valued and heard.

Teamwork in a veterinary practice often involves multitasking and prioritizing tasks based on urgency and importance. Veterinary technicians can enhance collaboration by developing strong organizational skills, enabling them to manage their workload effectively while supporting their colleagues. This may involve delegating tasks when appropriate, assisting team members during busy periods, and ensuring that patient care remains the top priority. By staying organized and adaptable, technicians can contribute to a seamless workflow that benefits both the team and the patients.

Shared goals and a common vision are powerful motivators for team collaboration. Veterinary technicians should align their efforts with the practice's mission and objectives, understanding how their contributions support the overall success of the clinic. By focusing on shared goals, such as improving patient outcomes or enhancing client satisfaction, team members can work together with a sense of purpose and dedication. Celebrating achievements and milestones as a team further reinforces this sense of unity and collective accomplishment.

Professional development and continuous learning are vital for fostering a collaborative team environment, as they equip team members with the skills and knowledge needed to excel in their roles. Veterinary technicians should seek opportunities for training and education, whether through workshops, conferences, or online courses, and share their insights with their colleagues. This commitment to learning not only enhances individual competencies but also strengthens the team's overall capabilities, enabling them to provide high-quality care and adapt to new challenges.

Technology plays an increasingly important role in facilitating team collaboration, offering tools and platforms that enhance communication, scheduling, and information sharing. Veterinary technicians should be proficient in using practice management software, electronic medical records, and other digital tools that streamline operations and support collaborative efforts. By leveraging technology effectively, technicians can improve efficiency, reduce the risk of miscommunication, and ensure that all team members have access to the information they need.

A positive workplace culture is essential for fostering effective team collaboration, as it creates an environment where team members feel supported, appreciated, and motivated to contribute their best efforts. Veterinary technicians can help cultivate a positive culture by promoting teamwork, recognizing the contributions of their colleagues, and encouraging open communication. Simple gestures, such as expressing gratitude, offering encouragement, and celebrating successes, can have a powerful impact on team morale and cohesion.

Adaptability and flexibility are key traits for successful team collaboration, particularly in a dynamic veterinary setting where priorities can shift rapidly. Veterinary technicians should be prepared to adjust their approach and support their colleagues as needed, whether in response to an unexpected emergency or changes in the schedule. By demonstrating adaptability, technicians can help the team navigate challenges with resilience and maintain a focus on patient care.

Leadership and mentorship are important aspects of team collaboration, providing guidance, support, and inspiration to team members. Veterinary technicians can exhibit leadership by taking initiative, setting a positive example, and offering mentorship to less experienced colleagues. Through mentorship, technicians can share their knowledge, skills, and experiences, helping to nurture the next generation of veterinary professionals and strengthen the team's capabilities.

In conclusion, effective team collaboration is vital for the success of a veterinary practice, enabling veterinary technicians to work seamlessly with their colleagues to deliver exceptional patient care. By embracing strategies such as open communication, conflict resolution, and professional development, technicians can foster a collaborative environment where team members are motivated, engaged, and aligned with the practice's goals. Through dedication and teamwork, veterinary technicians play a pivotal role in creating a supportive and efficient practice that benefits both patients and clients.

CHAPTER 11
EFFECTIVE STUDY TECHNIQUES AND EXAM PREPARATION

Time Management Strategies

Preparing for the VTNE (Veterinary Technician National Examination) demands a strategic approach to time management, as it involves mastering a broad range of topics and skills. Effective time management is essential for balancing study sessions, work commitments, and personal life, ensuring that you are well-prepared for the exam. This chapter provides practical strategies specifically tailored for VTNE candidates to help optimize their study time and enhance their exam readiness.

The foundation of effective time management begins with setting clear, realistic goals. For VTNE preparation, define both short-term and long-term objectives to guide your study plan. Consider the exam date and work backward to create a timeline that allocates time for each subject area. Break down these goals into specific tasks, such as reviewing anatomy, pharmacology, or clinical procedures, and set deadlines to keep yourself on track. This structured approach provides direction and motivation, helping you focus on what needs to be accomplished.

Crafting a detailed study schedule is critical for efficient time management. Utilize calendars or planners to block out study sessions, and be sure to include breaks and personal time to maintain balance. When designing your schedule, consider your peak productivity times and allocate your most challenging tasks to these periods. Consistency in your routine can help reinforce study habits and reduce the chances of procrastination as the exam date approaches.

Prioritization plays a key role in managing your time effectively. As you prepare for the VTNE, not all topics will require the same level of attention. Identify areas where you feel less confident and allocate additional time to these subjects. The Pareto Principle, or the 80/20 rule, can be helpful here: focus on the 20% of topics that will likely yield 80% of the results on the exam. By channeling your energy into high-impact areas, you can maximize your study efficiency.

Incorporating the Pomodoro Technique into your study routine can help maintain concentration and prevent burnout. This method involves working in focused intervals—typically 25 minutes—followed by a short, 5-minute break. After completing four intervals, take a longer break to recharge. This structured cycle encourages deep focus while allowing time for rest, enhancing overall productivity during study sessions.

Minimizing distractions is essential for maintaining focus during VTNE preparation. Identify potential sources of distraction, such as mobile devices, social media, or a noisy environment, and take steps to mitigate them. Creating a dedicated, quiet study space can help foster concentration. Additionally, consider using apps that block distracting websites during study hours to keep your attention focused on the material.

Batch processing is an effective strategy for managing related tasks together, reducing the cognitive load of switching between different types of work. For example, dedicate specific time blocks to reviewing notes, taking practice tests, or memorizing terminology. By grouping similar tasks, you can maintain a steady workflow and improve efficiency, making better use of your study time.

Time blocking is another valuable technique for organizing your study schedule. Divide your day into fixed blocks of time, each dedicated to a specific task or subject. This method ensures that all important topics are covered while preventing any single area from monopolizing your time. Time blocking can also help create a balanced schedule that includes study, work, and leisure activities, reducing the risk of burnout.

Regular reflection on your time management practices is crucial for continuous improvement. Periodically assess how you are spending your study time and identify any patterns or habits that may be hindering your progress. Keeping a time log or journal can provide insights into your study habits and highlight areas for refinement. This reflection allows you to make necessary adjustments and optimize your approach as the exam date nears.

Building time buffers into your schedule can help accommodate unexpected events or delays. By allowing extra time for each task, you reduce stress and increase flexibility, adapting more easily to unforeseen circumstances. This strategy is particularly useful during the final weeks of preparation, when unexpected challenges may arise.

Self-care is an integral part of effective time management, ensuring that you maintain the physical and mental stamina required for exam preparation. Prioritize regular breaks, exercise, and relaxation to support your well-being. Adequate sleep is also crucial for memory retention and cognitive function, so make rest a non-negotiable part of your routine. By taking care of yourself, you enhance your ability to focus and perform well on the VTNE.

Collaboration and delegation can also support your time management efforts, especially if you are studying as part of a group. Sharing resources, discussing challenging topics, and dividing tasks can reduce the individual workload and enhance collective understanding. Be open to asking for help when needed and leverage the strengths of your peers to improve study outcomes.

By incorporating these time management strategies into your VTNE preparation, you can increase your productivity, focus, and confidence. Setting clear goals, creating a structured schedule, and prioritizing tasks will help you make the most of your study time, while self-care and collaboration ensure that you remain balanced and motivated. Through diligent planning and reflection, you can cultivate the skills necessary for success on the VTNE and in your future career as a veterinary technician.

Stress Reduction Techniques

Stress is an inevitable companion on the journey to mastering the VTNE, but it doesn't have to be an overwhelming force. Managing stress effectively is crucial for maintaining focus, enhancing performance, and ensuring that the study experience remains positive and productive. This chapter delves into practical stress reduction techniques tailored specifically for those preparing for the VTNE, offering insights and strategies to help candidates maintain equilibrium during this demanding time.

The first step in managing stress is recognizing its presence and understanding its sources. Stress often arises from a feeling of being overwhelmed by the volume of material, approaching deadlines, or self-imposed pressure to excel. By identifying specific stressors, you can begin to address them directly. Consider keeping a journal to track moments of heightened stress and reflect on their triggers. This self-awareness can guide you in adapting your study habits and lifestyle to minimize these stressors.

Breathing exercises are a simple yet powerful tool for reducing stress and regaining a sense of control. Deep, intentional breathing can activate the body's relaxation response, counteracting the physical symptoms of stress. Techniques such as diaphragmatic breathing or the 4-7-8 method can be practiced anywhere and offer immediate relief. Dedicate a few minutes each day to focus on your breath, using this time to center your thoughts and calm your mind.

Mindfulness and meditation are practices that cultivate awareness of the present moment, reducing anxiety and enhancing concentration. For those preparing for the VTNE, incorporating mindfulness techniques into daily routines can improve focus and resilience. Begin with short, guided meditations or mindfulness exercises, gradually increasing the duration as you become more comfortable. Apps and online resources can provide guided sessions, making it easy to integrate mindfulness into your study regimen.

Physical activity is a proven stress reliever that offers both mental and physical benefits. Regular exercise can boost mood, improve sleep, and increase energy levels, all of which contribute to a more effective study experience. Find an activity that you enjoy, whether it's walking, yoga, or weightlifting, and make it a regular part of your routine. Even short bursts of movement, like a quick walk around the block, can provide a mental reset and reduce stress.

A balanced diet and proper hydration are essential for managing stress and maintaining cognitive function. Nutrient-rich foods support brain health, while dehydration can exacerbate feelings of stress and fatigue. Aim for a diet that includes a variety of fruits, vegetables, whole grains, and lean proteins, and remember to drink water throughout the day. Avoid excessive caffeine and sugar, as these can lead to energy crashes and increased anxiety.

Quality sleep is fundamental to stress management and cognitive performance. Adequate rest allows the brain to process information, consolidate memories, and recharge for the next day. Establish a regular sleep schedule by going to bed and waking up at the same time each day, even on weekends. Create a calming bedtime routine that may include reading, listening to soothing music, or practicing relaxation exercises. Limit screen time before bed to enhance the quality of your sleep.

Time management can mitigate stress by providing a sense of control over your study schedule. Break down study sessions into manageable chunks, and set realistic goals for each session. Prioritize tasks based on importance and deadlines, and use tools like planners or digital calendars to keep track of your progress. By organizing your time effectively, you can reduce the anxiety associated with looming deadlines and last-minute cramming.

Social support is a valuable resource for stress reduction. Connecting with friends, family, or fellow students can provide encouragement, perspective, and a sense of solidarity. Share your experiences and concerns with those who understand the pressures of exam preparation, and don't hesitate to reach out when you need support. Study groups can offer both academic assistance and emotional encouragement, making the preparation process less isolating.

Engaging in hobbies and leisure activities is important for maintaining balance and reducing stress. Allocate time for activities that bring you joy, whether it's reading, painting, playing an instrument, or spending time in nature. These pursuits offer a break from the demands of studying and can rejuvenate your mind, leaving you better equipped to tackle your academic responsibilities.

Laughter and humor are natural stress relievers that can lighten the atmosphere and shift your perspective. Seek out opportunities to laugh, whether through funny videos, books, or spending time with people who make you smile. Humor can provide a mental escape from stress and remind you not to take things too seriously, helping to maintain a positive outlook during your preparation.

Visualization and positive affirmations can bolster confidence and reduce exam-related anxiety. Spend a few minutes each day visualizing yourself successfully completing the VTNE, focusing on the feelings of accomplishment and relief. Combine this practice with positive affirmations, repeating phrases that reinforce your self-worth and capability. Over time, these mental exercises can build resilience and reduce stress.

By incorporating these stress reduction techniques into your daily routine, you can create a more balanced and focused approach to VTNE preparation. Recognizing stress, practicing mindfulness, and maintaining healthy habits will not only enhance your study experience but also equip you with valuable skills for managing stress in your future career. Through intentional practice and self-care, you can navigate the demands of exam preparation with confidence and poise.

Memory Enhancement: WAKEUPMEMORY

Memory enhancement is a critical component of effective study techniques, especially for a comprehensive exam like the VTNE, where retaining vast amounts of information is essential. The "WAKEUPMEMORY" strategy offers a multifaceted approach to boosting memory retention, leveraging various cognitive techniques that can be seamlessly integrated into your study routine. This chapter explores these strategies, providing practical advice on how to enhance your memory and optimize your preparation for the exam.

The "W" in WAKEUPMEMORY stands for "Write it Down." Writing by hand has been shown to improve memory retention more effectively than typing. The act of writing engages multiple senses and cognitive processes, which can help encode information into long-term memory. As you study, take handwritten notes, summarizing key concepts and creating diagrams to visualize complex information. This practice not only reinforces your learning but also provides a valuable resource for later review.

"A" represents "Active Engagement." Passive reading or listening often results in limited retention. Instead, engage actively with the material by asking questions, discussing topics with peers, or teaching concepts to someone else. The process of articulating your understanding requires deeper cognitive processing, which strengthens memory. Additionally, using techniques like self-quizzing can test your recall and highlight areas that need further study.

"K" stands for "Keyword Mnemonics." Mnemonics are memory aids that use associations to help recall information. Create vivid and memorable keywords or phrases that represent complex concepts. For instance, you might use "ROYGBIV" to remember the colors of the rainbow. By forming these associations, you can make information more accessible and easier to retrieve during the exam.

"E" is for "Elaboration." This technique involves expanding on the information you are learning by connecting it to what you already know. Elaborative interrogation, where you ask "why" and "how" questions about the material, promotes a deeper understanding and retention. By making these connections, you enhance the integration of new knowledge with existing cognitive frameworks, making it easier to recall when needed.

"U" stands for "Utilize Visualization." Visualization involves creating mental images to represent information. This technique is particularly useful for remembering procedures, anatomical structures, or sequences. As you study, close your eyes and visualize the process or structure in detail, imagining each step or component vividly. Visualization can strengthen memory by engaging the brain's visual processing areas, making abstract concepts more concrete.

"P" represents "Practice Retrieval." Retrieval practice involves recalling information from memory, rather than simply reviewing it. This process strengthens neural pathways associated with the material and improves long-term retention. Use flashcards, practice tests, or quizzes to regularly test your knowledge. By challenging yourself to retrieve information, you solidify your memory and identify areas that require additional focus.

The first "M" in MEMORY is for "Mind Mapping." Mind maps are visual tools that organize information hierarchically, showing relationships between concepts. Creating a mind map for each topic can help you see the big picture and understand how individual pieces fit together. This technique encourages active learning, as you must decide how to categorize and connect information, enhancing both understanding and recall.

"E" stands for "Encoding Variability." Encoding variability involves studying material in different contexts or environments. This variability can improve recall by allowing the brain to form multiple associations with the information. Try studying in different locations, at different times of day, or using varied methods, such as reading, listening, or discussing. By diversifying your study experiences, you increase the chances of retrieving the information in different situations.

"M" is for "Mnemonics and Chunking." Chunking involves breaking down large amounts of information into smaller, manageable units. This technique is especially useful for memorizing lists, sequences, or procedures. Combine chunking with mnemonics to create meaningful associations for each chunk, further enhancing recall. For example, break a list of veterinary drugs into categories based on their use and create a mnemonic for each category.

"O" represents "Organized Review." Regular, structured review sessions help reinforce memory and prevent forgetting. Implement a spaced repetition system, where you review material at increasing intervals, to optimize retention. Schedule periodic review sessions for each topic, ensuring that you revisit information multiple times before the exam. This method capitalizes on the spacing effect, which suggests that information is better retained when reviewed over time.

"R" stands for "Rest and Sleep." Adequate rest is crucial for memory consolidation, the process by which short-term memories are transformed into long-term ones. During sleep, the brain processes and organizes information, strengthening memory traces. Prioritize regular, restful sleep as part of your study routine, and consider short naps after intensive study sessions to enhance memory consolidation.

"Y" is for "Your Own Pace." Everyone learns differently, and it's important to find a pace that suits your individual needs. Avoid comparing your progress to others and focus on your own understanding and retention. Take breaks when needed, and adjust your study schedule to align with your natural rhythms and energy levels. By personalizing your approach, you can create an optimal learning environment that supports memory enhancement.

Integrating the WAKEUPMEMORY strategies into your study routine can significantly improve memory retention and recall, providing a solid foundation for VTNE success. By writing down information, actively engaging with the material, and employing techniques like visualization and retrieval practice, you can enhance your cognitive abilities and approach the exam with confidence. Through deliberate practice and mindfulness, memory enhancement becomes a powerful tool in your academic arsenal.

Exam Day Tips and Tricks

The day of the VTNE is a culmination of all your hard work and preparation, and while nerves are natural, having a strategic plan can make a significant difference in your performance. This chapter provides practical tips and tricks to help you navigate exam day with confidence and poise, ensuring that you can showcase your knowledge effectively.

Preparation begins before exam day. Start by ensuring that all logistical details are in order. Confirm the exam location, time, and any required materials or identification you need to bring. Pack your bag the night before with essentials such as your ID, admission ticket, and any allowed stationery. Having everything ready will minimize last-minute stress and allow you to focus entirely on the exam.

A good night's sleep is crucial for optimal cognitive function and performance. Aim to get at least seven to eight hours of restful sleep the night before the exam. Establish a calming bedtime routine, avoiding screens and stimulating activities in the hour leading up to bedtime. A well-rested mind is better equipped to process information, maintain focus, and think critically under pressure.

On the morning of the exam, fuel your body with a balanced breakfast that provides sustained energy. Opt for a meal that includes protein, complex carbohydrates, and healthy fats, such as eggs with whole-grain toast and avocado. Stay hydrated, but avoid excessive caffeine or sugar, which can lead to energy crashes and increased anxiety.

Arrive at the exam location early to allow yourself time to acclimate to the environment. Familiarize yourself with the layout, locate the restroom, and find a comfortable place to wait. Use this time to engage in relaxation techniques, such as deep breathing or visualization, to calm any nerves. Visualize yourself confidently navigating the exam, reinforcing a positive mindset.

As the exam begins, carefully read and follow all instructions provided. Skim through the entire exam to get a sense of its structure and allocate time appropriately. Prioritize questions that seem manageable, tackling them first to build momentum and confidence. If you encounter a challenging question, make a note of it and return to it later, rather than getting stuck and wasting valuable time.

Manage your time wisely throughout the exam. Keep an eye on the clock, but avoid checking it obsessively, which can increase stress. Divide the available time by the number of questions to establish a rough guideline for how long to spend on each one. Allocate extra time at the end for reviewing your answers, ensuring that you haven't overlooked any details or made careless mistakes.

When answering multiple-choice questions, read each question and all answer choices thoroughly before selecting an answer. Look for keywords or phrases that provide context or clues. Eliminate obviously incorrect options to narrow down your choices, increasing the probability of selecting the correct answer. Trust your instincts, as your first choice is often the right one.

For questions that require written responses, organize your thoughts before you begin writing. Outline your answer to ensure that it is structured logically and includes all necessary points. Be concise and clear, using technical terminology where appropriate. If time permits, review your written responses for clarity, coherence, and completeness.

Stay focused and maintain a positive attitude throughout the exam. If you feel your concentration waning, take a brief mental break by closing your eyes and taking a few deep breaths. Remind yourself of your preparation and capabilities, countering any negative self-talk with affirmations of your strengths. Maintaining a positive mindset can boost your confidence and performance.

If you finish the exam with time to spare, use the remaining time to review your answers. Check for any questions you might have missed or marked for review, and ensure that your responses are as accurate and complete as possible. Be cautious about changing answers unless you are certain of an error, as second-guessing can lead to unnecessary mistakes.

After the exam, take time to decompress and reflect on your performance. Acknowledge the effort and dedication you put into preparing, regardless of the outcome. Engage in activities that bring you joy and relaxation, allowing yourself to unwind. Reflect on any lessons learned from the experience, which can inform future exam strategies.

Remember that the VTNE is just one step in your journey as a veterinary technician. Regardless of the result, your passion and commitment to the field will continue to guide your career. Trust in your preparation and abilities, and approach the exam with the confidence that you are well-equipped to succeed.

CHAPTER 12
FULL PRACTICE TESTS

Full Test 1 with Detailed Explanations

Question 1: What electrolyte change can occur if you leave a blood sample sitting too long with red blood cells (RBCs) in contact with the serum?

a. Phosphorus increases
b. Bicarbonate decreases
c. Potassium decreases
d. Sodium increases

Correct Answer: a. Phosphorus increases.
Explanation: Over time, phosphate can leach out of cells into the serum if not processed promptly, making phosphorus levels falsely appear elevated. This emphasizes the need for timely sample processing.

Question 2: A client brings in her dog who ate a box of rat poison in the last 2 days. What symptoms would be expected?

a. Bleeding, weakness
b. Seizures, vomiting
c. Unconscious, rapid heartbeat
d. Severe pain, depression

Correct Answer: a. Bleeding, weakness.
Explanation: Rat poison often contains anticoagulants, leading to bleeding disorders. Symptoms like bleeding and weakness are common as the poison inhibits vitamin K recycling, crucial for blood clotting.

Question 3: Which color is a gram-positive bacteria on the microscopic slide?

a. Red
b. Blue
c. Orange
d. Green

Correct Answer: b. Blue.
Explanation: Gram-positive bacteria retain the crystal violet stain during the Gram staining process, appearing blue or purple under a microscope. This is due to their thick peptidoglycan cell wall.

Question 4: What lab result would you expect to find in a cat with Diabetes mellitus?

a. Increased urine glucose; Decreased blood glucose
b. Low urine glucose; Normal blood glucose
c. Increased urine glucose, Increased blood glucose
d. Urinary infection; Low blood glucose

Correct Answer: c. Increased urine glucose, Increased blood glucose.
Explanation: In diabetes mellitus, insufficient insulin leads to high blood glucose levels, which spill over into the urine, causing glucosuria. Monitoring these values is key for diabetes management.

Question 5: Which forceps secure drapes to the patient by penetrating the skin?

a. Backhaus
b. Roeder
c. Brown-Adson
d. Crile

Correct Answer: a. Backhaus.

Explanation: Backhaus forceps are specifically designed for holding drapes in place during surgical procedures by penetrating the skin, ensuring a sterile field is maintained.

Question 6: A rare Albanian hairy iguana has been prescribed "Iggy-cote" medicated shampoo q.o.d. for dandruff. How often does the iguana get treated?

a. Once a day
b. Four times a day
c. Every other day
d. As needed

Correct Answer: c. Every other day.

Explanation: The abbreviation "q.o.d." stands for "every other day." This dosing schedule helps manage the condition without over-treatment, which can be crucial for skin health in reptiles.

Question 7: Which two white blood cells are phagocytic (eat foreign cells and material by engulfing them)?

a. B-Lymphocyte, Eosinophil
b. Monocyte, Neutrophil
c. Basophil, Lymphocyte
d. Neutrophil, Thrombocyte

Correct Answer: b. Monocyte, Neutrophil.

Explanation: Monocytes and neutrophils are key phagocytic cells in the immune system, responsible for engulfing and digesting pathogens and debris, playing a central role in the body's defense mechanisms.

Question 8: What is a band neutrophil?

a. An old neutrophil
b. Immature neutrophil
c. A depleted neutrophil
d. A toxic neutrophil
e. A neutrophil that plays the drums

Correct Answer: b. Immature neutrophil.

Explanation: Band neutrophils are immature forms of neutrophils, identified by their non-segmented, band-shaped nucleus. Their presence often indicates an active response to infection.

Question 9: How do you prevent laryngospasm in cats before inducing anesthesia?

a. Pre-medicate with acepromazine
b. 1-2% Lidocaine spray
c. Pre-medicate with atropine or glycopyrrolate
d. Avoid halothane

Correct Answer: b. 1-2% Lidocaine spray.

Explanation: Applying lidocaine spray to the laryngeal area helps prevent laryngospasm, a reflex closure of the larynx, which can complicate intubation during anesthesia in cats.

Question 10: Which term describes inflammation of the testicle?

a. Orchitis
b. Phimosis
c. Phlebitis
d. Cryptorchid

Correct Answer: a. Orchitis.
Explanation: Orchitis refers to the inflammation of the testicles, which can result from infection or injury. Recognizing and treating this condition is essential to prevent complications.

Question 11: Which choice is often used in combination with ketamine or thiopental to induce anesthesia in horses?

a. Halothane
b. Phenobarbital
c. Naloxone
d. Guaifenesin

Correct Answer: d. Guaifenesin.
Explanation: Guaifenesin is commonly used as a muscle relaxant in combination with ketamine or thiopental to induce anesthesia in horses, helping to provide a smooth induction.

Question 12: What does it mean if a cat is azotemic?

a. Blood urea nitrogen (BUN) is increased
b. Blood urea nitrogen (BUN) is decreased
c. Creatinine is high
d. Sodium-Potassium ratio is too low

Correct Answer: a. Blood urea nitrogen (BUN) is increased.
Explanation: Azotemia is characterized by elevated blood urea nitrogen (BUN) and often creatinine, indicating impaired kidney function or dehydration, necessitating further investigation.

Question 13: Which drug can reverse the effects of xylazine (alpha2-adrenergic agonist with analgesic and sedative effects)?

a. Yohimbine
b. Pralidoxime
c. Atropine
d. Diazepam (Valium®)

Correct Answer: a. Yohimbine.
Explanation: Yohimbine acts as an antagonist to reverse the sedative and analgesic effects of xylazine, allowing for recovery from sedation more quickly and safely.

Question 14: Which one of the following dog breeds is classified as brachycephalic?

a. Golden retriever
b. Greyhound
c. English bulldog
d. Great Dane

Correct Answer: c. English bulldog.
Explanation: Brachycephalic breeds like the English bulldog have shortened skulls, leading to specific respiratory and health considerations that must be managed appropriately.

Question 15: Which kind of tissue causes the most x-ray scatter?

a. Thick body parts
b. Thin body parts
c. Joints 8 cm thick or less
d. Delicate bone, like nasal area

Correct Answer: a. Thick body parts.
Explanation: Thick tissues such as muscle and fat can cause more x-ray scatter due to increased absorption and scattering of x-ray photons, affecting image quality.

Question 16: You are called to a farm to help do a routine dental exam and float the teeth of an 8-year old Standardbred mare. What parts get filed down with the rasp when a horse gets its teeth floated?

a. Lingual aspect-upper molar arcade, Buccal aspect-lower molar arcade
b. Buccal aspect-upper molar arcade, rostral points of wolf teeth
c. Lingual aspect-upper molar arcade, Lingual aspect-lower molar arcade
d. Buccal aspect-upper molar arcade, Buccal aspect-lower molar arcade
e. Buccal aspect-upper molar arcade, Lingual aspect-lower molar arcade

Correct Answer: e. Buccal aspect-upper molar arcade, Lingual aspect-lower molar arcade.
Explanation: Floating involves filing down sharp enamel points on the buccal (cheek) side of the upper molars and the lingual (tongue) side of the lower molars to prevent discomfort and improve chewing efficiency.

Question 17: A 3-year-old domestic longhair female spayed cat is presented at your clinic with hypersalivation, vomiting, diarrhea, tremors, stumbling, and a temperature of 105.2 F (40.7 C). Her pupils are normal size and responsive to light. While the vet examines the animal, she has a seizure. The owner relates that he had treated her the night before with a flea dip he had originally bought for his dog. What toxic ingredient do you suspect most highly?

a. D-Limonene
b. Carbamate
c. Permethrin
d. Organophosphate

Correct Answer: c. Permethrin.
Explanation: Permethrin, found in some dog flea treatments, is highly toxic to cats and can cause severe neurological symptoms like seizures. Immediate veterinary intervention is required.

Question 18: Which choice lists these species in order of gestation length, from longest to shortest pregnancy?

a. Cow, Horse, Pig, Dog, Goat
b. Cow, Horse, Pig, Goat, Dog
c. Llama, Pig, Sheep, Ferret, Cat
d. Horse, Cow, Goat, Pig, Dog

Correct Answer: d. Horse, Cow, Goat, Pig, Dog.
Explanation: Horses have the longest gestation period among these animals, followed by cows, goats, pigs, and dogs, reflecting different reproductive strategies and developmental needs.

Question 19: What is a nosocomial infection?

a. A sinusitis, typically found in horses
b. An upper respiratory infection
c. An infection acquired in a hospital
d. An infection acquired secondary to injury

Correct Answer: c. An infection acquired in a hospital.
Explanation: Nosocomial infections, or hospital-acquired infections, occur in healthcare settings and are often resistant to antibiotics, necessitating stringent infection control measures.

Question 20: Why is the brachioradialis muscle clinically significant in dogs and cats?

a. Adjacent to the tibial nerve
b. Associated with brachial plexus avulsion
c. Lies above axillary artery
d. Implicated in medial patellar luxation
e. Can be mistaken for cephalic vein in venipuncture

Correct Answer: e. Can be mistaken for cephalic vein in venipuncture.
Explanation: The brachioradialis muscle can obscure the cephalic vein during venipuncture, leading to potential complications in blood sampling or intravenous access.

Question 21: What is the clinical significance of the femoral triangle in dogs and cats?

a. Associated with brachial plexus avulsion
b. Good place to take pulse from femoral artery
c. Often damaged with anterior cruciate injuries
d. Pulse oximeters attach there
e. Surgical approach for hip dysplasia repair

Correct Answer: b. Good place to take pulse from femoral artery.
Explanation: The femoral triangle is a prominent anatomical landmark for palpating the femoral pulse, crucial for assessing cardiovascular health in veterinary examinations.

Question 22: How long after birth does gut closure typically occur in calves and foals? (when protective maternal antibodies can no longer be absorbed from the gut to the bloodstream)

a. 1-3 hours
b. 3-6 hours
c. 9-12 hours
d. 15-18 hours
e. 18-24 hours

Correct Answer: e. 18-24 hours.
Explanation: Gut closure, the process by which the gut loses its ability to absorb maternal antibodies, occurs within 18-24 hours, highlighting the importance of timely colostrum intake in newborns.

Question 23: Vaccine-associated sarcomas in cats are primarily linked to which two vaccines?

a. FeLV and Feline Panleukopenia vaccines
b. FeLV and Rabies vaccines
c. Feline Calici/Herpes and Panleukopenia vaccines
d. FeLV and Feline Calici/Herpes vaccines
e. Rabies and Feline Panleukopenia vaccines

Correct Answer: b. FeLV and Rabies vaccines.
Explanation: Vaccine-associated sarcomas are linked with FeLV and Rabies vaccines, necessitating careful administration protocols and sites to minimize risk.

Question 24: How long after the first rabies vaccination is a dog, cat or ferret considered to be immunized and protected against rabies?

a. After 14 days
b. Same day
c. After 28 days
d. After 7 days

Correct Answer: c. After 28 days.
Explanation: After the first rabies vaccination, it takes about 28 days for the animal's immune system to mount a full protective response against the rabies virus.

Question 25: What is the function of a thrombocyte?

a. Cause blood clotting
b. Prevent blood clotting
c. Remove red blood cell parasites
d. Prevent phagocytosis

Correct Answer: a. Cause blood clotting.

Explanation: Thrombocytes, or platelets, are essential for blood clotting, preventing excessive bleeding during injury by forming a platelet plug and activating the clotting cascade.

Question 26: A 6-month-old mixed breed dog presents with a focal area of alopecia with comedones. A skin scraping is shown below. Which one of the following choices is the most likely diagnosis?

a. Demodecosis
b. Cheyletiellosis
c. Sarcoptic mange
d. Dermatophytosis
e. Microsporosis

Correct Answer: a. Demodecosis.

Explanation: Demodecosis is a common mite infestation in dogs characterized by hair loss and comedones, often diagnosed through skin scraping and microscopic examination.

Question 27: What is the normal amount of expected moisture on a paper testing strip in Schirmer's tear test?

a. 18-25 mm
b. 10-15 mm
c. 5-10 mm
d. 0-5 mm

Correct Answer: a. 18-25 mm.

Explanation: Schirmer's tear test measures tear production, with 18-25 mm of moisture on the strip indicating normal tear production, essential for diagnosing dry eye conditions.

Question 28: Which color is a gram-negative bacteria on the microscopic slide?

a. Red
b. Blue
c. Orange
d. Green

Correct Answer: a. Red.

Explanation: Gram-negative bacteria appear red or pink after Gram staining due to their thin peptidoglycan layer, which does not retain the crystal violet stain.

Question 29: Which of the following is the predominant white blood cell type seen on this peripheral blood smear from a dog?

a. Eosinophil
b. Basophil
c. Macrophage
d. Lymphocyte
e. Monocyte

Correct Answer: a. Eosinophil.

Explanation: Eosinophils are prominent in allergic reactions and parasitic infections, recognizable by their bilobed nucleus and large granules, and are a key component of the immune response.

Question 30: How common are dental caries (cavities) in dogs?

a. Common
b. Seen in 35% of adults older than 5 years
c. Uncommon
d. Seen in 75% of adults older than 5 years

Correct Answer: c. Uncommon.

Explanation: Dental caries are relatively rare in dogs compared to humans, due to differences in oral bacteria and diet, although other dental issues like periodontal disease are more prevalent.

Question 31: What is the most common malignant oral tumor in cats?

a. Osteosarcoma
b. Squamous cell carcinoma
c. Melanoma
d. Fibrosarcoma

Correct Answer: b. Squamous cell carcinoma.

Explanation: Squamous cell carcinoma is the most common malignant oral tumor in cats, characterized by aggressive local invasion and poor prognosis if not treated early.

Question 32: Which is more severe, periodontitis or gingivitis?

a. No difference in severity
b. Depends on patient
c. Periodontitis
d. Gingivitis

Correct Answer: c. Periodontitis.

Explanation: Periodontitis is more severe than gingivitis, involving deeper tissue structures and potentially leading to tooth loss and systemic health issues if untreated.

Question 33: What is the total serum protein level in a dog with an albumin of 4.0 g/dl and a globulin level of 3.5 g/dl?

a. 1.5 g/dl
b. 3.5 g/dl
c. 7.5 g/dl
d. Cannot calculate with this information

Correct Answer: c. 7.5 g/dl.

Explanation: Total serum protein is the sum of albumin and globulin levels. In this case, 4.0 g/dl (albumin) + 3.5 g/dl (globulin) = 7.5 g/dl, reflecting protein levels in the blood.

Question 34: How might you roughly calculate the hemoglobin concentration in a blood sample from a normal dog if you know the red blood cell (RBC) packed cell volume (PCV, %)?

a. Double the PCV
b. Divide PCV by half
c. Multiply PCV by one quarter (0.25)
d. Multiply PCV by one third (0.33)

Correct Answer: d. Multiply PCV by one third (0.33).

Explanation: Hemoglobin concentration can be estimated by multiplying the PCV by 0.33, providing a quick method to assess oxygen-carrying capacity in blood.

Now, let's continue by creating additional questions to reach a total of 170:

Question 35: What is the primary function of alveoli in the respiratory system?

a. Filter dust and particles
b. Exchange gases between air and blood
c. Produce mucus to trap inhaled contaminants
d. Control the rate of breathing

Correct Answer: b. Exchange gases between air and blood.
Explanation: Alveoli are tiny air sacs in the lungs where oxygen and carbon dioxide are exchanged between the air and the bloodstream, a critical function for respiration.

Question 36: Which type of muscle is responsible for voluntary movements?

a. Cardiac muscle
b. Smooth muscle
c. Skeletal muscle
d. Connective tissue

Correct Answer: c. Skeletal muscle.
Explanation: Skeletal muscles are attached to bones and are under voluntary control, enabling movement of the body and maintaining posture.

Question 37: What is the term for the process by which white blood cells engulf and digest foreign particles?

a. Exocytosis
b. Endocytosis
c. Phagocytosis
d. Pinocytosis

Correct Answer: c. Phagocytosis.
Explanation: Phagocytosis is the process by which certain white blood cells, like macrophages and neutrophils, engulf and digest pathogens and debris, crucial for immune defense.

Question 38: What is the primary role of the liver in digestion?

a. Absorb nutrients
b. Produce insulin
c. Produce bile
d. Store glucose

Correct Answer: c. Produce bile.
Explanation: The liver produces bile, which is stored in the gallbladder and released into the small intestine to aid in the digestion and absorption of fats.

Question 39: Which hormone is primarily responsible for regulating metabolism?

a. Insulin
b. Thyroxine
c. Cortisol
d. Melatonin

Correct Answer: b. Thyroxine.
Explanation: Thyroxine, produced by the thyroid gland, plays a crucial role in regulating metabolism, affecting how the body uses energy.

Question 40: What is the function of the myelin sheath?

a. Protect the brain from injury
b. Insulate nerve fibers
c. Connect neurons to blood vessels
d. Generate electrical impulses

Correct Answer: b. Insulate nerve fibers.
Explanation: The myelin sheath insulates nerve fibers, increasing the speed of nerve impulse conduction and ensuring efficient communication within the nervous system.

Question 41: Which vitamin is essential for blood clotting?

a. Vitamin A
b. Vitamin C
c. Vitamin D
d. Vitamin K

Correct Answer: d. Vitamin K.
Explanation: Vitamin K is essential for the synthesis of clotting factors, which are necessary for blood coagulation and preventing excessive bleeding.

Question 42: What is the main function of the large intestine in the digestive system?

a. Absorb nutrients
b. Absorb water and electrolytes
c. Produce digestive enzymes
d. Store bile

Correct Answer: b. Absorb water and electrolytes.
Explanation: The large intestine absorbs water and electrolytes from indigestible food matter, forming and storing feces until elimination.

Question 43: Which structure in the heart ensures one-way blood flow from the left atrium to the left ventricle?

a. Aortic valve
b. Mitral valve
c. Tricuspid valve
d. Pulmonary valve

Correct Answer: b. Mitral valve.
Explanation: The mitral valve, located between the left atrium and left ventricle, prevents backflow and ensures one-way blood flow during the cardiac cycle.

Question 44: What is the primary function of the renal glomerulus?

a. Concentrate urine
b. Filter blood
c. Reabsorb nutrients
d. Secrete hormones

Correct Answer: b. Filter blood.
Explanation: The glomerulus is a network of capillaries in the kidney that filters blood, removing waste products and excess substances to form urine.

Question 45: Which part of the brain is responsible for coordinating voluntary movements and balance?

a. Cerebrum
b. Cerebellum
c. Medulla oblongata
d. Hypothalamus

Correct Answer: b. Cerebellum.
Explanation: The cerebellum coordinates voluntary movements, balance, and posture, playing a vital role in motor control and precision.

Question 46: What is the primary function of hemoglobin in red blood cells?

a. Transport nutrients
b. Carry oxygen

c. Defend against infections
d. Store calcium

Correct Answer: b. Carry oxygen.
Explanation: Hemoglobin is a protein in red blood cells that binds to oxygen in the lungs and transports it to tissues throughout the body, facilitating respiration.

Question 47: Which of the following is a function of the spleen?

a. Produce insulin
b. Filter blood
c. Store bile
d. Produce red blood cells

Correct Answer: b. Filter blood.
Explanation: The spleen filters blood, removing old or damaged red blood cells and pathogens, and plays a role in immune response by producing lymphocytes.

Question 48: What is the primary role of the pancreas in digestion?

a. Produce bile
b. Absorb nutrients
c. Produce digestive enzymes
d. Store glycogen

Correct Answer: c. Produce digestive enzymes.
Explanation: The pancreas produces digestive enzymes that are secreted into the small intestine, aiding in the breakdown of carbohydrates, proteins, and fats.

Question 49: Which hormone regulates the sleep-wake cycle?

a. Cortisol
b. Insulin
c. Melatonin
d. Thyroxine

Correct Answer: c. Melatonin.
Explanation: Melatonin, produced by the pineal gland, regulates the sleep-wake cycle by responding to light and darkness cues, promoting sleep.

Question 50: What is the function of the epiglottis during swallowing?

a. Produce sound
b. Prevent food from entering the trachea
c. Open the esophagus
d. Stimulate saliva production

Correct Answer: b. Prevent food from entering the trachea.
Explanation: The epiglottis is a flap of tissue that covers the trachea during swallowing, preventing food and liquid from entering the airway and causing choking.

Question 51: What is the primary function of the lymphatic system?

a. Transport oxygen
b. Produce hormones
c. Return excess interstitial fluid to the bloodstream
d. Store glycogen

Correct Answer: c. Return excess interstitial fluid to the bloodstream.
Explanation: The lymphatic system returns excess interstitial fluid to the bloodstream, aids in fat absorption, and plays a crucial role in immune defense.

Question 52: Which type of cell is primarily responsible for antibody production?

a. Macrophage
b. Neutrophil
c. B lymphocyte
d. T lymphocyte

Correct Answer: c. B lymphocyte.
Explanation: B lymphocytes, or B cells, produce antibodies in response to antigens, marking pathogens for destruction by other immune cells.

Question 53: What is the role of the hypothalamus in the endocrine system?

a. Produce digestive enzymes
b. Regulate blood pressure
c. Control the pituitary gland
d. Store calcium

Correct Answer: c. Control the pituitary gland.
Explanation: The hypothalamus regulates the endocrine system by controlling the pituitary gland, influencing hormone release and maintaining homeostasis.

Question 54: Which part of the eye is responsible for focusing light onto the retina?

a. Cornea
b. Lens
c. Iris
d. Pupil

Correct Answer: b. Lens.
Explanation: The lens focuses light onto the retina, adjusting its shape to accommodate near and distant vision, essential for clear sight.

Question 55: What is the function of the auditory ossicles in the ear?

a. Convert sound waves into nerve impulses
b. Equalize pressure between the ear and atmosphere
c. Transmit sound vibrations to the inner ear
d. Produce earwax

Correct Answer: c. Transmit sound vibrations to the inner ear.
Explanation: The auditory ossicles (malleus, incus, and stapes) transmit sound vibrations from the eardrum to the inner ear, amplifying sound.

Question 56: What is the primary function of the small intestine in the digestive system?

a. Absorb nutrients
b. Produce bile
c. Store feces
d. Filter blood

Correct Answer: a. Absorb nutrients.
Explanation: The small intestine absorbs nutrients from digested food into the bloodstream, utilizing a large surface area for efficient absorption.

Question 57: Which structure in the human body is responsible for producing insulin?

a. Liver
b. Pancreas
c. Kidney
d. Spleen

Correct Answer: b. Pancreas.
Explanation: The pancreas produces insulin, a hormone that regulates blood glucose levels by facilitating the uptake of glucose into cells.

Question 58: A calf with pinkeye is being treated with an injection of long-acting oxytetracycline. The calf weighs 100 lbs and the dose is 10mg/kg. How many milligrams will be needed for one dose?

a. 454.5 milligrams
b. 22 milligrams
c. 2200 milligrams
d. 4.5 milligrams
e. 75 milligrams

Correct Answer: a. 454.5 milligrams.
Explanation: First, convert the calf's weight to kilograms (100 lbs = 45.45 kg). Then, multiply the weight by the dose per kg (45.45 kg x 10 mg/kg = 454.5 mg).

Question 59: Why are most antibiotics contraindicated in rabbits and hamsters?

a. Highly permeable blood-brain barrier
b. Their little hearts just can't take it
c. Disrupts gram-positive gut flora
d. Highly sensitive to renal toxicity

Correct Answer: c. Disrupts gram-positive gut flora.
Explanation: Antibiotics like penicillins and cephalosporins disrupt the gram-positive gut flora in rabbits and hamsters, leading to dysbiosis and potentially fatal enterotoxemia.

Question 60: Which drug causes vomiting in cats?

a. Xylazine
b. Phenobarbital
c. Ketamine
d. Diazepam

Correct Answer: a. Xylazine.
Explanation: Xylazine, an alpha-2 adrenergic agonist, is used as an emetic in cats to induce vomiting, often for decontaminating the gastrointestinal tract.

Question 61: The major active ingredient in most IV euthanasia solutions is:

a. Phenobarbital
b. Potassium chloride
c. Pentobarbital
d. Thiopental

Correct Answer: c. Pentobarbital.
Explanation: Pentobarbital is a barbiturate used in euthanasia solutions for its rapid and humane induction of unconsciousness and cardiac arrest.

Question 62: How would you change exposure settings to make an x-ray film lighter?

a. Decrease kVp, increase mA, increase time
b. Increase kVp, decrease mA, increase time
c. Decrease kVp, decrease mA, decrease time
d. Increase kVp, increase mA, increase time

Correct Answer: c. Decrease kVp, decrease mA, decrease time.
Explanation: Reducing kVp, mA, and exposure time decreases the amount of x-ray exposure, resulting in a lighter image on the film.

Question 63: What is the rule of thumb for how long an x-ray film should stay in the fixer bath?

a. Twice as long as film was in developer
b. Half as long as film was in developer
c. Five minutes
d. One minute

Correct Answer: a. Twice as long as film was in developer.
Explanation: This ensures proper removal of unexposed silver halide crystals, stabilizing the image and preventing fading over time.

Question 64: Which choice correctly lists the order in which gases pass through a typical circular anesthetic circuit?

a. Pressure regulator, vaporizer, patient, CO2 canister, flowmeter
b. Vaporizer, pressure regulator, flowmeter, CO2 canister, patient
c. Pressure regulator, flowmeter, vaporizer, patient, CO2 canister
d. Flowmeter, pressure regulator, vaporizer, patient, CO2 canister

Correct Answer: c. Pressure regulator, flowmeter, vaporizer, patient, CO2 canister.
Explanation: This sequence ensures accurate delivery of anesthetic gases, maintaining consistent pressure and concentration for safe anesthesia.

Question 65: Which of the following choices is a side effect that you should be aware of when using ketamine for anesthesia in cats?

a. Eyes stay open
b. Dose-dependent respiratory depression
c. Cardiac arrest
d. Laryngospasm

Correct Answer: a. Eyes stay open.
Explanation: Ketamine causes dissociative anesthesia, where cats maintain reflexes and muscle tone, including open eyes, necessitating lubrication to prevent corneal drying.

Question 66: What is the purpose of a curette?

a. Scrape hard tissues
b. Highly absorbent surgical sponge
c. Holds intramedullary bone pins
d. Cauterizes blood vessels

Correct Answer: a. Scrape hard tissues.
Explanation: Curettes are surgical instruments used to scrape or debride tissue, commonly used in dental, orthopedic, and dermatological procedures.

Question 67: Which anatomic area do these three surgical approaches access in the horse? Modified Whitehouse, Viborg's triangle, Hyovertebrotomy

a. Maxillary sinus
b. Soft palate
c. Atlanto-occipital joint
d. Osseous bullae
e. Guttural pouch

Correct Answer: e. Guttural pouch.

Explanation: These approaches provide access to the guttural pouch, a large air-filled sac in horses, often involved in infections and requiring surgical intervention.

Question 68: The vet has asked you to prepare for a pyometra surgery on a 7-year-old intact female schnauzer. What are you about to remove from the dog?

a. Uterus
b. Kidney
c. Gall bladder
d. Mammary glands

Correct Answer: a. Uterus.

Explanation: In pyometra, an infected and enlarged uterus is surgically removed (ovariohysterectomy) to prevent systemic infection and potential rupture.

Question 69: You are looking at a canine vaginal smear through a microscope. At what stage of the estrous cycle is this dog?

a. Cannot tell from this slide
b. Anestrus
c. Estrus
d. Diestrus

Correct Answer: d. Diestrus.

Explanation: Diestrus is characterized by significant cellular changes in vaginal smears, including increased neutrophils and fewer superficial cells, indicating post-ovulation.

Question 70: Where would a dog or cat be likely to encounter arsenic around the house?

a. De-icer crystals
b. Anti-mildew paint
c. Ant baits
d. Silver-polish
e. Snail baits

Correct Answer: c. Ant baits.

Explanation: Ant baits often contain arsenic as an active ingredient, posing a risk of poisoning if ingested by pets, necessitating careful placement and monitoring.

Question 71: How long is a practice required to maintain client medical records?

a. Years
b. Weeks
c. Months
d. Decades
e. A practice is not legally required to preserve medical records

Correct Answer: a. Years.

Explanation: Veterinary practices are typically required to maintain medical records for several years, varying by jurisdiction, to ensure continuity of care and legal compliance.

Question 72: Which choice correctly describes apnea?

a. No breathing
b. Difficult breathing
c. Heart murmur
d. Atopic allergy

Correct Answer: a. No breathing.
Explanation: Apnea refers to the complete cessation of breathing, a potentially life-threatening condition requiring immediate medical intervention.

Question 73: Which drug family is associated with tooth enamel problems?

a. Aminoglycosides
b. Quinolones
c. Macrolides
d. Tetracyclines
e. Cephalosporins

Correct Answer: d. Tetracyclines.
Explanation: Tetracyclines can cause permanent discoloration and enamel hypoplasia in developing teeth, making them contraindicated in young animals and pregnant females.

Question 74: Which statement about the proper storage of fresh or frozen plasma is most correct?

a. Can be frozen for up to 1 year
b. Must be used within 48 h
c. Should be stored above 98.6 F (37 C)
d. Can be stored at 39.2 F - 50 F (4 C - 10 C) for up to 3 weeks

Correct Answer: a. Can be frozen for up to 1 year.
Explanation: Fresh or frozen plasma can be stored in a frozen state for up to one year, preserving clotting factors and proteins for therapeutic use.

Now, let's continue creating questions until we reach a total of 170:

Question 75: What is the primary purpose of a pulse oximeter?

a. Measure blood pressure
b. Assess heart rate
c. Evaluate oxygen saturation in blood
d. Monitor respiratory rate

Correct Answer: c. Evaluate oxygen saturation in blood.
Explanation: A pulse oximeter non-invasively measures the oxygen saturation of hemoglobin in arterial blood, essential for monitoring respiratory function during anesthesia and critical care.

Question 76: Which of the following is a zoonotic disease?

a. Canine parvovirus
b. Feline leukemia
c. Rabies
d. Equine influenza

Correct Answer: c. Rabies.
Explanation: Rabies is a viral zoonotic disease that affects the central nervous system of mammals, including humans, transmitted through bites from infected animals.

Question 77: What is the main function of the gallbladder?

a. Produce digestive enzymes
b. Store bile
c. Absorb nutrients
d. Filter toxins

Correct Answer: b. Store bile.
Explanation: The gallbladder stores and concentrates bile produced by the liver, releasing it into the small intestine to aid in fat digestion.

Question 78: Which organ is primarily responsible for detoxifying harmful substances in the body?

a. Kidney
b. Liver
c. Spleen
d. Pancreas

Correct Answer: b. Liver.
Explanation: The liver metabolizes and detoxifies drugs and harmful substances, producing bile for digestion and regulating metabolic processes.

Question 79: What is the role of the autonomic nervous system?

a. Control voluntary muscle movements
b. Regulate involuntary body functions
c. Maintain balance and posture
d. Process sensory information

Correct Answer: b. Regulate involuntary body functions.
Explanation: The autonomic nervous system controls involuntary functions like heart rate, digestion, and respiratory rate, maintaining homeostasis.

Question 80: What is the primary component of a cell membrane?

a. Proteins
b. Carbohydrates
c. Lipids
d. Nucleic acids

Correct Answer: c. Lipids.
Explanation: Cell membranes are primarily composed of a phospholipid bilayer, providing structure and regulating the passage of substances into and out of cells.

Question 81: Which part of the brain controls temperature regulation?

a. Thalamus
b. Cerebrum
c. Hypothalamus
d. Cerebellum

Correct Answer: c. Hypothalamus.
Explanation: The hypothalamus regulates body temperature by controlling mechanisms like sweating and shivering, crucial for maintaining homeostasis.

Question 82: What is the primary function of the respiratory system?

a. Produce red blood cells
b. Exchange gases between air and blood
c. Regulate blood pressure
d. Filter toxins from blood

Correct Answer: b. Exchange gases between air and blood.
Explanation: The respiratory system facilitates the exchange of oxygen and carbon dioxide between the air and bloodstream, essential for cellular respiration.

Question 83: Which hormone is primarily involved in the fight-or-flight response?

a. Insulin
b. Thyroxine
c. Cortisol
d. Epinephrine

Correct Answer: d. Epinephrine.
Explanation: Epinephrine, released by the adrenal glands, prepares the body for rapid action by increasing heart rate, blood flow, and energy availability during stress.

Question 84: What is the primary function of red blood cells?

a. Fight infections
b. Transport oxygen
c. Regulate blood pressure
d. Produce antibodies

Correct Answer: b. Transport oxygen.
Explanation: Red blood cells contain hemoglobin, which binds to oxygen in the lungs and transports it to tissues throughout the body, facilitating cellular respiration.

Question 85: What structure in the eye adjusts the size of the pupil?

a. Lens
b. Cornea
c. Retina
d. Iris

Correct Answer: d. Iris.
Explanation: The iris is a ring of muscle that adjusts the size of the pupil in response to light, controlling the amount of light entering the eye.

Question 86: Which vitamin is important for vision and immune function?

a. Vitamin A
b. Vitamin C
c. Vitamin D
d. Vitamin E

Correct Answer: a. Vitamin A.
Explanation: Vitamin A is crucial for maintaining vision, particularly in low light, and supports immune function by maintaining skin and mucosal barriers.

Question 87: What is the primary function of the kidneys?

a. Produce bile
b. Filter blood and form urine
c. Store vitamins and minerals
d. Synthesize proteins

Correct Answer: b. Filter blood and form urine.
Explanation: The kidneys filter blood to remove waste products and excess substances, forming urine for excretion, and regulate electrolyte balance and blood pressure.

Question 88: What is the role of neurotransmitters in the nervous system?

a. Protect neurons from damage
b. Transmit electrical signals between neurons
c. Provide structural support to neurons
d. Generate action potentials

Correct Answer: b. Transmit electrical signals between neurons.
Explanation: Neurotransmitters are chemical messengers that transmit signals across synapses between neurons, enabling communication within the nervous system.

Question 89: Which part of the heart receives oxygenated blood from the lungs?

a. Left atrium
b. Right atrium
c. Left ventricle
d. Right ventricle

Correct Answer: a. Left atrium.
Explanation: The left atrium receives oxygenated blood from the pulmonary veins, which is then pumped into the left ventricle and distributed to the body.

Question 90: What is the primary function of the endocrine system?

a. Protect against infection
b. Produce movement
c. Regulate body functions through hormones
d. Exchange gases

Correct Answer: c. Regulate body functions through hormones.
Explanation: The endocrine system secretes hormones into the bloodstream, regulating various physiological processes, including growth, metabolism, and reproduction.

Question 91: Which mineral is essential for bone health and blood clotting?

a. Iron
b. Calcium
c. Potassium
d. Sodium

Correct Answer: b. Calcium.
Explanation: Calcium is vital for maintaining bone density and structure, and it plays a key role in blood clotting and nerve transmission.

Question 92: What is the function of the synovial fluid in joints?

a. Provide structural support
b. Absorb shock
c. Nourish cartilage and lubricate joints
d. Connect bones

Correct Answer: c. Nourish cartilage and lubricate joints.
Explanation: Synovial fluid reduces friction between joint surfaces during movement and provides nutrients to the cartilage, maintaining joint health and function.

Question 93: Which part of the digestive system is primarily responsible for nutrient absorption?

a. Stomach
b. Small intestine
c. Large intestine
d. Esophagus

Correct Answer: b. Small intestine.
Explanation: The small intestine is the main site for nutrient absorption, utilizing its extensive surface area and specialized cells to absorb digested food into the bloodstream.

Question 94: What is the main function of the lymph nodes?

a. Produce red blood cells
b. Filter lymph and fight infections
c. Store energy
d. Transport oxygen

Correct Answer: b. Filter lymph and fight infections.
Explanation: Lymph nodes filter lymphatic fluid, trapping pathogens and foreign particles, and are sites where immune cells can respond to infections.

Question 95: Which hormone lowers blood glucose levels?

a. Glucagon
b. Cortisol
c. Insulin
d. Thyroxine

Correct Answer: c. Insulin.
Explanation: Insulin, produced by the pancreas, lowers blood glucose levels by facilitating the uptake of glucose into cells for energy use or storage.

Question 96: Which part of the brain is responsible for processing visual information?

a. Temporal lobe
b. Frontal lobe
c. Occipital lobe
d. Parietal lobe

Correct Answer: c. Occipital lobe.
Explanation: The occipital lobe, located at the back of the brain, processes visual information received from the eyes, enabling sight and perception.

Question 97: What is the role of the adrenal glands in the body?

a. Filter blood
b. Produce digestive enzymes
c. Secrete hormones like adrenaline and cortisol
d. Store vitamins

Correct Answer: c. Secrete hormones like adrenaline and cortisol.
Explanation: The adrenal glands produce hormones that regulate metabolism, immune response, blood pressure, and stress response, including adrenaline and cortisol.

Question 98: What is the primary function of the esophagus?

a. Absorb nutrients
b. Transport food from mouth to stomach
c. Produce digestive enzymes
d. Store food

Correct Answer: b. Transport food from mouth to stomach.
Explanation: The esophagus is a muscular tube that moves food from the mouth to the stomach through peristaltic contractions, initiating the digestive process.

Question 99: Which organ is primarily responsible for producing bile?

a. Pancreas
b. Liver
c. Gallbladder
d. Spleen

Correct Answer: b. Liver.
Explanation: The liver produces bile, a digestive fluid that emulsifies fats in the small intestine, facilitating their digestion and absorption.

Question 100: Which vitamin is essential for calcium absorption in the body?

a. Vitamin A
b. Vitamin B12
c. Vitamin C
d. Vitamin D

Correct Answer: d. Vitamin D.
Explanation: Vitamin D enhances calcium absorption in the gut, crucial for maintaining healthy bones and preventing disorders like rickets and osteoporosis.

Question 101: What is the primary function of the cerebrum in the brain?

a. Control balance and coordination
b. Process sensory information and voluntary movement
c. Regulate heart rate and breathing
d. Control endocrine functions

Correct Answer: b. Process sensory information and voluntary movement.
Explanation: The cerebrum is the largest part of the brain, responsible for processing sensory inputs, voluntary movements, reasoning, emotions, and language comprehension.

Question 102: A cat that weighs 11 lb (5 kg) is prescribed antibiotics at a dosage of 0.2 mg/lb (0.44 mg/kg). The medication is available only in 2 mg tablets. How many tablets should the cat receive in a single dose?

a. ~1/4 tablet
b. ~1/2 tablet
c. ~1 tablet
d. ~1 1/2 tablets

Correct Answer: c. ~1 tablet.
Explanation: The cat requires 2.2 mg (0.2 mg/lb x 11 lb) or 2.2 mg (0.44 mg/kg x 5 kg). Since the medication is available in 2 mg tablets, the cat would need approximately 1 tablet to reach the prescribed dosage.

Question 103: What does it mean if a cow is multiparous?

a. Has given birth more than once
b. Pregnant with twins
c. Has been pregnant, then aborted
d. Is a twin and other animal is male
e. She is good at math

Correct Answer: a. Has given birth more than once.
Explanation: A multiparous cow is one that has had more than one pregnancy resulting in live births, indicating its reproductive history and capabilities.

Question 104: The vet has asked you to prepare for an onychectomy on a cat. What kind of surgery is this?

a. Declaw
b. Spay
c. Cesarean delivery
d. Castration

Correct Answer: a. Declaw.
Explanation: An onychectomy refers to the surgical removal of a cat's claws, commonly known as declawing, which involves amputating part of the distal phalanges.

Question 105: A basset hound with galloping halitosis has been prescribed with medicated mint dog treats prn for bad breath. How often does the dog get treated?

a. Every other day
b. Once a day
c. Four times a day
d. As needed

Correct Answer: d. As needed.
Explanation: "Prn" stands for "pro re nata," a Latin phrase meaning "as the situation arises" or "as needed," implying the dog treats are given whenever bad breath occurs.

Question 106: Which choice indicates that the soda lime granules in a CO2 absorbent canister have become exhausted?

a. Color stays pink, regardless of exposure
b. Color change from white to purple
c. Color change from purple to white
d. Color stays white, regardless of exposure

Correct Answer: b. Color change from white to purple.
Explanation: Soda lime granules turn from white to purple when they are exhausted and cannot absorb more CO2, signaling the need for replacement or reactivation.

Question 107: What is an iatrogenic medical or surgical problem?

a. A disease secondary to inbreeding
b. A genetic predisposition
c. A disease that gets better without treatment
d. A bad outcome, inflicted by the therapy itself

Correct Answer: d. A bad outcome, inflicted by the therapy itself.
Explanation: Iatrogenic problems are adverse conditions or complications caused unintentionally by medical treatment or diagnostic procedures, highlighting the importance of cautious practice.

Question 108: Which one of the following choices does not produce energy when ingested?

a. Mineral
b. Carbohydrate
c. Protein
d. Sucrose
e. Cellulose

Correct Answer: a. Mineral.
Explanation: Minerals provide no caloric energy; they are essential micronutrients involved in various physiological processes, but they don't contribute to energy metabolism like carbohydrates, proteins, or fats.

Question 109: While examining a high-producing dairy cow that is off-feed, the vet puts her stethoscope on the left side in a line between the left elbow and the cow's hip bones and starts flicking her fingers against the side of the cow while listening to the stethoscope. What is she listening for?

a. The characteristic dead spot of an impacted omasum
b. The dull thud of rumen stasis
c. The musical ping of a left displaced abomasum
d. The regular movement of rumen contraction waves

Correct Answer: c. The musical ping of a left displaced abomasum.
Explanation: The vet listens for a "ping," a distinct sound indicating a left displaced abomasum, where the abomasum has moved from its normal position, impacting digestion and health.

Question 110: Which direction is plantar?

a. The bottom of the hindfoot
b. The top of the hoof
c. The top of the hind foot
d. The bottom of the fore foot

Correct Answer: a. The bottom of the hindfoot.
Explanation: "Plantar" refers to the sole of the hindfoot, akin to the bottom of human feet, and is an anatomical term used to describe location and movement in veterinary medicine.

Question 111: What treatment in the clinic will make the cat vomit as soon as possible?

a. Fomepizole (4-MP) IV
b. Clofazimine SQ
c. Yohimbine IM
d. Xylazine IV

Correct Answer: d. Xylazine IV.
Explanation: Xylazine is an alpha-2 adrenergic agonist that can induce vomiting in cats when administered intravenously, often used in cases of toxin ingestion.

Question 112: Which commonly-used anesthetic circuit is made up of a tube within a tube?

a. Bain system
b. Closed circle system
c. Semi-closed circle system
d. Universal Y circuit

Correct Answer: a. Bain system.
Explanation: The Bain system, a modification of the Mapleson D circuit, features a coaxial design with fresh gas flow delivered through an inner tube, reducing dead space and warming inspired gases.

Question 113: Which choice best describes the process of repairing a clean wound within a few hours of injury by first intention?

a. Suture the wound closed
b. Delayed primary closure
c. Allow wound to contract and epithelialize
d. Allow wound to granulate closed

Correct Answer: a. Suture the wound closed.
Explanation: First intention healing involves suturing a clean, recent wound, facilitating rapid healing with minimal scarring by approximating tissue edges.

Question 114: How long after a booster rabies vaccination is a dog, cat, or ferret considered to be currently vaccinated and protected against rabies?

a. Immediately
b. After 24 hours
c. After 48 hours
d. After 7 days
e. After 14 days

Correct Answer: a. Immediately.
Explanation: Animals are considered currently vaccinated and protected against rabies immediately after receiving a booster, as per standard veterinary guidelines and vaccine manufacturer recommendations.

Question 115: Which electrolyte imbalance can lead to cardiac arrest?

a. Hypernatremia
b. Hypokalemia

c. Hyperkalemia
d. Hypocalcemia

Correct Answer: c. Hyperkalemia.
Explanation: Hyperkalemia, an elevated level of potassium in the blood, can disrupt normal cardiac electrical activity, leading to potentially fatal arrhythmias and cardiac arrest.

Question 116: What is the primary cause of feline infectious peritonitis (FIP)?

a. Feline herpesvirus
b. Feline coronavirus
c. Feline calicivirus
d. Feline leukemia virus

Correct Answer: b. Feline coronavirus.
Explanation: Feline infectious peritonitis is caused by a mutation of the feline coronavirus, leading to a fatal systemic inflammatory disease affecting various organ systems.

Question 117: Which of the following is a common sign of hypothyroidism in dogs?

a. Hyperactivity
b. Weight gain
c. Increased appetite
d. Diarrhea

Correct Answer: b. Weight gain.
Explanation: Hypothyroidism in dogs often results in weight gain due to decreased metabolism, along with lethargy and skin issues, as the thyroid gland's hormone production is insufficient.

Question 118: What is the role of insulin in the body?

a. Increase blood glucose levels
b. Lower blood glucose levels
c. Stimulate fat breakdown
d. Inhibit protein synthesis

Correct Answer: b. Lower blood glucose levels.
Explanation: Insulin, produced by the pancreas, lowers blood glucose levels by facilitating cellular uptake of glucose, promoting glycogen storage, and reducing gluconeogenesis.

Question 119: Which animal is most commonly associated with the transmission of Lyme disease?

a. Dog
b. Cat
c. Deer
d. Tick

Correct Answer: d. Tick.
Explanation: Lyme disease is primarily transmitted through the bite of infected black-legged ticks (Ixodes species), with deer and rodents serving as reservoir hosts for the bacterium Borrelia burgdorferi.

Question 120: What is the term for the surgical removal of a kidney in animals?

a. Nephrectomy
b. Cystectomy
c. Splenectomy
d. Cholecystectomy

Correct Answer: a. Nephrectomy.
Explanation: Nephrectomy is the surgical procedure for removing a kidney, often performed in cases of severe kidney disease, trauma, or neoplasia.

Question 121: Which of the following is a common cause of anemia in dogs?

a. Hyperglycemia
b. Hypothyroidism
c. Hemolysis
d. Hyperlipidemia

Correct Answer: c. Hemolysis.
Explanation: Hemolysis, the destruction of red blood cells, is a common cause of anemia in dogs, occurring due to immune-mediated disease, toxins, or infections.

Question 122: Which disease is characterized by the destruction of the adrenal cortex?

a. Cushing's disease
b. Addison's disease
c. Diabetes mellitus
d. Hyperthyroidism

Correct Answer: b. Addison's disease.
Explanation: Addison's disease, or hypoadrenocorticism, is characterized by inadequate production of adrenal hormones due to adrenal cortex destruction, leading to electrolyte imbalances and fatigue.

Question 123: What is the primary function of the pancreas in digestion?

a. Produce bile
b. Secrete digestive enzymes
c. Absorb nutrients
d. Break down cellulose

Correct Answer: b. Secrete digestive enzymes.
Explanation: The pancreas produces digestive enzymes like amylase, lipase, and proteases, released into the small intestine to aid in the breakdown of carbohydrates, fats, and proteins.

Question 124: Which of the following is a non-steroidal anti-inflammatory drug (NSAID)?

a. Prednisone
b. Meloxicam
c. Dexamethasone
d. Triamcinolone

Correct Answer: b. Meloxicam.
Explanation: Meloxicam is an NSAID used to reduce inflammation and pain in animals, particularly for musculoskeletal disorders, without the immunosuppressive effects of steroids.

Question 125: What is a common symptom of hyperthyroidism in cats?

a. Lethargy
b. Weight loss despite increased appetite
c. Hair loss
d. Constipation

Correct Answer: b. Weight loss despite increased appetite.
Explanation: Hyperthyroidism in cats leads to increased metabolism, causing weight loss despite increased appetite, along with hyperactivity and tachycardia.

Question 126: What does the term "brachycephalic" refer to in dogs?

a. Long-legged body type
b. Short-nosed and flat-faced skull
c. Large body size
d. Curly coat

Correct Answer: b. Short-nosed and flat-faced skull.

Explanation: Brachycephalic refers to dogs with a shortened skull, such as Bulldogs and Pugs, often resulting in respiratory challenges due to compressed airways.

Question 127: Which parasite is known for causing heartworm disease in dogs and cats?

a. Dirofilaria immitis
b. Toxocara canis
c. Ancylostoma caninum
d. Trichuris vulpis

Correct Answer: a. Dirofilaria immitis.

Explanation: Dirofilaria immitis is a parasitic worm transmitted by mosquitoes, causing heartworm disease, which affects the heart and lungs of infected animals.

Question 128: What is the purpose of a tourniquet in veterinary practice?

a. Immobilize a broken limb
b. Reduce blood flow to a limb
c. Administer intravenous fluids
d. Monitor heart rate

Correct Answer: b. Reduce blood flow to a limb.

Explanation: A tourniquet is used to temporarily reduce or stop blood flow to a limb, often during surgical procedures or to control bleeding.

Question 129: Which zoonotic disease is caused by a protozoan parasite and can be transmitted through cat feces?

a. Toxoplasmosis
b. Leptospirosis
c. Brucellosis
d. Giardiasis

Correct Answer: a. Toxoplasmosis.

Explanation: Toxoplasmosis is caused by Toxoplasma gondii, a protozoan parasite that can be transmitted to humans through cat feces or undercooked meat, posing risks especially to pregnant women.

Question 130: Which of the following is a symptom of feline lower urinary tract disease (FLUTD)?

a. Vomiting
b. Increased thirst
c. Straining to urinate
d. Diarrhea

Correct Answer: c. Straining to urinate.

Explanation: FLUTD is characterized by difficulty urinating, often due to inflammation, obstruction, or infection of the urinary tract, requiring prompt veterinary attention.

Question 131: What is the main cause of kennel cough in dogs?

a. Parainfluenza virus
b. Bordetella bronchiseptica
c. Canine distemper virus
d. Canine adenovirus

Correct Answer: b. Bordetella bronchiseptica.

Explanation: Kennel cough is a highly contagious respiratory disease in dogs primarily caused by the bacterium Bordetella bronchiseptica, often in conjunction with viral infections.

Question 132: What is the primary function of the spleen in the body?

a. Produce bile
b. Filter blood and recycle red blood cells
c. Store glucose
d. Secrete hormones

Correct Answer: b. Filter blood and recycle red blood cells.
Explanation: The spleen filters and removes old or damaged red blood cells, stores white blood cells and platelets, and plays a role in the immune response.

Question 133: Which of the following is a common fungal infection in cats?

a. Ringworm
b. Parvovirus
c. Giardia
d. Ehrlichiosis

Correct Answer: a. Ringworm.
Explanation: Ringworm is a fungal infection affecting the skin, hair, and nails, causing circular lesions and hair loss, and is transmissible to humans and other animals.

Question 134: What is the function of alveoli in the lungs?

a. Produce mucus
b. Exchange gases between air and blood
c. Filter out dust particles
d. Strengthen the respiratory muscles

Correct Answer: b. Exchange gases between air and blood.
Explanation: Alveoli are tiny air sacs in the lungs where oxygen is exchanged for carbon dioxide in the blood, essential for respiratory function and oxygenation of the body.

Question 135: Which of the following is a symptom of Cushing's disease in dogs?

a. Hypoglycemia
b. Hyperpigmentation
c. Increased thirst and urination
d. Muscle hypertrophy

Correct Answer: c. Increased thirst and urination.
Explanation: Cushing's disease, or hyperadrenocorticism, is characterized by excessive cortisol production, leading to symptoms like increased thirst, urination, panting, and a pot-bellied appearance.

Question 136: Which type of immunity is acquired through vaccination?

a. Passive immunity
b. Innate immunity
c. Adaptive immunity
d. Natural immunity

Correct Answer: c. Adaptive immunity.
Explanation: Vaccination stimulates adaptive immunity by exposing the body to antigens, prompting the immune system to develop memory cells and antibodies for future protection.

Question 137: What is the primary cause of feline immunodeficiency virus (FIV)?

a. Retrovirus
b. Herpesvirus
c. Calicivirus
d. Coronavirus

Correct Answer: a. Retrovirus.
Explanation: FIV is caused by a retrovirus that compromises the immune system in cats, similar to HIV in humans, transmitted mainly through bite wounds.

Question 138: Which body system is primarily affected by Lyme disease?

a. Respiratory system
b. Nervous system
c. Musculoskeletal system
d. Endocrine system

Correct Answer: c. Musculoskeletal system.
Explanation: Lyme disease primarily affects the musculoskeletal system, causing symptoms like joint pain, lameness, and arthritis, though it can also impact other systems if untreated.

Question 139: Which of the following is a symptom of feline asthma?

a. Diarrhea
b. Coughing and wheezing
c. Increased appetite
d. Weight gain

Correct Answer: b. Coughing and wheezing.
Explanation: Feline asthma is characterized by coughing, wheezing, and difficulty breathing due to airway inflammation and constriction, often requiring medical management.

Question 140: What is the term for the surgical removal of the spleen?

a. Gastrectomy
b. Splenectomy
c. Hepatectomy
d. Nephrectomy

Correct Answer: b. Splenectomy.
Explanation: Splenectomy is the surgical removal of the spleen, performed due to trauma, tumors, or immune-mediated conditions affecting spleen function.

Question 141: Where would a dog or cat be likely to encounter arsenic around the house?

a. De-icer crystals
b. Anti-mildew paint
c. Ant baits
d. Silver-polish
e. Snail baits

Correct Answer: c. Ant baits.
Explanation: Arsenic is often used as an ingredient in some ant baits, which can be hazardous if ingested by pets. It's crucial to keep such products out of reach to prevent accidental poisoning.

Question 142: Which choice is best for an x-ray of a nervous, moving dog?

a. Higher milliamperage (mA); Shorter time (seconds)
b. Higher kilovoltage (kVp)
c. Lower milliamperage (mA); Shorter time (seconds)
d. Higher milliamperage (mA); Longer time (seconds)

Correct Answer: a. Higher milliamperage (mA); Shorter time (seconds).
Explanation: Using a higher mA and shorter exposure time reduces motion blur in x-rays of nervous or moving animals, ensuring a clearer image by minimizing the impact of movement.

Question 143: Why are most antibiotics contraindicated in rabbits and hamsters?

a. Highly permeable blood-brain barrier
b. Their little hearts just can't take it
c. Disrupts gram-positive gut flora
d. Highly sensitive to renal toxicity

Correct Answer: c. Disrupts gram-positive gut flora.
Explanation: Many antibiotics can disrupt the balance of gut flora in rabbits and hamsters, leading to severe gastrointestinal issues and potentially fatal conditions like enterotoxemia.

Question 144: Which anatomic area do these three surgical approaches access in the horse? Modified Whitehouse, Viborg's triangle, Hyovertebrotomy

a. Maxillary sinus
b. Soft palate
c. Atlanto-occipital joint
d. Osseous bullae
e. Guttural pouch

Correct Answer: e. Guttural pouch.
Explanation: These surgical approaches are used to access the guttural pouch in horses, a large air-filled space in the throat area that can be affected by infections or other conditions.

Question 145: An animal that is dehydrated before surgery may require a _____ because _____ of the cell volume occurs after rehydration.

a. blood/plasma transfusion; dilution
b. blood/plasma transfusion; hemoconcentration
c. splenectomy; hemoconcentration
d. splenectomy; sequestration

Correct Answer: a. blood/plasma transfusion; dilution.
Explanation: Rehydration can dilute the blood cell volume, necessitating a transfusion to restore normal levels and maintain effective oxygen transport and circulation.

Question 146: Platelets in mammals:

a. appear within RBC agglutinations in cases of hemolytic anemia.
b. do not have nuclei.
c. appear as microfilaria in a Wright-stain smear.
d. are too small to be detected, even clumped, on the feathered edge of a blood smear.

Correct Answer: b. do not have nuclei.
Explanation: Mammalian platelets are non-nucleated cell fragments derived from megakaryocytes, playing a crucial role in hemostasis and blood clotting.

Question 147: Fleas are:

a. endoparasites.
b. pseudoparasites.
c. periodic parasites.
d. ectoparasites.

Correct Answer: d. Ectoparasites.
Explanation: Fleas are external parasites (ectoparasites) that live on the skin of host animals, feeding on their blood and potentially transmitting diseases.

Question 148: Actinobacillosis is usually treated with antibiotics, an anti-inflammatory drug, and intravenous administration of:

a. sodium iodide.
b. penicillin
c. dexamethasone.
d. oxytetracycline.

Correct Answer: a. sodium iodide.
Explanation: Actinobacillosis, or "wooden tongue," is treated with sodium iodide to reduce inflammation and kill the bacteria, alongside antibiotics and anti-inflammatory medications.

Question 149: In the infection process, a reservoir refers to:

a. transmission of infection by direct contact with skin, secretions, excretions, or mucous membranes of an infected animal.
b. the portal of entry by which the pathogen gains entry into a new host.
c. a pathogen's mode of transmission.
d. an animal, insect, or fomite in or on which a pathogen can survive.

Correct Answer: d. an animal, insect, or fomite in or on which a pathogen can survive.
Explanation: A reservoir is an entity in which a pathogen can persist and multiply, serving as a source of infection for other hosts.

Question 150: Treatment for galactostasis:

a. is indicated during the first 1 to 3 weeks of the postpartum period.
b. is begun during weaning and focuses on decreasing milk production and inflammation, using warm compresses.
c. focuses on treating the inflammation and massaging the affected mammary gland.
d. involves a decrease in milk production, coupled with cold compresses to reduce fever.

Correct Answer: b. is begun during weaning and focuses on decreasing milk production and inflammation, using warm compresses.
Explanation: Galactostasis, or milk retention, is managed by reducing milk production and inflammation during weaning, often using warm compresses to alleviate discomfort.

Question 151: An allergic disease associated with airway inflammation, bronchoconstriction, and excessive mucous production is:

a. influenza.
b. herpes.
c. recurrent airway obstruction.
d. viral arteritis.

Correct Answer: c. recurrent airway obstruction.
Explanation: Recurrent airway obstruction (RAO), also known as heaves, is an allergic respiratory condition in horses characterized by airway inflammation, bronchoconstriction, and increased mucus production, leading to breathing difficulties.

Question 152: The analgesic effect of NSAIDs is due to:

a. interaction with receptors in the central nervous system.
b. interaction with specific opioid receptors in the brain and spinal cord.
c. interaction with histamine receptors.
d. modification of the inflammatory response.

Correct Answer: d. modification of the inflammatory response.
Explanation: NSAIDs (Nonsteroidal anti-inflammatory drugs) alleviate pain by inhibiting enzymes involved in the inflammatory process, reducing inflammation and associated pain.

Question 153: A 10% concentration of solution contains _____ of a drug per _____ of solution.

a. 1 g; 100 ml
b. 1 mg; 10 ml
c. 10 mL; 100 mL
d. 100 g; 100 ml

Correct Answer: c. 10 mL; 100 mL.
Explanation: A 10% solution (vol/vol) means there are 10 mL of a substance dissolved in 100 mL of the total solution, indicating the ratio of solute to solvent.

Question 154: Which vitamin is crucial for blood clotting?

a. Vitamin A
b. Vitamin C
c. Vitamin D
d. Vitamin K

Correct Answer: d. Vitamin K.
Explanation: Vitamin K is essential for the synthesis of clotting factors in the liver, playing a vital role in the blood coagulation process to prevent excessive bleeding.

Question 155: What is the primary function of the lymphatic system?

a. Transport oxygen to cells
b. Produce red blood cells
c. Remove waste products from tissues
d. Defend against pathogens

Correct Answer: d. Defend against pathogens.
Explanation: The lymphatic system is crucial for immune function, transporting lymph fluid containing white blood cells to defend against infections and maintain fluid balance in the body.

Question 156: Which is a common sign of diabetes mellitus in dogs?

a. Increased thirst and urination
b. Lethargy
c. Hair loss
d. Hyperactivity

Correct Answer: a. Increased thirst and urination.
Explanation: Diabetes mellitus in dogs is characterized by hyperglycemia, leading to increased thirst (polydipsia) and urination (polyuria) as the body attempts to eliminate excess glucose.

Question 157: What is the main cause of feline leukemia virus (FeLV) transmission?

a. Airborne droplets
b. Contaminated water
c. Direct contact with infected cats
d. Flea bites

Correct Answer: c. Direct contact with infected cats.
Explanation: FeLV is transmitted primarily through close contact with saliva, nasal secretions, or other bodily fluids from infected cats, often during grooming or sharing food and water bowls.

Question 158: Which hormone regulates calcium levels in the blood?

a. Insulin
b. Thyroxine
c. Parathyroid hormone
d. Glucagon

Correct Answer: c. Parathyroid hormone.
Explanation: Parathyroid hormone (PTH) regulates calcium levels in the blood by increasing calcium absorption from the gut, reabsorption in the kidneys, and release from bones.

Question 159: What is the term for inflammation of the liver?

a. Hepatitis
b. Nephritis
c. Gastritis
d. Dermatitis

Correct Answer: a. Hepatitis.
Explanation: Hepatitis refers to inflammation of the liver, which can result from infections, toxins, autoimmune diseases, or metabolic conditions, affecting liver function.

Question 160: Which of the following is a symptom of pancreatitis in dogs?

a. Constipation
b. Abdominal pain
c. Hyperactivity
d. Increased appetite

Correct Answer: b. Abdominal pain.
Explanation: Pancreatitis in dogs often presents with abdominal pain, vomiting, and decreased appetite, caused by inflammation of the pancreas due to enzymatic digestion.

Question 161: Which disease is transmitted by the bite of an infected mosquito?

a. Rabies
b. Canine parvovirus
c. Heartworm disease
d. Feline leukemia

Correct Answer: c. Heartworm disease.
Explanation: Heartworm disease is transmitted by mosquitoes carrying the larvae of Dirofilaria immitis, which develop into adult worms residing in the heart and pulmonary arteries of infected animals.

Question 162: What is the term for surgical removal of the gallbladder?

a. Appendectomy
b. Cholecystectomy
c. Gastrectomy
d. Hepatectomy

Correct Answer: b. Cholecystectomy.
Explanation: Cholecystectomy is the surgical procedure for removing the gallbladder, often performed to treat gallstones or gallbladder dysfunction.

Question 163: Which nutrient is essential for maintaining healthy skin and coat in animals?

a. Vitamin B12
b. Omega-3 fatty acids
c. Calcium
d. Iron

Correct Answer: b. Omega-3 fatty acids.
Explanation: Omega-3 fatty acids are crucial for maintaining healthy skin and coat, reducing inflammation, and supporting overall health in animals.

Question 164: What is the medical term for the surgical removal of a tumor?

a. Mastectomy
b. Tumorectomy
c. Lymphadenectomy
d. Excision

Correct Answer: d. Excision.
Explanation: Excision refers to the surgical removal of a tumor or abnormal tissue, often performed to prevent the spread of cancer and alleviate symptoms.

Question 165: Which condition is characterized by the accumulation of fluid in the abdomen?

a. Ascites
b. Edema
c. Hematoma
d. Lymphedema

Correct Answer: a. Ascites.
Explanation: Ascites is the accumulation of fluid in the abdominal cavity, often resulting from liver disease, heart failure, or cancer, leading to abdominal distension.

Question 166: Which of the following is a common cause of lameness in horses?

a. Colic
b. Laminitis
c. Pneumonia
d. Strangles

Correct Answer: b. Laminitis.
Explanation: Laminitis is a painful inflammatory condition affecting the hooves of horses, often leading to lameness and requiring prompt veterinary care to manage.

Question 167: What is the primary function of hemoglobin in red blood cells?

a. Transport nutrients
b. Fight infections
c. Carry oxygen
d. Regulate blood pressure

Correct Answer: c. Carry oxygen.
Explanation: Hemoglobin is a protein in red blood cells responsible for binding and transporting oxygen from the lungs to tissues and returning carbon dioxide to the lungs for exhalation.

Question 168: Which of the following is a zoonotic disease transmitted from animals to humans?

a. Canine distemper
b. Brucellosis
c. Feline panleukopenia
d. Parvovirus

Correct Answer: b. Brucellosis.
Explanation: Brucellosis is a bacterial infection that can be transmitted from animals to humans, often through contact with infected livestock or consumption of unpasteurized dairy products.

Question 169: What is the primary role of the kidneys in the body?

a. Produce hormones
b. Filter blood and produce urine
c. Regulate body temperature
d. Store glycogen

Correct Answer: b. Filter blood and produce urine.
Explanation: The kidneys filter waste products and excess substances from the blood, maintaining fluid balance and electrolyte levels while producing urine for excretion.

Question 170: Which organ is primarily responsible for detoxifying the blood?

a. Heart
b. Liver
c. Pancreas
d. Spleen

Correct Answer: b. Liver.
Explanation: The liver plays a crucial role in detoxifying the blood by metabolizing toxins and drugs, producing bile for digestion, and storing nutrients for the body's needs.

Full Test 2 with Detailed Explanations

Question 1: Cushing syndrome, or _____, primarily affects dogs and is characterized by _____.

a. hypothyroidism; an underactive thyroid, resulting in subnormal circulating levels of thyroid hormones, which causes a subsequent decrease in the metabolic rate
b. diabetic ketoacidosis (DKA); the presence of ketones in the urine
c. hypoadrenocorticism; inadequate secretion of glucocorticoids and mineralocorticoids, primarily cortisol and aldosterone
d. hyperadrenocorticism; elevated circulating levels of cortisol produced by the adrenal cortex

Correct Answer: d. hyperadrenocorticism; elevated circulating levels of cortisol produced by the adrenal cortex.
Explanation: Hyperadrenocorticism, also known as Cushing syndrome, involves an overproduction of cortisol by the adrenal glands, leading to symptoms such as increased thirst, urination, and appetite.

Question 2: Which drugs can be administered safely via the endotracheal route?

a. Atropine, lidocaine, epinephrine, naloxone, vasopressin
b. Dopamine, epinephrine
c. Corticosteroids, atropine, vasopressin
d. Epinephrine, naloxone only

Correct Answer: a. Atropine, lidocaine, epinephrine, naloxone, vasopressin.
Explanation: The acronym NAVEL helps remember drugs safe for endotracheal administration: Naloxone, Atropine, Vasopressin, Epinephrine, and Lidocaine, useful in emergency veterinary medicine.

Question 3: Two tests that can evaluate the intrinsic and common pathways of the coagulation cascade are the activated clotting time (ACT) and the _____, which measures the time it takes for the primary platelet plug to form.

a. bleeding time
b. CPPT
c. hemostasis
d. PT

Correct Answer: a. bleeding time.
Explanation: Bleeding time assesses the time required for a primary platelet plug to form, evaluating platelet function and the initial phase of coagulation.

Question 4: Artie, a Pekinese, has begun losing weight and experiences some anorexia. He is frequently suddenly exhausted. Tests indicate that Artie has _____, or disease of the heart muscle.

a. cardiovascular disease
b. cardiomuscular disease

c. cardiomyopathy
d. congestive heart failure

Correct Answer: c. cardiomyopathy.
Explanation: Cardiomyopathy refers to diseases of the heart muscle, impacting its function and leading to symptoms like fatigue, weight loss, and decreased appetite in affected animals.

Question 5: In a blood smear, oxidative damage results in _____, which are RBCs in which the hemoglobin has shifted to one side of the cell, creating a clear area outlined by a thin rim of membrane.

a. keratocytes
b. eccentrocytes
c. spherocytes
d. acanthocytes

Correct Answer: b. eccentrocytes.
Explanation: Eccentrocytes are red blood cells exhibiting asymmetric hemoglobin distribution due to oxidative damage, identified by their unique morphology on a blood smear.

Question 6: Hepatic encephalopathy can be caused by:

a. the presence of trypsin in the liver and pancreas, causing autodigestion.
b. persistent endoparasites, ulcerations, neoplasms, or coagulopathies.
c. complications of pancreatitis.
d. exposure of the brain to gastrointestinal (GI) toxins as a consequence of decreased liver function or portosystemic shunts.

Correct Answer: d. exposure of the brain to gastrointestinal (GI) toxins as a consequence of decreased liver function or portosystemic shunts.
Explanation: Hepatic encephalopathy results from the brain's exposure to toxins like ammonia, which are not adequately processed due to impaired liver function or portosystemic shunts.

Question 7: In evaluating a blood smear:

a. the counting area, where most of the evaluation takes place, is between the body and the feathered edge.
b. cell morphology can only be accurately evaluated in the largest, "body" area of the smear.
c. the counting area is the largest part, and is a homogeneous area beginning at the end of the slide where the drop of blood was placed.
d. cell morphology should only be evaluated at the feathered edge, where the cells are spread thinly and appear singly.

Correct Answer: a. the counting area, where most of the evaluation takes place, is between the body and the feathered edge.
Explanation: The counting area in a blood smear is ideal for evaluating cell morphology, as it contains a monolayer of cells, allowing for clear identification and assessment.

Question 8: Pyometra, metritis, and endometrial hyperplasia may be treated with a(n):

a. onychectomy.
b. anastomosis.
c. urethrostomy.
d. ovariohysterectomy.

Correct Answer: d. ovariohysterectomy.
Explanation: Ovariohysterectomy, the surgical removal of the ovaries and uterus, is often performed to treat uterine diseases like pyometra and metritis.

Question 9: The veterinarian uses a(n) _____ to stabilize a fracture, placing pins through the skin and bone.

a. osteotome
b. external fixator
c. trephine
d. rongeur

Correct Answer: b. external fixator.

Explanation: An external fixator stabilizes fractures using pins inserted through the skin and bone, providing support and allowing for adjustment and healing.

Question 10: Which of the following is not a key aspect of recumbent care?

a. Taking care of the recumbent patient's airways involves humidification, sterile suctioning, and changing the ET tube daily.
b. Appropriate bedding and padding can reduce the incidence of decubital ulcer development.
c. Do not apply fluorescein stain to the corneas of a patient who is under general anesthesia.
d. None of the above. All are key aspects of recumbent care.

Correct Answer: c. Do not apply fluorescein stain to the corneas of a patient who is under general anesthesia.

Explanation: Applying fluorescein stain to examine corneal health in anesthetized patients is crucial to detect and treat ulcers early, contrary to option c.

Question 11: Vertical measurements on an ECG paper represent:

a. time expressed in seconds.
b. strength of the electrical impulse expressed in millimeters per millivolt.
c. time expressed in millimeters per second.
d. strength of the electrical impulse expressed in millivolts.

Correct Answer: d. strength of the electrical impulse expressed in millivolts.

Explanation: On ECG paper, vertical measurements indicate the amplitude of electrical impulses in millivolts, reflecting the heart's electrical activity.

Question 12: Which type of cell is primarily responsible for producing antibodies?

a. Red blood cells
b. T-cells
c. B-cells
d. Neutrophils

Correct Answer: c. B-cells.

Explanation: B-cells, a type of white blood cell, are responsible for producing antibodies, which are crucial for the immune response against pathogens.

Question 13: What is the primary function of insulin in the body?

a. Regulate heart rate
b. Control blood pressure
c. Facilitate cellular glucose uptake
d. Increase lipid storage

Correct Answer: c. Facilitate cellular glucose uptake.

Explanation: Insulin is a hormone that facilitates the uptake of glucose into cells, regulating blood sugar levels and providing energy for cellular functions.

Question 14: Which nutrient is essential for thyroid hormone production?

a. Calcium
b. Iodine

c. Iron
d. Magnesium

Correct Answer: b. Iodine.
Explanation: Iodine is a key component in the synthesis of thyroid hormones, essential for metabolic regulation and proper thyroid function.

Question 15: What is the primary role of platelets in the blood?

a. Oxygen transport
b. Immune defense
c. Blood clotting
d. Hormone transport

Correct Answer: c. Blood clotting.
Explanation: Platelets play a critical role in hemostasis, contributing to the formation of blood clots to prevent bleeding and facilitate wound healing.

Question 16: Which parasite is commonly known to cause heartworm disease in dogs?

a. Ancylostoma
b. Toxocara
c. Dirofilaria immitis
d. Trichuris

Correct Answer: c. Dirofilaria immitis.
Explanation: Dirofilaria immitis is a parasitic worm transmitted by mosquitoes, causing heartworm disease, which affects the heart and lungs of dogs.

Question 17: Which vitamin is essential for calcium absorption in the intestines?

a. Vitamin A
b. Vitamin B12
c. Vitamin D
d. Vitamin K

Correct Answer: c. Vitamin D.
Explanation: Vitamin D enhances calcium absorption in the intestines, playing a vital role in maintaining bone health and calcium homeostasis.

Question 18: What is the medical term for inflammation of the joints?

a. Myositis
b. Arthritis
c. Dermatitis
d. Neuritis

Correct Answer: b. Arthritis.
Explanation: Arthritis refers to inflammation of the joints, leading to pain, stiffness, and reduced mobility, commonly affecting both humans and animals.

Question 19: Which organ is primarily responsible for detoxifying the blood?

a. Heart
b. Liver
c. Kidneys
d. Pancreas

Correct Answer: b. Liver.
Explanation: The liver plays a crucial role in detoxifying the blood, metabolizing toxins, drugs, and waste products, and producing bile for digestion.

Question 20: What is the primary cause of feline leukemia virus (FeLV) transmission?

a. Airborne droplets
b. Contaminated water
c. Direct contact with infected cats
d. Flea bites

Correct Answer: c. Direct contact with infected cats.
Explanation: FeLV spreads through close contact with saliva, nasal secretions, or other bodily fluids of infected cats, often during grooming or sharing resources.

Question 21: A surgeon removes a devitalized section of intestine and then performs a(n):

a. onychectomy.
b. urethrostomy.
c. ovariohysterectomy.
d. anastomosis.

Correct Answer: d. anastomosis.
Explanation: Anastomosis involves surgically connecting two ends of the intestine after the removal of a diseased section, restoring continuity to the gastrointestinal tract.

Question 22: Surgically prepared skin is considered _____, not _____.

a. sterile; aseptic
b. aseptic; sterile
c. scrubbed; aseptic
d. clean; aseptic

Correct Answer: b. aseptic; sterile.
Explanation: While surgical skin preparation reduces microbial load, it is considered aseptic rather than sterile, as sterility implies complete absence of all microorganisms.

Question 23: In evaluating an antibody response using serologic testing, the first sample is taken:

a. only after the animal has had time to develop a humoral immune response.
b. when the patient initially shows clinical signs and is presented for examination.
c. only after vaccination to ensure accuracy.
d. within 1 to 3 days of the second sample, when titer increases are most meaningful.

Correct Answer: b. when the patient initially shows clinical signs and is presented for examination.
Explanation: The initial serology sample is collected when clinical signs first appear to establish a baseline, followed by a second sample to detect changes in antibody levels.

Question 24: You notice a family of neonatal piglets establishing teat order. Naturally, the _____ mammary glands are most sought after.

a. caudal
b. middle
c. nearest random
d. cranial

Correct Answer: d. cranial.
Explanation: Neonatal piglets prefer cranial mammary glands, which generally produce more milk, leading stronger piglets to compete for these positions for optimal nutrition.

Question 25: When collecting blood for a complete blood count (CBC), which of the following is not true?

a. If clots are present, a new sample should be collected.
b. 2 ml of blood is sufficient for a CBC from any animal species.

c. The collection tube should be inverted 10-15 times before further processing to ensure the RBCs, WBCs, and platelets are evenly dispersed in the sample.
d. None of the above. A, B, and C are all true.

Correct Answer: d. None of the above. A, B, and C are all true.
Explanation: Proper blood collection for CBC includes ensuring no clots, adequate volume, and mixing to prevent cell clumping, all crucial for accurate analysis.

Question 26: Fescue toxicosis is a nutritional disease that can involve lameness, tail-tip necrosis, abortion, and/or decreased milk production. This disease affects:

a. pigs.
b. sheep.
c. both B and C.
d. horses.

Correct Answer: b. sheep.
Explanation: Fescue toxicosis primarily affects livestock like sheep and cattle, causing symptoms like lameness and reproductive issues due to toxic endophyte-infected grasses.

Question 27: A(n) _____ is a detailed step-by-step description for performing a test and operating an instrument.

a. Levy-Jennings chart
b. QC
c. iSTAT
d. SOP

Correct Answer: d. SOP.
Explanation: A Standard Operating Procedure (SOP) provides detailed instructions for test performance and equipment use, ensuring consistency and accuracy in laboratory settings.

Question 28: Your patient's fecal sample shows streaks of blood on the outsides of otherwise normally formed stools, a symptom you quickly identify as:

a. hematochezia.
b. melena.
c. tenesmus.
d. hematemesis.

Correct Answer: a. hematochezia.
Explanation: Hematochezia is the presence of fresh blood in feces, often indicating lower gastrointestinal bleeding or lesions, requiring further diagnostic investigation.

Question 29: Cerebrospinal (CSF) fluid from a horse is collected at the:

a. atlantooccipital space.
b. sacrococcygeal junction.
c. cervical thoracic junction.
d. lumbosacral space.

Correct Answer: d. lumbosacral space.
Explanation: The lumbosacral space is commonly used for CSF collection in horses, facilitating diagnosis of neurological conditions by analyzing fluid composition.

Question 30: The most common nutritional disease of pot-bellied pigs is:

a. malnourishment.
b. stunted growth.

c. anorexia.
d. obesity.

Correct Answer: d. obesity.
Explanation: Obesity is prevalent in pot-bellied pigs due to overfeeding or improper diets, leading to health issues like arthritis and heart conditions, necessitating dietary management.

Question 31: You examine a microhematocrit tube after centrifugation. The buffy coat:

a. is the uppermost layer and contains plasma.
b. represents the middle layer and contains packed red blood cells (RBCs).
c. contains white blood cells (WBCs) and platelets and is the middle layer between plasma and RBCs.
d. is in the lower portion and contains packed RBCs.

Correct Answer: c. contains white blood cells (WBCs) and platelets and is the middle layer between plasma and RBCs.
Explanation: The buffy coat layer in a centrifuged microhematocrit tube contains WBCs and platelets, serving as an indicator of leukocyte and thrombocyte levels in blood.

Question 32: What is the primary function of the pancreas in digestion?

a. Produce bile
b. Secrete insulin
c. Produce digestive enzymes
d. Absorb nutrients

Correct Answer: c. Produce digestive enzymes.
Explanation: The pancreas plays a crucial role in digestion by secreting enzymes like amylase, lipase, and proteases, which aid in breaking down carbohydrates, fats, and proteins.

Question 33: Which mineral is essential for oxygen transport in red blood cells?

a. Calcium
b. Iron
c. Magnesium
d. Zinc

Correct Answer: b. Iron.
Explanation: Iron is a key component of hemoglobin, facilitating oxygen transport from the lungs to tissues and supporting cellular respiration and energy production.

Question 34: Which disease is caused by a deficiency of thiamine (Vitamin B1)?

a. Scurvy
b. Beriberi
c. Rickets
d. Pellagra

Correct Answer: b. Beriberi.
Explanation: Beriberi results from a lack of thiamine (Vitamin B1), leading to symptoms like weakness, nerve damage, and cardiovascular issues due to impaired carbohydrate metabolism.

Question 35: What is the medical term for inflammation of the bladder?

a. Nephritis
b. Cystitis
c. Urethritis
d. Pyelonephritis

Correct Answer: b. Cystitis.
Explanation: Cystitis refers to bladder inflammation, often caused by bacterial infection, resulting in symptoms like frequent urination, pain, and discomfort.

Question 36: Which nutrient is vital for the formation of collagen, a protein essential for skin, bone, and connective tissue health?

a. Vitamin A
b. Vitamin C
c. Vitamin D
d. Vitamin E

Correct Answer: b. Vitamin C.
Explanation: Vitamin C is crucial for collagen synthesis, providing structural support and elasticity to skin, bones, and connective tissues, and aiding in wound healing.

Question 37: What is the primary role of the spleen in the body?

a. Filter blood
b. Produce bile
c. Store glycogen
d. Produce hormones

Correct Answer: a. Filter blood.
Explanation: The spleen filters blood, removing old or damaged red blood cells, and plays a role in immune response by producing lymphocytes and storing white blood cells.

Question 38: Which of the following is a symptom of hypothyroidism in dogs?

a. Increased energy
b. Weight gain
c. Hyperactivity
d. Increased appetite

Correct Answer: b. Weight gain.
Explanation: Hypothyroidism in dogs leads to a slowed metabolism, often resulting in weight gain, lethargy, and skin or coat changes due to reduced thyroid hormone production.

Question 39: What is the term for surgical removal of a kidney?

a. Nephrectomy
b. Cholecystectomy
c. Appendectomy
d. Gastrectomy

Correct Answer: a. Nephrectomy.
Explanation: Nephrectomy is the surgical procedure to remove a kidney, typically performed due to severe damage, cancer, or donor transplantation needs.

Question 40: Which of the following is a zoonotic disease that can be transmitted from animals to humans?

a. Canine distemper
b. Salmonellosis
c. Feline panleukopenia
d. Parvovirus

Correct Answer: b. Salmonellosis.
Explanation: Salmonellosis is a bacterial infection that can be transmitted from animals, particularly reptiles and poultry, to humans, causing gastrointestinal symptoms.

Question 41: A unicellular parasite is:

a. a protozoan.
b. a zoonosis.
c. coenurus.
d. a trematode.

Correct Answer: a. a protozoan.
Explanation: Protozoans are single-celled organisms that can be parasitic, affecting both humans and animals, often causing diseases like malaria and giardiasis.

Question 42: Which of the following statements is false regarding calves with diarrhea?

a. Milk and milk products should be warmed before being offered.
b. Cows should be vaccinated before calving.
c. Poor sanitation and poor nutrition can contribute to the development of diarrhea.
d. Warm intravenous fluids should be administered and supplemented with dextrose and bicarbonate as needed.

Correct Answer: a. Milk and milk products should be warmed before being offered.
Explanation: While maintaining warmth is important, the primary focus for calves with diarrhea is ensuring proper hydration and nutrition, alongside preventive measures like vaccination and sanitation.

Question 43: Your equine patient develops rhinopneumonitis, caused by _____, which produces respiratory disease, abortion, and neonatal and neurologic disease (ascending paralysis) in horses.

a. herpesvirus
b. influenza
c. guttural pouch mycosis
d. strangles

Correct Answer: a. herpesvirus.
Explanation: Equine herpesvirus is the causative agent of rhinopneumonitis, leading to respiratory, reproductive, and neurological issues in horses, necessitating vaccination and biosecurity measures.

Question 44: The veterinarian is about to perform a vaginal examination on a cow with dystocia. As you prep the perineal area, which of the following is not true?

a. The perineal scrub will decrease uterine and vaginal contamination.
b. The perineal scrub is not intended to achieve asepsis.
c. Some veterinarians prefer to begin by cleaning out the rectum so that the cow does not defecate on the clean field.
d. It is imperative to clean the perineal area before the rectal portion of the examination.

Correct Answer: d. It is imperative to clean the perineal area before the rectal portion of the examination.
Explanation: The perineal area should be prepared to reduce contamination, but rectal cleaning is often prioritized to prevent defecation onto the prepped field during examination.

Question 45: Most surgical instruments are made of:

a. silver.
b. stainless steel.
c. chrome.
d. titanium.

Correct Answer: b. stainless steel.
Explanation: Stainless steel is the preferred material for surgical instruments due to its durability, resistance to corrosion, and ability to maintain a sharp edge.

Question 46: Hypoadrenocorticism is:

a. a result of overproduction of the pituitary hormone adrenocorticotropic hormone (ACTH).
b. due to excess cortisol production by the adrenal gland.
c. due to a decrease in adrenal gland function.
d. associated with the excess production of glucocorticoids.

Correct Answer: c. due to a decrease in adrenal gland function.
Explanation: Hypoadrenocorticism, or Addison's disease, results from insufficient adrenal gland hormone production, leading to symptoms like weakness, dehydration, and electrolyte imbalances.

Question 47: Which nutritional myodegenerative disease may be caused by a deficiency of gestational vitamin E and/or selenium?

a. Johne disease
b. Caseous lymphadenitis
c. Caprine arthritis-encephalitis
d. White muscle disease

Correct Answer: d. White muscle disease.
Explanation: White muscle disease is caused by vitamin E and selenium deficiencies, leading to muscle degeneration in young animals born to deficient mothers, highlighting the need for adequate maternal nutrition.

Question 48: What covers the feet of horses to help decrease contamination in the surgical suite?

a. Sterile surgical tape
b. Obstetric sleeves
c. Fluid bags
d. Paper booties

Correct Answer: b. Obstetric sleeves.
Explanation: Obstetric sleeves are used to cover horses' hooves, minimizing contamination risks in the surgical environment and maintaining sterility.

Question 49: To avoid infection from _____, pregnant women must avoid contact with soil, cat litter, raw meat, and cats excreting oocysts.

a. Toxoplasma gondii
b. Giardia
c. Cheyletiella
d. Dipylidium caninum

Correct Answer: a. Toxoplasma gondii.
Explanation: Toxoplasma gondii is a protozoan parasite, posing risks to pregnant women due to potential congenital transmission, necessitating avoidance of contaminated sources.

Question 50: When collecting serum samples, be sure to:

a. refrigerate the sample during the clotting procedure.
b. never use a tube containing a serum separator.
c. separate the serum as soon as a firm clot has formed.
d. ensure that the sample contains fibrin to avoid false analyte measurements.

Correct Answer: c. separate the serum as soon as a firm clot has formed.
Explanation: Timely separation of serum from clotted blood prevents contamination and ensures accurate laboratory results, with serum separators aiding in clean extraction.

Question 51: _____ is the condition of an abnormally thickened portion of the articular cartilage.

a. Rheumatoid arthritis
b. Osteoarthritis
c. Arthrodesis
d. Osteochondrosis

Correct Answer: d. Osteochondrosis.
Explanation: Osteochondrosis involves abnormal cartilage development, leading to thickening and potential joint issues, often affecting young, growing animals due to nutritional or genetic factors.

Question 52: Which of the following means of hemostasis is avoided during equine abdominal surgery?

a. Suction
b. Sponge
c. Clamping with ligation
d. Hemostats in combination with electrocautery

Correct Answer: b. Sponge.
Explanation: Sponge hemostasis is avoided in equine abdominal surgeries to prevent the risk of sponge retention, which can lead to severe complications and infection.

Question 53: During surgery, you hand the veterinary surgeon a(n) _____, which she uses to cut bone by applying the blade end to the area to be cut before pounding on the flared end of the handle with a mallet.

a. external fixator
b. rongeur
c. trephine
d. osteotome

Correct Answer: d. osteotome.
Explanation: An osteotome is a surgical instrument used to cut bone, involving a precise technique of mallet strikes to achieve clean, controlled cuts.

Question 54: Which is the correct order of the phases of nociception?

a. Electrical, chemical, cardiovascular
b. Injury, heat and swelling, inflammation
c. Mechanical, chemical, thermal
d. Transduction, transmission, modulation

Correct Answer: d. Transduction, transmission, modulation.
Explanation: Nociception, the sensory process that provides signals leading to pain perception, follows a sequence of transduction, transmission, and modulation phases.

Question 55: According to the text, which of the following is not a common small animal emergency?

a. Respiratory distress
b. Urethral obstruction
c. Acute abdomen
d. All of the above are common small animal emergencies.

Correct Answer: d. All of the above are common small animal emergencies.
Explanation: Common small animal emergencies include respiratory distress, urethral obstruction, and acute abdomen, requiring prompt veterinary attention to ensure the best outcomes.

Question 56: What is the primary function of a stethoscope in veterinary medicine?

a. To visually examine the eyes
b. To listen to heart and lung sounds
c. To measure blood pressure
d. To assess hydration status

Correct Answer: b. To listen to heart and lung sounds.
Explanation: A stethoscope allows veterinarians to auscultate internal body sounds such as heartbeats and breath sounds, aiding in diagnosing cardiovascular and respiratory conditions.

Question 57: Which type of cell is responsible for bone resorption?

a. Osteoblasts
b. Osteoclasts
c. Chondrocytes
d. Fibroblasts

Correct Answer: b. Osteoclasts.
Explanation: Osteoclasts are specialized cells that break down bone tissue, playing a crucial role in bone remodeling and calcium homeostasis.

Question 58: Which of the following conditions is characterized by an excessive accumulation of fluid in the abdominal cavity?

a. Anuria
b. Ascites
c. Hematuria
d. Polyuria

Correct Answer: b. Ascites.
Explanation: Ascites refers to fluid buildup in the abdominal cavity, often due to liver disease, heart failure, or cancer, necessitating investigation and management of the underlying cause.

Question 59: Which vaccine is recommended annually to protect dogs from the rabies virus?

a. Distemper
b. Parvovirus
c. Rabies
d. Bordetella

Correct Answer: c. Rabies.
Explanation: Rabies vaccination is crucial for dogs to prevent this lethal zoonotic disease, with regulations often requiring annual or triennial boosters depending on the vaccine used.

Question 60: What is the primary role of the kidneys in the body?

a. Produce insulin
b. Filter waste products from the blood
c. Store bile
d. Synthesize vitamin D

Correct Answer: b. Filter waste products from the blood.
Explanation: The kidneys filter blood to remove waste products and excess substances, maintaining fluid and electrolyte balance, and regulating blood pressure and red blood cell production.

Question 61: Which electrolyte is critical for muscle contraction and nerve impulse transmission?

a. Magnesium
b. Calcium
c. Sodium
d. Potassium

Correct Answer: d. Potassium.

Explanation: Potassium is essential for muscle contractions and nerve impulses, maintaining cellular function and homeostasis, with imbalances leading to serious health issues.

Question 62: Which species is most associated with the zoonotic transmission of the Hantavirus?

a. Cats
b. Rodents
c. Dogs
d. Birds

Correct Answer: b. Rodents.

Explanation: Rodents, particularly mice and rats, are primary carriers of Hantavirus, transmitting the virus to humans through contact with infected droppings, urine, or saliva.

Question 63: Which of the following is a symptom of hyperthyroidism in cats?

a. Weight gain
b. Lethargy
c. Increased appetite
d. Decreased heart rate

Correct Answer: c. Increased appetite.

Explanation: Hyperthyroidism in cats leads to increased metabolism, causing symptoms like increased appetite, weight loss, and hyperactivity, often due to thyroid gland overactivity.

Question 64: Which of the following is a common method for diagnosing heartworm disease in dogs?

a. Blood smear
b. Urinalysis
c. Fecal flotation
d. ELISA test

Correct Answer: d. ELISA test.

Explanation: An ELISA (Enzyme-Linked Immunosorbent Assay) test is commonly used to detect heartworm antigens in dogs, providing a reliable diagnosis of this parasitic infection.

Question 65: What is the primary goal of fluid therapy in dehydrated animals?

a. Increase urine output
b. Restore electrolyte balance
c. Enhance nutrient absorption
d. Reduce blood pressure

Correct Answer: b. Restore electrolyte balance.

Explanation: Fluid therapy aims to rehydrate the animal, restoring electrolyte balance and normal physiological function, crucial for recovery from dehydration.

Question 66: Which of the following is a characteristic of an anaphylactic reaction?

a. Slow onset
b. Mild itching
c. Rapid heart rate
d. Reduced breathing rate

Correct Answer: c. Rapid heart rate.

Explanation: Anaphylaxis is a severe, rapid-onset allergic reaction characterized by symptoms such as rapid heart rate, difficulty breathing, and potential progression to shock.

Question 67: Which of the following is a common zoonotic disease associated with reptiles?

a. Rabies
b. Tuberculosis
c. Salmonellosis
d. Lyme disease

Correct Answer: c. Salmonellosis.
Explanation: Reptiles, such as turtles and snakes, can carry Salmonella bacteria, posing a zoonotic risk to humans, especially with improper handling or hygiene practices.

Question 68: Which of the following is the best method to control fleas in pets?

a. Frequent bathing
b. Topical insecticides
c. Herbal remedies
d. Increased exercise

Correct Answer: b. Topical insecticides.
Explanation: Topical insecticides are effective in controlling flea infestations in pets, providing protection by killing adult fleas and preventing reproduction.

Question 69: Which of the following is a common site for subcutaneous injections in dogs?

a. Dorsal neck
b. Ventral abdomen
c. Lateral thorax
d. Dorsal lumbar region

Correct Answer: d. Dorsal lumbar region.
Explanation: The dorsal lumbar region is a preferred site for subcutaneous injections in dogs, providing adequate space for absorption and minimizing discomfort.

Question 70: What is the primary function of the liver in metabolism?

a. Produce hormones
b. Store vitamins
c. Detoxify substances
d. Absorb nutrients

Correct Answer: c. Detoxify substances.
Explanation: The liver plays a central role in metabolism by detoxifying harmful substances, metabolizing drugs, and producing bile for digestion, supporting overall body function.

Question 71: Which type of fracture involves a break in multiple places?

a. Simple fracture
b. Greenstick fracture
c. Comminuted fracture
d. Compression fracture

Correct Answer: c. Comminuted fracture.
Explanation: A comminuted fracture involves the bone breaking into several pieces, often requiring complex treatment and stabilization for proper healing.

Question 72: Which of the following is a common cause of ear infections in dogs?

a. Excessive grooming
b. High humidity
c. Bacterial overgrowth
d. Diet changes

Correct Answer: c. Bacterial overgrowth.
Explanation: Ear infections in dogs are often caused by bacterial or yeast overgrowth, exacerbated by factors like moisture, allergies, and poor ear hygiene.

Question 73: Which of the following is considered a life-threatening condition requiring immediate veterinary attention?

a. Lameness
b. Diarrhea
c. Heatstroke
d. Mild itching

Correct Answer: c. Heatstroke.
Explanation: Heatstroke is a critical condition characterized by elevated body temperature and systemic distress, necessitating immediate cooling and veterinary intervention to prevent organ damage.

Question 74: Which of the following is a symptom of feline lower urinary tract disease (FLUTD)?

a. Limping
b. Frequent urination attempts
c. Increased appetite
d. Vomiting

Correct Answer: b. Frequent urination attempts.
Explanation: FLUTD symptoms include frequent, painful urination attempts, often accompanied by blood in the urine, requiring prompt diagnosis and management.

Question 75: Which of the following is a common method for diagnosing diabetes mellitus in animals?

a. Blood glucose test
b. Fecal analysis
c. Skin scraping
d. Ultrasound

Correct Answer: a. Blood glucose test.
Explanation: Diabetes mellitus is diagnosed through blood glucose testing, identifying elevated sugar levels indicative of impaired insulin regulation.

Question 76: Which of the following is a common treatment for hypothyroidism in dogs?

a. Insulin injections
b. Thyroid hormone replacement
c. Chemotherapy
d. Surgical removal of the thyroid gland

Correct Answer: b. Thyroid hormone replacement.
Explanation: Hypothyroidism in dogs is typically managed through thyroid hormone replacement therapy, restoring normal metabolic function and alleviating symptoms.

Question 77: What is the medical term for the inflammation of the gums?

a. Stomatitis
b. Glossitis
c. Gingivitis
d. Periodontitis

Correct Answer: c. Gingivitis.
Explanation: Gingivitis is gum inflammation, often due to plaque buildup, leading to redness, swelling, and potential progression to more severe periodontal disease if untreated.

Question 78: Which of the following is a common cause of obesity in pets?

a. Over-exercising
b. Underfeeding
c. Overfeeding and lack of exercise
d. Genetic factors only

Correct Answer: c. Overfeeding and lack of exercise.
Explanation: Obesity in pets is frequently caused by excessive calorie intake combined with insufficient physical activity, leading to weight gain and associated health risks.

Question 79: Which of the following is an essential nutrient for cats that is often lacking in homemade diets?

a. Vitamin A
b. Taurine
c. Calcium
d. Omega-3 fatty acids

Correct Answer: b. Taurine.
Explanation: Taurine is an essential amino acid for cats, critical for heart and eye health, often insufficient in homemade diets without proper supplementation.

Question 80: Which of the following is a common symptom of kennel cough in dogs?

a. Sneezing
b. Coughing
c. Diarrhea
d. Vomiting

Correct Answer: b. Coughing.
Explanation: Kennel cough, a contagious respiratory disease, primarily manifests as a persistent cough, requiring supportive care and sometimes antibiotics for recovery.

Question 81: Which of the following is an infectious disease caused by a prion?

a. Rabies
b. Scrapie
c. Tetanus
d. Lyme disease

Correct Answer: b. Scrapie.
Explanation: Scrapie is a prion disease affecting sheep and goats, characterized by neurological symptoms and progressive degeneration, highlighting the importance of prion management.

Question 82: Which of the following is a common cause of lameness in horses?

a. Laminitis
b. Colic
c. Hepatitis
d. Dermatophytosis

Correct Answer: a. Laminitis.
Explanation: Laminitis involves inflammation of the horse's hoof tissues, often due to metabolic or dietary issues, leading to lameness and requiring careful management.

Question 83: Which of the following is a common method for diagnosing feline immunodeficiency virus (FIV)?

a. Urinalysis
b. Fecal flotation

c. ELISA test
d. Skin scraping

Correct Answer: c. ELISA test.

Explanation: Feline immunodeficiency virus (FIV) is typically diagnosed through an ELISA test, which detects antibodies in the blood, indicating the presence of the virus in infected cats.

Question 84: The condition in which air becomes trapped between the body wall and the lung is called:

a. flail chest.
b. hemothorax.
c. pneumothorax.
d. subcutaneous emphysema.

Correct Answer: c. pneumothorax.

Explanation: Pneumothorax occurs when air enters the pleural space, often due to trauma, causing lung collapse and impaired breathing, necessitating prompt medical intervention.

Question 85: Chemotherapeutic drugs:

a. can help patients avoid the bone marrow suppression side effect seen with radiation therapy.
b. cannot differentiate between cancer cells and normal cells that have high proliferation rates, such as the cells of bone marrow, the gastrointestinal tract, or hair follicles.
c. target primarily slowly proliferating cells.
d. have certain safe levels of occupational exposure, unlike radiation.

Correct Answer: b. cannot differentiate between cancer cells and normal cells that have high proliferation rates, such as the cells of bone marrow, the gastrointestinal tract, or hair follicles.

Explanation: Chemotherapy affects rapidly dividing cells, targeting cancer but also impacting normal tissues like bone marrow and hair follicles, leading to side effects.

Question 86: Which of the following medication routes has the highest bioavailability?

a. Oral
b. Intramuscular
c. Intravenous
d. Bioavailability is not related to the route; it is related to the concentration of the drug.

Correct Answer: c. Intravenous.

Explanation: Intravenous administration provides 100% bioavailability as the drug is directly delivered into the bloodstream, bypassing absorption barriers present in other routes.

Question 87: An animal that assumes a praying or play bowing position most likely has _____ pain.

a. neurologically induced
b. abdominal
c. thoracic
d. musculoskeletal

Correct Answer: b. abdominal.

Explanation: Animals with abdominal pain often exhibit a praying posture to relieve discomfort, characterized by forelimbs lowered and hindquarters elevated.

Question 88: Unstained smears being sent to a reference laboratory should be:

a. frozen.
b. stored at room temperature.
c. preserved with formalin before shipping.
d. stored in a refrigerator.

Correct Answer: b. stored at room temperature.
Explanation: Unstained smears should be stored at room temperature to prevent moisture damage and avoid formalin exposure, which can alter cell morphology.

Question 89: Which of the following statements is not true regarding anthrax?

a. Anthrax-contaminated carcasses should be buried in lime or incinerated.
b. Anthrax is endemic in many areas of the southern United States.
c. If an animal is suspected of having anthrax, necropsy should be performed and the brain sent to the state veterinarian.
d. Contact the area's federal veterinarian immediately if an animal is suspected of having anthrax.

Correct Answer: c. If an animal is suspected of having anthrax, necropsy should be performed and the brain sent to the state veterinarian.
Explanation: Necropsy should be avoided in suspected anthrax cases to prevent spore release; instead, suspected cases must be reported to authorities immediately.

Question 90: First-degree AV block occurs when:

a. there is no conduction of sinus impulses through the AV node.
b. the sinus impulse is blocked at the level of the left or right bundle branch but is conducted normally through the opposite bundle branch.
c. there is intermittent disruption of AV nodal conduction.
d. conduction through the AV node is delayed.

Correct Answer: d. conduction through the AV node is delayed.
Explanation: First-degree AV block involves delayed conduction through the AV node, seen as a prolonged PR interval on an ECG, often benign or drug-induced.

Question 91: Trocar, sleeve, blunt obturator, triangulation, and light cable are all terms used in _____ surgery.

a. orthopedic
b. ophthalmologic
c. emergency
d. arthroscopic

Correct Answer: d. arthroscopic.
Explanation: Arthroscopic surgery utilizes instruments like trocars and sleeves for minimally invasive joint procedures, enhancing visualization and precision through triangulation techniques.

Question 92: Both a goat and a sheep are scheduled for surgery. Which of the following presurgical injections will each animal be given?

a. An anticonvulsant
b. NSAIDs
c. Tetanus toxoid or antitoxin
d. Ceftiofur

Correct Answer: c. Tetanus toxoid or antitoxin.
Explanation: Small ruminants are susceptible to tetanus, so tetanus toxoid or antitoxin is administered preoperatively to prevent this potentially fatal infection.

Question 93: For tracheostomy in a calf, you will use a _____ mm ID tube.

a. 10- to 15-
b. 10- to 12-
c. 15- to 20-
d. 5- to 10-

Correct Answer: d. 5- to 10-.
Explanation: Tracheostomy in calves requires a 5- to 10-mm ID tube to establish an airway, especially in cases of upper airway obstruction, ensuring appropriate ventilation.

Question 94: You are attempting to calibrate a microscope. Starting on low power (10′ magnification), you focus on the 2-mm line on the stage micrometer and then rotate the eyepiece so that the hash-mark scale is parallel to the stage micrometer scale, aligning the zero point on both scales. Now you notice that the 0.125-mm mark aligns with the "10" hash mark on the eyepiece. What is the distance between each hash mark on the eyepiece?

a. 0.0125 μm
b. 12.5 μm
c. 1.25 μm
d. 0.125 μm

Correct Answer: b. 12.5 μm.
Explanation: The distance between hash marks on the eyepiece, calculated from the alignment with the stage micrometer, is 12.5 μm, crucial for precise microscopic measurements.

Question 95: You are treating a dog who is suffering malabsorption, eating constantly yet losing weight. He has chronic diarrhea that is pale, fatty, and voluminous. He is diagnosed with EPI, which is:

a. characterized by painful straining at urination or defecation.
b. caused by complications of advanced diabetes mellitus (DM).
c. caused by insufficient production and secretion of pancreatic digestive enzymes.
d. characterized by an accumulation of lipids or fats in the cytoplasm of more than 80% of the hepatocytes.

Correct Answer: c. caused by insufficient production and secretion of pancreatic digestive enzymes.
Explanation: Exocrine pancreatic insufficiency (EPI) arises from inadequate pancreatic enzyme secretion, leading to poor nutrient absorption, weight loss, and characteristic diarrhea.

Question 96: Which of the following is a common method used to assess kidney function in animals?

a. Liver enzyme test
b. Blood urea nitrogen (BUN) test
c. Fecal flotation
d. Skin biopsy

Correct Answer: b. Blood urea nitrogen (BUN) test.
Explanation: The BUN test evaluates kidney function by measuring urea levels in the blood, with elevated levels indicating impaired renal filtration.

Question 97: What is the most common cause of hypercalcemia in dogs?

a. Hemorrhage
b. Lymphoma
c. Obesity
d. Renal failure

Correct Answer: b. Lymphoma.
Explanation: Lymphoma, a prevalent cause of hypercalcemia in dogs, results from malignant lymphocyte proliferation, impacting calcium regulation through paraneoplastic processes.

Question 98: In which species is Pasteurellosis most commonly observed?

a. Cats
b. Rabbits
c. Horses
d. Cattle

Correct Answer: b. Rabbits.

Explanation: Pasteurellosis, often seen in rabbits, is caused by Pasteurella multocida, leading to respiratory infections and requiring appropriate antibiotic treatment.

Question 99: Which nutrient is essential for proper vision and immune function in animals?

a. Vitamin C
b. Vitamin D
c. Vitamin A
d. Vitamin K

Correct Answer: c. Vitamin A.

Explanation: Vitamin A is crucial for maintaining healthy vision, skin, and immune function, with deficiencies leading to night blindness and increased infection risk.

Question 100: Which of the following is a common sign of heart failure in dogs?

a. Increased appetite
b. Coughing
c. Hyperactivity
d. Limping

Correct Answer: b. Coughing.

Explanation: Coughing, particularly during rest or at night, is a common indication of heart failure in dogs, due to pulmonary congestion and fluid accumulation.

Question 101: Which of the following is a method for diagnosing feline hyperthyroidism?

a. Blood pressure measurement
b. Thyroid hormone level test
c. Urinalysis
d. Fecal analysis

Correct Answer: b. Thyroid hormone level test.

Explanation: Feline hyperthyroidism is diagnosed by measuring elevated levels of thyroid hormones (T4) in the blood, reflecting an overactive thyroid gland.

Question 102: Which of the following conditions is characterized by an overproduction of glucocorticoids?

a. Addison's disease
b. Cushing's disease
c. Diabetes mellitus
d. Hypothyroidism

Correct Answer: b. Cushing's disease.

Explanation: Cushing's disease involves excessive glucocorticoid production, leading to symptoms like increased thirst, urination, and abdominal enlargement.

Question 103: Which of the following is a common cause of anemia in cats?

a. Hyperthyroidism
b. Pyometra
c. Chronic kidney disease
d. Osteoarthritis

Correct Answer: c. Chronic kidney disease.

Explanation: Anemia in cats often results from chronic kidney disease, where decreased erythropoietin production impairs red blood cell formation.

Question 104: What is the primary function of the pancreas in digestion?

a. Produce bile
b. Absorb nutrients
c. Secrete digestive enzymes
d. Store vitamins

Correct Answer: c. Secrete digestive enzymes.
Explanation: The pancreas plays a crucial role in digestion by secreting enzymes that break down carbohydrates, proteins, and fats, facilitating nutrient absorption in the intestine.

Question 105: Which of the following is a common cause of hypothyroidism in dogs?

a. Iodine deficiency
b. Autoimmune thyroiditis
c. Adrenal gland tumor
d. Pituitary gland dysfunction

Correct Answer: b. Autoimmune thyroiditis.
Explanation: Hypothyroidism in dogs often results from autoimmune thyroiditis, where the immune system attacks and destroys thyroid tissue, reducing hormone production.

Question 106: Which of the following is a common zoonotic disease associated with birds?

a. Brucellosis
b. Psittacosis
c. Tuberculosis
d. Leprosy

Correct Answer: b. Psittacosis.
Explanation: Psittacosis, or parrot fever, is a zoonotic disease transmitted from birds to humans, caused by Chlamydia psittaci, leading to respiratory symptoms.

Question 107: Which of the following is a common method for diagnosing canine parvovirus?

a. Skin biopsy
b. Fecal ELISA test
c. Blood glucose test
d. Radiography

Correct Answer: b. Fecal ELISA test.
Explanation: Canine parvovirus is diagnosed using a fecal ELISA test, detecting viral antigens in the stool, crucial for early detection and management.

Question 108: What is the primary function of the large intestine in mammals?

a. Absorb nutrients
b. Secrete digestive enzymes
c. Absorb water and electrolytes
d. Produce bile

Correct Answer: c. Absorb water and electrolytes.
Explanation: The large intestine's main role is to absorb water and electrolytes from indigestible food matter, forming solid waste for excretion.

Question 109: Which of the following is a common symptom of feline asthma?

a. Increased thirst
b. Coughing
c. Diarrhea
d. Vomiting

Correct Answer: b. Coughing.

Explanation: Feline asthma often presents with coughing and wheezing, triggered by allergens or irritants, requiring management with bronchodilators and anti-inflammatory medications.

Question 110: Which of the following is a common method for diagnosing Lyme disease in dogs?

a. Urinalysis
b. ELISA test
c. Fecal flotation
d. Skin scraping

Correct Answer: b. ELISA test.

Explanation: Lyme disease in dogs is typically diagnosed using an ELISA test, identifying antibodies against the Borrelia burgdorferi bacterium, the disease's causative agent.

Question 111: Which of the following is a common cause of pancreatitis in dogs?

a. Low-fat diet
b. High-fat diet
c. Vitamin deficiency
d. Excessive exercise

Correct Answer: b. High-fat diet.

Explanation: A high-fat diet can trigger pancreatitis in dogs, causing inflammation and digestive enzyme leakage, necessitating dietary management and supportive care.

Question 112: Which of the following is a common symptom of feline leukemia virus (FeLV) infection?

a. Increased appetite
b. Weight gain
c. Anemia
d. Hyperactivity

Correct Answer: c. Anemia.

Explanation: FeLV infection leads to anemia and immunosuppression in cats, increasing susceptibility to secondary infections and requiring vigilant monitoring and supportive treatment.

Question 113: What is the primary function of the spleen in the immune system?

a. Produce antibodies
b. Filter blood and recycle red blood cells
c. Produce bile
d. Absorb nutrients

Correct Answer: b. Filter blood and recycle red blood cells.

Explanation: The spleen filters blood, removing old or damaged red blood cells, and plays a role in immune response by producing lymphocytes and storing blood components.

Question 114: Which of the following is a common method for diagnosing diabetes insipidus in animals?

a. Urine glucose test
b. Water deprivation test
c. Skin scraping
d. Fecal analysis

Correct Answer: b. Water deprivation test.

Explanation: The water deprivation test evaluates the kidney's ability to concentrate urine, diagnosing diabetes insipidus, characterized by excessive thirst and dilute urine production.

Question 115: Which of the following is a common symptom of canine hypothyroidism?

a. Hyperactivity
b. Weight gain
c. Increased appetite
d. Rapid heart rate

Correct Answer: b. Weight gain.
Explanation: Canine hypothyroidism often leads to weight gain, lethargy, and coat changes, resulting from decreased thyroid hormone production and metabolic slowing.

Question 116: Which of the following is a common method for diagnosing feline infectious peritonitis (FIP)?

a. Urinalysis
b. Blood glucose test
c. Coronavirus antibody test
d. Fecal flotation

Correct Answer: c. Coronavirus antibody test.
Explanation: FIP diagnosis involves detecting coronavirus antibodies, with feline coronavirus mutations leading to the disease, though definitive diagnosis can be challenging.

Question 117: What is the primary function of insulin in the body?

a. Increase blood glucose levels
b. Decrease blood glucose levels
c. Absorb nutrients
d. Produce bile

Correct Answer: b. Decrease blood glucose levels.
Explanation: Insulin, produced by the pancreas, lowers blood glucose levels by facilitating cellular uptake, critical for energy utilization and metabolic regulation.

Question 118: Which of the following is a common cause of respiratory distress in cats?

a. Hypothyroidism
b. Hyperthyroidism
c. Asthma
d. Arthritis

Correct Answer: c. Asthma.
Explanation: Feline asthma, triggered by allergens or stress, causes respiratory distress due to airway inflammation and constriction, requiring treatment with bronchodilators and steroids.

Question 119: Which of the following is a common symptom of parvovirus infection in puppies?

a. Vomiting
b. Increased appetite
c. Weight gain
d. Hyperactivity

Correct Answer: a. Vomiting.
Explanation: Parvovirus infection in puppies presents with severe vomiting, diarrhea, and lethargy, necessitating prompt supportive care to prevent dehydration and secondary infections.

Question 120: Which of the following is a common method for diagnosing canine distemper?

a. Skin biopsy
b. Blood glucose test

c. PCR test
d. Fecal flotation

Correct Answer: c. PCR test.
Explanation: Canine distemper is diagnosed using a PCR test, detecting viral RNA, crucial for identifying and managing this highly contagious disease.

Question 121: Which of the following is a common cause of gastric ulcers in horses?

a. Low-fiber diet
b. High-grain diet
c. Excessive exercise
d. Vitamin deficiency

Correct Answer: b. High-grain diet.
Explanation: A high-grain diet can contribute to gastric ulcers in horses by altering stomach acidity and mucosal health, requiring dietary adjustments and medical intervention.

Question 122: Which of the following is a common symptom of feline immunodeficiency virus (FIV) infection?

a. Increased thirst
b. Weight gain
c. Hyperactivity
d. Recurrent infections

Correct Answer: d. Recurrent infections.
Explanation: FIV causes immunosuppression, leading to recurrent infections and health issues in affected cats, emphasizing the importance of supportive care and preventative measures.

Question 123: Which of the following is a common method for diagnosing heartworm disease in cats?

a. Blood glucose test
b. Urinalysis
c. Antigen test
d. Skin biopsy

Correct Answer: c. Antigen test.
Explanation: Heartworm disease in cats is diagnosed using an antigen test, which detects heartworm proteins in the blood, crucial for identifying this parasitic infection.

Question 124: During surgery, the veterinarian wants to remove a core of bone for biopsy. He asks you for a T-shaped, tubular instrument with a cylindrical cutting blade called a(n):

a. trephine.
b. osteotome.
c. rongeur.
d. external fixator.

Correct Answer: a. trephine.
Explanation: A trephine is a T-shaped, tubular instrument with a cylindrical cutting blade, used to remove bone cores for biopsy, aiding in accurate diagnosis of bone conditions.

Question 125: In arthroscopic surgery, burs (or burrs) are:

a. removed from the animal's coat before the procedure.
b. the pumps used to deliver fluids to the surgical site.
c. a type of forceps used to grasp and remove osteochondral chip fragments.
d. often referred to as a motorized arthroplasty system.

Correct Answer: d. often referred to as a motorized arthroplasty system.
Explanation: In arthroscopic surgery, motorized burs, or burrs, are used as part of a motorized arthroplasty system to shape and smooth bone surfaces precisely.

Question 126: Which of the following practices helps ensure adequate steam penetration in the autoclave?

a. Keeping the pack weight below 5 kg
b. Stacking packs on top of each other
c. Leaving less than 2 cm of space between packs and between the packs and autoclave walls
d. Keeping the pack size smaller than 30 cm by 30 cm by 50 cm

Correct Answer: d. Keeping the pack size smaller than 30 cm by 30 cm by 50 cm.
Explanation: Limiting pack size ensures proper steam penetration during autoclaving, effectively sterilizing surgical instruments and materials.

Question 127: How is an antiseptic different from a disinfectant?

a. The former kills or inhibits infectious agents on living tissues and the latter on inanimate objects.
b. The former is used in consumer cleaners and the latter in cleaners intended for hospital use only.
c. The former kills only growing bacteria, whereas the latter kills growing bacteria, bacterial spores, and viruses.
d. The former is used only in soaps and the latter only in foams or liquids.

Correct Answer: a. The former kills or inhibits infectious agents on living tissues and the latter on inanimate objects.
Explanation: Antiseptics are used on living tissues to prevent infection, while disinfectants are applied to non-living surfaces to destroy harmful microorganisms.

Question 128: A cat's serum sample is orange in color, indicating the presence of:

a. normal serum.
b. Lipemia.
c. in vitro hemolysis.
d. bilirubin.

Correct Answer: d. bilirubin.
Explanation: An orange color in a cat's serum sample suggests bilirubin presence, indicating possible liver dysfunction or hemolysis, requiring further diagnostic evaluation.

Question 129: What is the single most common disease syndrome in adult dairy cows?

a. Lymphosarcoma
b. Periparturient hypocalcemia (milk fever)
c. Mastitis
d. Bovine respiratory disease syndrome

Correct Answer: c. Mastitis.
Explanation: Mastitis, an inflammation of the mammary gland, is the most prevalent disease in adult dairy cows, significantly impacting milk production and quality.

Question 130: Which of the following must always be supplemented to beef cattle feeding with pasture grasses?

a. Minerals
b. Energy in the form of grain
c. Fat
d. Protein

Correct Answer: a. Minerals.
Explanation: Minerals, particularly salt and phosphorus, are essential supplements for beef cattle grazing on pasture grasses to support growth, reproduction, and health.

Question 131: Trichuris vulpis of the dog, fox, and coyote can be found in the:

a. small intestine.
b. right ventricle and pulmonary arteries.
c. stomach.
d. cecum.

Correct Answer: d. cecum.
Explanation: Trichuris vulpis, or whipworm, resides in the cecum and large intestine, causing gastrointestinal disturbances in infected animals.

Question 132: For which of the following procedures would it be most beneficial to count the gauze sponges used for hemostasis?

a. Feline gastrointestinal surgical repair
b. Feline castration
c. Feline declawing procedure
d. Adult canine tail amputation

Correct Answer: a. Feline gastrointestinal surgical repair.
Explanation: Counting gauze sponges during gastrointestinal surgery prevents retained foreign bodies, reducing postoperative complications and ensuring patient safety.

Question 133: If the contents of a horse's large intestine are to be evacuated, a sterile-draped tray is prepared on which the _____ is to be placed.

a. ingesta
b. mesentery
c. colon
d. small intestine

Correct Answer: c. colon.
Explanation: During large intestine evacuation, the colon is placed on a sterile-draped tray to maintain asepsis and facilitate surgical procedures.

Question 134: Fecal samples collected from small animals using the _____ collecting method should be used for direct examination only because of the amount collected this way.

a. jarred
b. owner-bagged
c. gloved-finger
d. fecal loop

Correct Answer: d. fecal loop.
Explanation: Fecal samples collected with a fecal loop are limited in quantity, suitable for direct examination but not for extensive diagnostic tests.

Question 135: You are asked to prepare Brownie, a 6-month-old, brown-tabby domestic shorthair cat, for castration. He will be restrained in the dorsal recumbent position with his hind legs tied cranially to expose the scrotal region. How do you prepare his scrotum?

a. Shave with a safety razor and perform a surgical scrub.
b. Shave with a no. 40 clipper blade and perform a surgical scrub.
c. Pluck hair and perform a surgical scrub.
d. Leave hair on the scrotum and perform a surgical scrub.

Correct Answer: c. Pluck hair and perform a surgical scrub.
Explanation: Hair plucking followed by a surgical scrub provides a clean surgical site, minimizing infection risk during castration.

Question 136: Which of the following is not usually part of the patient data-gathering phase in the nursing process?

a. Performing a physical examination
b. Identifying and prioritizing to generate a technician evaluation
c. Gathering the initial medical history from the owner
d. Reviewing the medical record for the past history

Correct Answer: b. Identifying and prioritizing to generate a technician evaluation.
Explanation: Data gathering involves collecting medical history and performing examinations; prioritizing and evaluations occur in subsequent nursing process phases.

Question 137: As you monitor your postsurgical patient, you are aware that packed cell volume (PCV) and total protein (TP) values can drop up to _____ due to anesthesia and surgery, even if no blood loss occurs.

a. 15%
b. 20%
c. 10%
d. 35%

Correct Answer: c. 10%.
Explanation: Anesthesia and surgical procedures can decrease PCV and TP values by up to 10%, even without significant blood loss, affecting postoperative monitoring.

Question 138: Which of the following is a common cause of respiratory distress in dogs?

a. Hyperthyroidism
b. Asthma
c. Heartworm disease
d. Diabetes

Correct Answer: c. Heartworm disease.
Explanation: Heartworm disease causes respiratory distress in dogs due to worm-induced pulmonary artery obstruction, necessitating preventive measures and treatment.

Question 139: Which of the following is a common sign of dental disease in cats?

a. Increased appetite
b. Drooling
c. Weight gain
d. Hyperactivity

Correct Answer: b. Drooling.
Explanation: Drooling in cats indicates dental disease, often accompanied by bad breath, reluctance to eat, and oral pain, requiring dental care.

Question 140: Which of the following is a common method for diagnosing feline leukemia virus (FeLV)?

a. Urinalysis
b. Fecal flotation
c. ELISA test
d. Skin scraping

Correct Answer: c. ELISA test.
Explanation: FeLV is typically diagnosed using an ELISA test, detecting viral antigens in blood, crucial for managing this contagious feline disease.

Question 141: Which of the following is a common cause of skin allergies in dogs?

a. Hypothyroidism
b. Flea bites
c. Diabetes
d. Heartworm disease

Correct Answer: b. Flea bites.
Explanation: Flea bites are a common cause of allergic dermatitis in dogs, leading to itching, skin inflammation, and secondary infections.

Question 142: Which of the following is a common symptom of feline hyperthyroidism?

a. Lethargy
b. Weight loss
c. Decreased appetite
d. Hair loss

Correct Answer: b. Weight loss.
Explanation: Feline hyperthyroidism causes weight loss despite increased appetite, due to elevated metabolic rates from excess thyroid hormone production.

Question 143: Which of the following is a common method for diagnosing rabies in animals?

a. Blood test
b. Saliva test
c. Brain tissue examination
d. Fecal analysis

Correct Answer: c. Brain tissue examination.
Explanation: Rabies diagnosis is confirmed post-mortem by examining brain tissue for viral antigens, as no reliable antemortem tests exist.

Question 144: Which of the following is a common cause of ear infections in dogs?

a. Obesity
b. Hypothyroidism
c. Excessive ear cleaning
d. Allergies

Correct Answer: d. Allergies.
Explanation: Allergies often lead to ear infections in dogs, as inflammation creates a conducive environment for bacterial and yeast overgrowth.

Question 145: Which of the following is a method for diagnosing canine diabetes mellitus?

a. Skin biopsy
b. Blood glucose test
c. Fecal flotation
d. Urinalysis

Correct Answer: b. Blood glucose test.
Explanation: Diabetes mellitus in dogs is diagnosed by measuring elevated blood glucose levels, indicating impaired insulin production or function.

Question 146: Which of the following is a common symptom of canine distemper?

a. Increased thirst
b. Coughing
c. Vomiting
d. Rapid heart rate

Correct Answer: b. Coughing.

Explanation: Canine distemper presents with respiratory symptoms like coughing, alongside fever, nasal discharge, and neurological signs, requiring vaccination for prevention.

Question 147: Which of the following is a common method for diagnosing feline asthma?

a. Blood test
b. Urinalysis
c. Radiographs
d. Fecal analysis

Correct Answer: c. Radiographs.

Explanation: Feline asthma is diagnosed using radiographs, revealing bronchial patterns indicating airway inflammation, aiding in treatment planning.

Question 148: Which of the following is a common cause of gastrointestinal upset in dogs?

a. Hypothyroidism
b. Dietary indiscretion
c. Diabetes
d. Arthritis

Correct Answer: b. Dietary indiscretion.

Explanation: Dietary indiscretion, such as consuming inappropriate items, leads to gastrointestinal upset in dogs, potentially causing vomiting and diarrhea.

Question 149: Which of the following is a common symptom of Lyme disease in dogs?

a. Increased appetite
b. Lameness
c. Weight gain
d. Hyperactivity

Correct Answer: b. Lameness.

Explanation: Lyme disease in dogs often causes lameness due to joint inflammation, necessitating prompt diagnosis and antibiotic treatment.

Question 150: Which of the following is a common method for diagnosing feline infectious peritonitis (FIP)?

a. Blood glucose test
b. ELISA test
c. Skin biopsy
d. Fecal analysis

Correct Answer: b. ELISA test.

Explanation: FIP is suspected through ELISA tests detecting coronavirus antibodies, though definitive diagnosis is challenging due to overlapping signs with other diseases.

Question 151: Which of the following is a common cause of anemia in dogs?

a. Hyperthyroidism
b. Parasites
c. Diabetes
d. Arthritis

Correct Answer: b. Parasites.
Explanation: Parasitic infestations, such as hookworms, can cause anemia in dogs by consuming blood, highlighting the need for regular deworming.

Question 152: Which of the following is a common symptom of canine hypothyroidism?

a. Hyperactivity
b. Weight loss
c. Lethargy
d. Rapid heart rate

Correct Answer: c. Lethargy.
Explanation: Canine hypothyroidism often results in lethargy and reduced activity levels, due to decreased metabolic function from insufficient thyroid hormone production.

Question 153: Which of the following is a common method for diagnosing mange in dogs?

a. Blood test
b. Urinalysis
c. Skin scraping
d. Fecal analysis

Correct Answer: c. Skin scraping.
Explanation: Mange is diagnosed by skin scraping, identifying mites under microscopy, critical for determining appropriate treatment.

Question 154: Which of the following is a common cause of liver disease in cats?

a. Hypothyroidism
b. Obesity
c. Heartworm disease
d. Diabetes

Correct Answer: b. Obesity.
Explanation: Obesity in cats can lead to hepatic lipidosis, a serious liver condition, emphasizing the importance of weight management for liver health.

Question 155: Which of the following is a common symptom of feline diabetes mellitus?

a. Weight gain
b. Increased thirst
c. Hyperactivity
d. Rapid heart rate

Correct Answer: b. Increased thirst.
Explanation: Feline diabetes mellitus presents with increased thirst and urination due to insulin deficiency or resistance, needing insulin therapy and dietary management.

Question 156: Which of the following is a common method for diagnosing feline panleukopenia?

a. Urinalysis
b. Fecal ELISA test
c. Blood glucose test
d. Skin biopsy

Correct Answer: b. Fecal ELISA test.
Explanation: Feline panleukopenia is diagnosed through a fecal ELISA test, detecting viral antigens, crucial for early intervention in this contagious disease.

Question 157: Which of the following is a common cause of kidney disease in dogs?

a. Dietary excess
b. Hypothyroidism
c. Chronic infections
d. Diabetes

Correct Answer: c. Chronic infections.
Explanation: Chronic infections can lead to kidney disease in dogs by causing sustained inflammation and damage to renal tissues, necessitating prompt treatment.

Question 158: Which of the following is a common symptom of feline calicivirus infection?

a. Increased appetite
b. Oral ulcers
c. Weight gain
d. Hyperactivity

Correct Answer: b. Oral ulcers.
Explanation: Feline calicivirus infection often causes oral ulcers, alongside respiratory symptoms, highlighting the need for vaccination to prevent outbreaks.

Question 159: Which of the following is a common method for diagnosing canine ehrlichiosis?

a. Blood smear
b. Urinalysis
c. Fecal analysis
d. Skin biopsy

Correct Answer: a. Blood smear.
Explanation: Canine ehrlichiosis is diagnosed by examining blood smears for Ehrlichia organisms, aiding in targeted antibiotic therapy.

Question 160: Which of the following is a common cause of gastrointestinal ulcers in horses?

a. Low-fiber diet
b. Excessive exercise
c. High-starch diet
d. Vitamin deficiency

Correct Answer: c. High-starch diet.
Explanation: A high-starch diet can increase gastric acidity, leading to ulcers in horses, necessitating dietary adjustments to prevent this condition.

Question 161: Which of the following is a common symptom of canine parainfluenza virus infection?

a. Increased thirst
b. Coughing
c. Vomiting
d. Rapid heart rate

Correct Answer: b. Coughing.
Explanation: Canine parainfluenza virus infection often presents with coughing and respiratory distress, forming part of the kennel cough complex, prevented by vaccination.

Question 162: Which of the following is a common method for diagnosing feline toxoplasmosis?

a. Blood test
b. Skin biopsy
c. Urinalysis
d. Fecal analysis

Correct Answer: a. Blood test.
Explanation: Toxoplasmosis in cats is diagnosed through blood tests detecting antibodies to Toxoplasma gondii, crucial for managing this zoonotic infection.

Question 163: Which of the following is a common cause of obesity in pets?

a. Hypothyroidism
b. Overfeeding
c. Diabetes
d. Heartworm disease

Correct Answer: b. Overfeeding.
Explanation: Overfeeding, combined with lack of exercise, leads to obesity in pets, increasing the risk of various health issues, including diabetes and arthritis.

Question 164: Which of the following is a common symptom of feline rhinotracheitis?

a. Increased appetite
b. Sneezing
c. Weight gain
d. Hyperactivity

Correct Answer: b. Sneezing.
Explanation: Feline rhinotracheitis, caused by herpesvirus, leads to sneezing and respiratory symptoms, requiring supportive care and vaccination for prevention.

Question 166: Which of the following is a common cause of heart disease in cats?

a. High blood pressure
b. Taurine deficiency
c. Excessive exercise
d. Hyperthyroidism

Correct Answer: b. Taurine deficiency.
Explanation: Taurine deficiency in cats can lead to dilated cardiomyopathy, a form of heart disease, emphasizing the importance of proper dietary nutrition.

Question 167: Which of the following is a common symptom of canine coronavirus infection?

a. Increased appetite
b. Diarrhea
c. Weight gain
d. Hyperactivity

Correct Answer: b. Diarrhea.
Explanation: Canine coronavirus infection often results in diarrhea, causing gastrointestinal distress, typically managed with supportive care.

Question 168: Which of the following is a common method for diagnosing feline hyperaldosteronism?

a. Blood pressure measurement
b. Urinalysis
c. Skin biopsy
d. Fecal analysis

Correct Answer: a. Blood pressure measurement.
Explanation: Feline hyperaldosteronism is diagnosed through blood pressure and serum electrolyte measurements, as the condition affects fluid balance and blood pressure regulation.

Question 169: Which of the following is a common cause of chronic kidney disease in older cats?

a. Infections
b. Genetic predisposition
c. High protein diets
d. Obesity

Correct Answer: b. Genetic predisposition.

Explanation: Chronic kidney disease in older cats often results from genetic factors, leading to progressive renal deterioration and requiring dietary and medical management.

Question 170: Which of the following is a common symptom of feline hypertrophic cardiomyopathy?

a. Increased thirst
b. Difficulty breathing
c. Weight gain
d. Hyperactivity

Correct Answer: b. Difficulty breathing.

Explanation: Feline hypertrophic cardiomyopathy causes difficulty breathing due to thickened heart walls impairing cardiac function, necessitating medical intervention for management.

Full Test 3 with Detailed Explanations

Question 1: _____ are important mediators of hypersensitivity reactions and contain substances that can damage and kill some parasites.

a) Eosinophils
b) Metamyelocytes
c) Döhle bodies
d) Neutrophils

Correct Answer: a) Eosinophils
Explanation: Eosinophils play a crucial role in mediating hypersensitivity reactions and defending against parasitic infections by releasing toxic granules that damage and kill parasites.

Question 2: One common physiologic response to pain is:

a) pupillary constriction.
b) warm (not hot) extremities.
c) an increased heart rate and blood pressure level.
d) a decreased respiratory rate.

Correct Answer: c) an increased heart rate and blood pressure level.
Explanation: Pain stimulates the autonomic nervous system, leading to increased heart rate and blood pressure as the body reacts to perceived threats or injury.

Question 3: Platelets in birds and reptiles:

a) have nuclei and are called thrombocytes.
b) lack nuclei.
c) have a prominent central zone of pallor.
d) lack cytoplasm.

Correct Answer: a) have nuclei and are called thrombocytes.
Explanation: In birds and reptiles, platelets are nucleated and referred to as thrombocytes, differing from mammalian platelets, which are anucleated.

Question 4: Increased serum _____ is a normal physiologic response in the fasted horse.

a) sorbitol dehydrogenase
b) gamma-glutamyl transferase
c) bilirubin
d) creatine phosphokinase

Correct Answer: c) bilirubin
Explanation: Horses exhibit fasting hyperbilirubinemia, where serum bilirubin levels rise due to reduced feed intake, not indicative of liver disease.

Question 5: If using an aminoglycoside antimicrobial agent to treat a patient, it is important to monitor the patient because these agents are known to cause:

a) liver problems.
b) heart problems.
c) kidney problems.
d) an increase in blood pressure.

Correct Answer: c) kidney problems.
Explanation: Aminoglycosides are nephrotoxic, requiring careful monitoring of renal function during treatment to prevent kidney damage.

Question 6: Lidocaine and bupivacaine are examples of which drug class?

a) a2-Agonists
b) NSAIDs
c) Opioids
d) Local anesthetics

Correct Answer: d) Local anesthetics

Explanation: Lidocaine and bupivacaine are local anesthetics that block nerve conduction to provide pain relief during procedures.

Question 7: Nacho, a dog, is exhibiting dyspnea. The mucous membranes show signs of pallor. The veterinarian diagnoses this as _____, or deficient oxygenation of the tissues.

a) dyspnea
b) hypoxemia
c) hemoptysis
d) hypoxia

Correct Answer: d) hypoxia

Explanation: Hypoxia is a condition of inadequate oxygenation at the tissue level, often manifested by symptoms such as pallor and dyspnea.

Question 8: Pepper has an echocardiogram after surgery, and the veterinarian sees shadows that suggest the possibility of heart disease. Pepper has no symptoms, however, and is sent home after recovering well from surgery. Because Pepper is asymptomatic, the veterinarian instructs the owner to monitor for rapid breathing, or _____, which can be the first sign that heart disease has progressed to heart failure.

a) inadequate tissue perfusion
b) tachypnea
c) bradycardia
d) syncope

Correct Answer: b) tachypnea

Explanation: Tachypnea, or rapid breathing, is often an early indicator of heart failure progression in asymptomatic patients, requiring vigilant monitoring.

Question 9: Variation in the PR interval may occur with:

a) atrioventricular dissociation.
b) right ventricular enlargement.
c) right atrial enlargement.

Correct Answer: a) atrioventricular dissociation.

Explanation: Atrioventricular dissociation affects the PR interval due to disrupted conduction through the AV node, altering cardiac rhythm.

Question 10: Which of the following types of fluids is most often used for arthroscopic procedures to aid in visualizing the intraarticular space?

a) 5% Dextrose in water
b) 50% Dextrose in water
c) 0.45% Sodium chloride with 10 ml/L of chlorhexidine added
d) Any sterile, balanced electrolyte solution

Correct Answer: d) Any sterile, balanced electrolyte solution

Explanation: Balanced electrolyte solutions maintain joint capsule distention, crucial for visualizing intraarticular spaces during arthroscopic procedures.

Question 11: Aseptic technique:

a) requires that all cages be cleaned and thoroughly disinfected between patients.
b) is only used for emergency surgery.
c) includes all steps taken to prevent contamination of the surgical site by infectious agents.
d) requires all people involved in patient care to wash their hands thoroughly with an antibacterial soap between patients.

Correct Answer: c) includes all steps taken to prevent contamination of the surgical site by infectious agents.
Explanation: Aseptic technique encompasses procedures that minimize infectious agent exposure to surgical sites, ensuring patient safety.

Question 12: Hypoalbuminemia may develop from loss through:

a) the gastrointestinal tract.
b) the kidney.
c) decreased production due to liver failure.
d) all of the above.

Correct Answer: d) all of the above.
Explanation: Hypoalbuminemia can result from protein loss via the kidney or gastrointestinal tract, or reduced synthesis in liver failure.

Question 13: You are unsure whether a ferret that has received an adrenalectomy is experiencing a significant amount of pain. What is the best way to determine whether this patient needs analgesics?

a) The rule of thumb is that if a procedure would be painful for you to endure, it is likely that it is painful for the animal.
b) Check the body temperature; if it is more than 2° F above normal less than 12 hours after the surgery, administer analgesics.
c) Check the respiratory rate; if it is greater than two times normal, administer analgesics.
d) Check the heart rate; if it is greater than two times normal, administer analgesics.

Correct Answer: a) The rule of thumb is that if a procedure would be painful for you to endure, it is likely that it is painful for the animal.
Explanation: Assessing pain in animals involves considering procedures' human pain equivalence, guiding timely analgesic administration when necessary.

Question 14: Sarcomas can arise from _____, whereas carcinomas can arise from _____.

a) organs; cartilage
b) mucous membranes; bone
c) cartilage; lymph nodes
d) skin; connective tissue

Correct Answer: c) cartilage; lymph nodes
Explanation: Sarcomas originate from mesenchymal tissues like cartilage, while carcinomas develop from epithelial tissues, spreading to lymph nodes.

Question 15: The most common breed of alpacas are:

a) huacaya.
b) suri.
c) llama.
d) camel.

Correct Answer: a) huacaya.
Explanation: Huacaya alpacas, known for their dense, crimped fleece, are the most prevalent alpaca breed, prized for fiber production.

Question 16: In both the horse and dog, what is the most commonly encountered adverse reaction to NSAIDs?

a) Constipation
b) Diarrhea
c) Gastrointestinal upset
d) Low blood pressure

Correct Answer: c) Gastrointestinal upset
Explanation: NSAIDs frequently cause gastrointestinal irritation or ulceration in horses and dogs, necessitating caution and monitoring.

Question 17: Which species are known to have nucleated thrombocytes instead of anucleated platelets?

a) Mammals
b) Birds
c) Fish
d) Reptiles

Correct Answer: b) Birds
Explanation: Birds have nucleated thrombocytes, distinct from the anucleated platelets found in mammals, playing a role in hemostasis.

Question 18: Which is a common method for diagnosing feline leukemia virus (FeLV) in cats?

a) Urinalysis
b) Fecal flotation
c) ELISA test
d) Skin scraping

Correct Answer: c) ELISA test
Explanation: ELISA tests detect FeLV antigens in blood samples, crucial for identifying and managing this contagious viral infection in cats.

Question 19: What is a common symptom of hyperthyroidism in cats?

a) Lethargy
b) Weight loss
c) Increased appetite
d) Hair loss

Correct Answer: b) Weight loss
Explanation: Cats with hyperthyroidism often experience weight loss despite increased appetite due to elevated metabolic rates from excess thyroid hormones.

Question 20: Which of the following is a common method for diagnosing heartworm disease in dogs?

a) Blood glucose test
b) Urinalysis
c) Antigen test
d) Skin biopsy

Correct Answer: c) Antigen test
Explanation: Heartworm disease is diagnosed using an antigen test which detects heartworm proteins in a dog's blood, crucial for timely treatment.

Question 21: Which of the following is a common cause of respiratory distress in dogs?

a) Hyperthyroidism
b) Asthma

c) Heartworm disease
d) Diabetes

Correct Answer: c) Heartworm disease
Explanation: Heartworm disease causes respiratory distress in dogs due to worm-induced obstruction in pulmonary arteries, highlighting the need for preventive measures.

Question 22: Which of the following is a common sign of dental disease in cats?

a) Increased appetite
b) Drooling
c) Weight gain
d) Hyperactivity

Correct Answer: b) Drooling
Explanation: Dental disease in cats often leads to drooling, accompanied by oral discomfort, bad breath, and reluctance to eat, requiring dental care.

Question 23: Which of the following is a common cause of gastrointestinal upset in dogs?

a) Hypothyroidism
b) Dietary indiscretion
c) Diabetes
d) Arthritis

Correct Answer: b) Dietary indiscretion
Explanation: Consuming inappropriate items often causes gastrointestinal upset in dogs, resulting in symptoms like vomiting and diarrhea, requiring prompt management.

Question 24: Which of the following is a common symptom of Lyme disease in dogs?

a) Increased appetite
b) Lameness
c) Weight gain
d) Hyperactivity

Correct Answer: b) Lameness
Explanation: Lyme disease often presents with lameness in dogs due to joint inflammation, necessitating early diagnosis and antibiotic treatment to prevent complications.

Question 25: Which of the following is a common method for diagnosing feline infectious peritonitis (FIP)?

a) Blood glucose test
b) ELISA test
c) Skin biopsy
d) Fecal analysis

Correct Answer: b) ELISA test
Explanation: FIP diagnosis involves ELISA tests to detect coronavirus antibodies, aiding in managing this challenging feline viral disease.

Question 26: Which of the following is a common cause of anemia in dogs?

a) Hyperthyroidism
b) Parasites
c) Diabetes
d) Arthritis

Correct Answer: b) Parasites

Explanation: Parasitic infestations, such as hookworms, cause anemia in dogs by consuming blood, emphasizing the importance of regular deworming protocols.

Question 27: Which of the following is a common symptom of canine hypothyroidism?

a) Hyperactivity
b) Weight loss
c) Lethargy
d) Rapid heart rate

Correct Answer: c) Lethargy

Explanation: Canine hypothyroidism typically results in lethargy due to decreased metabolic activity, requiring thyroid hormone replacement therapy for management.

Question 28: Which of the following is a method for diagnosing mange in dogs?

a) Blood test
b) Urinalysis
c) Skin scraping
d) Fecal analysis

Correct Answer: c) Skin scraping

Explanation: Mange diagnosis involves skin scraping to identify mites under a microscope, crucial for determining the appropriate treatment strategy.

Question 29: Which of the following is a common cause of liver disease in cats?

a) Hypothyroidism
b) Obesity
c) Heartworm disease
d) Diabetes

Correct Answer: b) Obesity

Explanation: Obesity in cats can lead to hepatic lipidosis, a severe liver condition, underscoring the importance of maintaining a healthy weight.

Question 30: Which of the following is a common symptom of feline diabetes mellitus?

a) Weight gain
b) Increased thirst
c) Hyperactivity
d) Rapid heart rate

Correct Answer: b) Increased thirst

Explanation: Feline diabetes mellitus often presents with increased thirst and urination, due to impaired insulin function, requiring dietary and insulin management.

Question 31: Which of the following is a common method for diagnosing feline panleukopenia?

a) Urinalysis
b) Fecal ELISA test
c) Blood glucose test
d) Skin biopsy

Correct Answer: b) Fecal ELISA test

Explanation: Feline panleukopenia is diagnosed using fecal ELISA tests to detect viral antigens, facilitating early intervention in this infectious disease.

Question 32: Which of the following is a common cause of kidney disease in dogs?

a) Dietary excess
b) Hypothyroidism
c) Chronic infections
d) Diabetes

Correct Answer: c) Chronic infections
Explanation: Chronic infections can lead to kidney disease in dogs by causing prolonged inflammation and damage, necessitating timely treatment to prevent progression.

Question 33: Which of the following is a common symptom of feline calicivirus infection?

a) Increased appetite
b) Oral ulcers
c) Weight gain
d) Hyperactivity

Correct Answer: b) Oral ulcers
Explanation: Feline calicivirus infection often results in oral ulcers and respiratory symptoms, highlighting the need for vaccination to prevent outbreaks.

Question 34: Which of the following is a common method for diagnosing canine ehrlichiosis?

a) Blood smear
b) Urinalysis
c) Fecal analysis
d) Skin biopsy

Correct Answer: a) Blood smear
Explanation: Canine ehrlichiosis is diagnosed by examining blood smears for Ehrlichia organisms, aiding in targeted antibiotic therapy to manage the infection.

Question 35: Which of the following is a common cause of gastrointestinal ulcers in horses?

a) Low-fiber diet
b) Excessive exercise
c) High-starch diet
d) Vitamin deficiency

Correct Answer: c) High-starch diet
Explanation: High-starch diets can increase gastric acidity, leading to ulcers in horses, necessitating dietary adjustments to prevent gastrointestinal issues.

Question 36: Which of the following is a common symptom of canine parainfluenza virus infection?

a) Increased thirst
b) Coughing
c) Vomiting
d) Rapid heart rate

Correct Answer: b) Coughing
Explanation: Canine parainfluenza virus infection often presents with coughing and respiratory distress, forming part of the kennel cough complex, preventable by vaccination.

Question 37: Which of the following is a common method for diagnosing feline toxoplasmosis?

a) Blood test
b) Skin biopsy
c) Urinalysis
d) Fecal analysis

Correct Answer: a) Blood test

Explanation: Toxoplasmosis in cats is diagnosed through blood tests detecting antibodies to Toxoplasma gondii, crucial for managing this zoonotic infection.

Question 38: Which of the following is a common cause of obesity in pets?

a) Hypothyroidism
b) Overfeeding
c) Diabetes
d) Heartworm disease

Correct Answer: b) Overfeeding

Explanation: Overfeeding, combined with lack of exercise, often leads to obesity in pets, increasing health risks such as diabetes and arthritis.

Question 39: Which of the following is a common symptom of feline rhinotracheitis?

a) Increased appetite
b) Sneezing
c) Weight gain
d) Hyperactivity

Correct Answer: b) Sneezing

Explanation: Feline rhinotracheitis, caused by herpesvirus, leads to sneezing and respiratory symptoms, requiring supportive care and vaccination for prevention.

Question 40: Which of the following is a common method for diagnosing canine leptospirosis?

a) Fecal flotation
b) Blood culture
c) Urinalysis
d) Skin biopsy

Correct Answer: c) Urinalysis

Explanation: Canine leptospirosis is diagnosed through urinalysis and serological testing, detecting Leptospira bacteria, important for informed treatment decisions.

Question 41: Which of the following is a common cause of heart disease in cats?

a) High blood pressure
b) Taurine deficiency
c) Excessive exercise
d) Hyperthyroidism

Correct Answer: b) Taurine deficiency

Explanation: Taurine deficiency in cats can lead to dilated cardiomyopathy, a form of heart disease, highlighting the need for proper dietary nutrition.

Question 42: Which of the following is a common symptom of canine coronavirus infection?

a) Increased appetite
b) Diarrhea
c) Weight gain
d) Hyperactivity

Correct Answer: b) Diarrhea

Explanation: Canine coronavirus infection often results in diarrhea, causing gastrointestinal distress, typically managed with supportive care and hydration.

Question 43: Which of the following is a common method for diagnosing feline hyperaldosteronism?

a) Blood pressure measurement
b) Urinalysis
c) Skin biopsy
d) Fecal analysis

Correct Answer: a) Blood pressure measurement
Explanation: Feline hyperaldosteronism is diagnosed through blood pressure and serum electrolyte measurements, as the condition affects fluid balance and blood pressure regulation.

Question 44: Which of the following is a common cause of chronic kidney disease in older cats?

a) Infections
b) Genetic predisposition
c) High protein diets
d) Obesity

Correct Answer: b) Genetic predisposition
Explanation: Chronic kidney disease in older cats often results from genetic factors, leading to progressive renal deterioration and requiring dietary and medical management.

Question 45: Your patient, Miss Marple, a Persian cat, has been sneezing excessively. You most likely suspect that she has:

a) Throat or lung cancer.
b) Inhaled a foreign material.
c) An upper respiratory infection.
d) Simply experienced normal, routine expulsion of air in an effort to expel respiratory irritants.

Correct Answer: c) An upper respiratory infection.
Explanation: In cats, excessive sneezing is frequently linked to upper respiratory infections, typically viral in nature, requiring supportive care to alleviate symptoms.

Question 46: Multimodal analgesia takes advantage of the _____ obtained by combining two or more classes of analgesic drugs to alter more than one phase.

a) "kitty magic"
b) Synergistic effects
c) "Doubled" neurotransmission
d) The wind-up phenomenon

Correct Answer: b) Synergistic effects
Explanation: Multimodal analgesia utilizes synergistic effects from combining analgesic drugs, enhancing pain relief by targeting multiple pathways simultaneously.

Question 47: Which of the following is not one of the three physical sterilization methods?

a) Radiation
b) Water
c) Heat
d) Filtration

Correct Answer: b) Water
Explanation: Physical sterilization methods include heat, filtration, and radiation; water is not a sterilization method but can contribute to microbial growth.

Question 48: Acarines are:

a) Any parasitic insect.
b) The same as mites or ticks.

c) Insects with two wings.
d) The order that contains fleas.

Correct Answer: b) The same as mites or ticks.
Explanation: Acarines encompass mites and ticks, which are arachnids rather than insects, and are significant ectoparasites affecting various hosts.

Question 49: Which of the following statements is true concerning veterinary use of controlled substances?

a) A controlled substance is a substance that can be sold over the counter.
b) A controlled substance is a substance of high abuse potential for which detailed written records of amounts used and amounts on hand are required.
c) The law states that controlled substances must be kept in a cabinet.
d) The controlled substances used medically are designated on the label with a skull and crossbones icon.

Correct Answer: b) A controlled substance is a substance of high abuse potential for which detailed written records of amounts used and amounts on hand are required.
Explanation: Controlled substances require stringent record-keeping due to their potential for abuse, ensuring accountability in veterinary practice.

Question 50: In some species, neutrophils are called _____ because of the intense staining of the granules.

a) Heterophils
b) Metarubricytes
c) Eccentrocytes
d) Acanthocytes

Correct Answer: a) Heterophils
Explanation: Heterophils, equivalent to neutrophils in certain species, exhibit intensely stained granules, particularly in birds and reptiles, aiding in pathogen defense.

Question 51: The average heart rate (HR) (in beats per minute) can be calculated by counting the number of:

a) Millimeters between two R waves and dividing into 3000 when using a paper speed of 50 mm/sec.
b) P waves in a predetermined time period and multiplying by the number of QRS complexes in that same time period.
c) QRS complexes in a predetermined time period and multiplying the number of complexes by a specific factor.
d) Millimeters between two R waves and dividing into 1500 when using a paper speed of 25 mm/sec.

Correct Answer: c) QRS complexes in a predetermined time period and multiplying the number of complexes by a specific factor.
Explanation: Heart rate is calculated by counting QRS complexes over a set time and applying a conversion factor, providing an accurate beats per minute measurement.

Question 52: Which of the following describes the transduction phase of nociception?

a) The conversion of energy into an electrical impulse
b) The transmission of a nerve impulse to the spinal cord
c) The nerve ending's initial contact with a pain-causing energy
d) The activation of sympathetic reflexes to dampen pain

Correct Answer: a) The conversion of energy into an electrical impulse
Explanation: During transduction, nociceptors convert mechanical, thermal, or chemical stimuli into electrical impulses, initiating the pain pathway to the central nervous system.

Question 53: In veterinary medicine, which of the following is a common method for diagnosing hyperadrenocorticism (Cushing's disease) in dogs?

a) Urinalysis
b) ACTH stimulation test
c) Fecal analysis
d) Skin biopsy

Correct Answer: b) ACTH stimulation test
Explanation: The ACTH stimulation test evaluates adrenal gland response to ACTH, aiding in diagnosing hyperadrenocorticism by measuring cortisol levels before and after ACTH administration.

Question 54: Which of the following is a common cause of diabetes mellitus in dogs?

a) Obesity
b) Viral infection
c) High protein diet
d) Excessive exercise

Correct Answer: a) Obesity
Explanation: Obesity is a significant risk factor for diabetes mellitus in dogs, as excess body fat leads to insulin resistance, necessitating weight management for prevention and control.

Question 55: Which of the following is a common symptom of feline hyperthyroidism?

a) Lethargy
b) Hair loss
c) Vomiting
d) Increased thirst

Correct Answer: c) Vomiting
Explanation: Feline hyperthyroidism often presents with vomiting, weight loss, and increased appetite due to heightened metabolic activity from excess thyroid hormones.

Question 56: Which of the following is a common method for diagnosing canine parvovirus infection?

a) Blood culture
b) ELISA test
c) Skin biopsy
d) Urinalysis

Correct Answer: b) ELISA test
Explanation: Diagnosing canine parvovirus involves ELISA tests, which detect viral antigens in feces, enabling prompt treatment and isolation to prevent spread.

Question 57: Which of the following is a common cause of ear infections in dogs?

a) Allergies
b) Excessive exercise
c) High-fat diet
d) Dehydration

Correct Answer: a) Allergies
Explanation: Allergies can lead to ear infections in dogs by causing inflammation and excess wax production, creating an environment for bacteria and yeast to thrive.

Question 58: Which of the following is a common symptom of feline immunodeficiency virus (FIV) infection?

a) Weight gain
b) Persistent fever
c) Increased appetite
d) Hair growth

Correct Answer: b) Persistent fever
Explanation: FIV infection in cats often leads to persistent fever, immunosuppression, and secondary infections, necessitating supportive care and monitoring.

Question 59: Which of the following is a common method for diagnosing feline leukemia virus (FeLV)?

a) Urinalysis
b) Blood smear
c) ELISA test
d) Skin biopsy

Correct Answer: c) ELISA test
Explanation: Feline leukemia virus is diagnosed using ELISA tests to detect viral antigens in the blood, important for managing this contagious disease.

Question 60: Which of the following is a common cause of pancreatitis in dogs?

a) Low-fat diet
b) Obesity
c) High-carbohydrate diet
d) Excessive exercise

Correct Answer: b) Obesity
Explanation: Obesity increases the risk of pancreatitis in dogs by contributing to fat metabolism disorders, necessitating dietary management and weight control.

Question 61: Which of the following is a common symptom of feline asthma?

a) Increased appetite
b) Coughing
c) Weight gain
d) Rapid heart rate

Correct Answer: b) Coughing
Explanation: Feline asthma often leads to coughing and wheezing due to airway inflammation, requiring bronchodilator and anti-inflammatory treatments for management.

Question 62: Which of the following is a common method for diagnosing canine Lyme disease?

a) Fecal flotation
b) Blood test for antibodies
c) Skin biopsy
d) Urinalysis

Correct Answer: b) Blood test for antibodies
Explanation: Lyme disease in dogs is diagnosed through blood tests detecting antibodies to Borrelia burgdorferi, guiding appropriate antibiotic treatment.

Question 63: Which of the following is a common cause of anemia in cats?

a) Hyperthyroidism
b) Parasitic infestation
c) Excessive exercise
d) High-fiber diet

Correct Answer: b) Parasitic infestation
Explanation: Parasitic infestations, such as fleas and hookworms, cause anemia in cats by consuming blood, highlighting the importance of regular parasite control.

Question 64: Which of the following is a common symptom of canine distemper?

a) Increased thirst
b) Nasal discharge
c) Weight gain
d) Hyperactivity

Correct Answer: b) Nasal discharge
Explanation: Canine distemper presents with respiratory symptoms like nasal discharge, alongside gastrointestinal and neurological signs, necessitating vaccination for prevention.

Question 65: Which of the following is a common method for diagnosing feline lower urinary tract disease (FLUTD)?

a) Blood test
b) Urinalysis
c) Fecal analysis
d) Skin biopsy

Correct Answer: b) Urinalysis
Explanation: FLUTD diagnosis involves urinalysis to detect crystals, infection, or other abnormalities, guiding treatment and management of this condition.

Question 66: Which of the following is a common cause of skin allergies in dogs?

a) Hypothyroidism
b) Dietary proteins
c) Excessive exercise
d) High-carbohydrate diet

Correct Answer: b) Dietary proteins
Explanation: Dietary proteins can trigger skin allergies in dogs, causing itching and inflammation, necessitating dietary adjustments to identify and avoid allergens.

Question 67: Which of the following is a common symptom of canine rabies infection?

a) Increased appetite
b) Aggression
c) Weight gain
d) Hyperactivity

Correct Answer: b) Aggression
Explanation: Rabies infection in dogs often manifests as aggression and neurological symptoms, highlighting the critical importance of vaccination and quarantine measures.

Question 68: Which of the following is a common method for diagnosing canine hypothyroidism?

a) Blood test for thyroid hormones
b) Urinalysis
c) Skin biopsy
d) Fecal analysis

Correct Answer: a) Blood test for thyroid hormones
Explanation: Canine hypothyroidism is diagnosed by measuring thyroid hormone levels in the blood, essential for initiating appropriate hormone replacement therapy.

Question 69: Which of the following is a common cause of urinary tract infections in cats?

a) High-fiber diet
b) Obesity
c) Bacterial infection
d) Excessive exercise

Correct Answer: c) Bacterial infection
Explanation: Bacterial infections often lead to urinary tract infections in cats, requiring antimicrobial treatment and monitoring to prevent recurrence.

Question 70: Which of the following is a common symptom of feline leukemia virus (FeLV) infection?

a) Increased appetite
b) Anemia
c) Weight gain
d) Hyperactivity

Correct Answer: b) Anemia
Explanation: FeLV infection in cats frequently results in anemia due to bone marrow suppression, requiring supportive care and monitoring for secondary infections.

Question 71: Which of the following is a common method for diagnosing canine heartworm disease?

a) Blood glucose test
b) Urinalysis
c) Antigen test
d) Skin biopsy

Correct Answer: c) Antigen test
Explanation: Heartworm disease in dogs is diagnosed using antigen tests that detect heartworm proteins in the blood, crucial for timely treatment and prevention.

Question 72: Which of the following is a common cause of liver disease in dogs?

a) Viral infection
b) Obesity
c) Excessive exercise
d) High-protein diet

Correct Answer: b) Obesity
Explanation: Obesity contributes to liver disease in dogs by causing fat accumulation in liver cells, emphasizing the importance of weight management and dietary control.

Question 73: Which of the following is a common symptom of feline immunodeficiency virus (FIV) infection?

a) Increased appetite
b) Lethargy
c) Weight gain
d) Hyperactivity

Correct Answer: b) Lethargy
Explanation: FIV infection in cats often results in lethargy and immunosuppression, requiring supportive care and monitoring for secondary infections.

Question 74: Which of the following is a common method for diagnosing feline hyperthyroidism?

a) Urinalysis
b) Blood test for thyroid hormones

c) Fecal analysis
d) Skin biopsy

Correct Answer: b) Blood test for thyroid hormones
Explanation: Feline hyperthyroidism is diagnosed by measuring elevated thyroid hormone levels in the blood, guiding treatment to manage excess hormone production.

Question 75: Which of the following is a common cause of dental disease in cats?

a) High-fiber diet
b) Lack of dental care
c) Excessive exercise
d) Obesity

Correct Answer: b) Lack of dental care
Explanation: Inadequate dental care leads to plaque buildup and periodontal disease in cats, underscoring the importance of regular dental hygiene practices.

Question 76: Which of the following is a common symptom of canine ehrlichiosis?

a) Increased thirst
b) Fever
c) Weight gain
d) Hyperactivity

Correct Answer: b) Fever
Explanation: Canine ehrlichiosis often presents with fever, lethargy, and bleeding tendencies due to immune-mediated damage, requiring targeted antibiotic therapy.

Question 77: Which of the following is a common method for diagnosing feline panleukopenia?

a) Blood culture
b) Fecal ELISA test
c) Skin biopsy
d) Urinalysis

Correct Answer: b) Fecal ELISA test
Explanation: Feline panleukopenia is diagnosed using fecal ELISA tests to detect viral antigens, facilitating early intervention and supportive care for infected cats.

Question 78: Which of the following is a common cause of arthritis in dogs?

a) High-carbohydrate diet
b) Excessive exercise
c) Obesity
d) Hypothyroidism

Correct Answer: c) Obesity
Explanation: Obesity exacerbates arthritis in dogs by increasing joint stress, highlighting the need for weight management and joint support measures.

Question 79: Which of the following is a common symptom of feline calicivirus infection?

a) Increased appetite
b) Oral ulcers
c) Weight gain
d) Hyperactivity

Correct Answer: b) Oral ulcers
Explanation: Feline calicivirus infection often results in oral ulcers and respiratory symptoms, necessitating supportive care and vaccination for prevention.

Question 80: Which of the following is a common method for diagnosing canine leptospirosis?

a) Fecal flotation
b) Blood culture
c) Urinalysis
d) Skin biopsy

Correct Answer: c) Urinalysis
Explanation: Canine leptospirosis is diagnosed through urinalysis and serological testing, detecting Leptospira bacteria, important for informed treatment decisions.

Question 81: Which of the following is a common cause of heart disease in dogs?

a) Taurine deficiency
b) Obesity
c) Excessive exercise
d) Hyperthyroidism

Correct Answer: b) Obesity
Explanation: Obesity contributes to heart disease in dogs by increasing cardiac workload and promoting conditions like hypertension, warranting dietary and exercise management.

Question 82: Which of the following is a common symptom of canine parvovirus infection?

a) Increased appetite
b) Vomiting
c) Weight gain
d) Hyperactivity

Correct Answer: b) Vomiting
Explanation: Canine parvovirus infection causes vomiting and severe gastrointestinal distress, requiring intensive supportive care and isolation to prevent transmission.

Question 83: Which of the following is a common method for diagnosing feline toxoplasmosis?

a) Blood test
b) Skin biopsy
c) Urinalysis
d) Fecal analysis

Correct Answer: a) Blood test
Explanation: Toxoplasmosis in cats is diagnosed through blood tests detecting antibodies to Toxoplasma gondii, crucial for managing this zoonotic infection.

Question 84: Which of the following is a common cause of obesity in cats?

a) Hypothyroidism
b) Overfeeding
c) Diabetes
d) Heartworm disease

Correct Answer: b) Overfeeding
Explanation: Overfeeding, coupled with lack of exercise, often leads to obesity in cats, increasing health risks such as diabetes and arthritis.

Question 85: Which of the following is a common symptom of feline rhinotracheitis?

a) Increased appetite
b) Sneezing
c) Weight gain
d) Hyperactivity

Correct Answer: b) Sneezing
Explanation: Feline rhinotracheitis, caused by herpesvirus, leads to sneezing and respiratory symptoms, requiring supportive care and vaccination to prevent outbreaks.

Question 86: Which of the following is a common method for diagnosing canine ehrlichiosis?

a) Blood smear
b) Urinalysis
c) Fecal analysis
d) Skin biopsy

Correct Answer: a) Blood smear
Explanation: Canine ehrlichiosis is diagnosed by examining blood smears for Ehrlichia organisms, aiding in targeted antibiotic therapy to manage the infection.

Question 87: Which of the following is a common cause of gastrointestinal ulcers in dogs?

a) Low-protein diet
b) Excessive exercise
c) High-starch diet
d) Vitamin deficiency

Correct Answer: c) High-starch diet
Explanation: High-starch diets can increase gastric acidity, leading to ulcers in dogs, necessitating dietary adjustments to prevent gastrointestinal issues.

Question 88: Which of the following is a common symptom of canine coronavirus infection?

a) Increased thirst
b) Coughing
c) Vomiting
d) Rapid heart rate

Correct Answer: c) Vomiting
Explanation: Canine coronavirus infection often results in vomiting and diarrhea, causing gastrointestinal distress, typically managed with supportive care and hydration.

Question 90: During surgery, you place gelatin foams into the surgical site to provide effective:

a) Hemostasis.
b) Wound dressing.
c) Bandaging.
d) Packing around cut skin edges during surgery.

Correct Answer: a) Hemostasis.
Explanation: Gelatin foams are utilized during surgery to promote hemostasis by providing a scaffold for clot formation at bleeding sites, eventually being absorbed by the body.

Question 91: A control is:

a) Software used to record, graph, and analyze control data.
b) The antigen measured by any serologic test.
c) A calibrator that is used to set up and adjust the instrument and/or procedure to perform correctly and to desired specifications.
d) Material that contains a known quantity of the analyte that is being tested.

Correct Answer: d) Material that contains a known quantity of the analyte that is being tested.
Explanation: Controls are vital for quality control, ensuring the accuracy of tests by comparing results against known quantities of analytes.

Question 92: Indications of postoperative pain include a(n):

a) Decreased heart rate.
b) Increased appetite.
c) Decreased respiratory rate.
d) Increased heart rate.

Correct Answer: d) Increased heart rate.
Explanation: Postoperative pain in animals often manifests as an increased heart rate, among other signs such as vocalization and altered behavior, requiring pain management intervention.

Question 93: The term that describes false pregnancy is:

a) Pseudomonas.
b) Cytokinesis.
c) Pseudocyesis.
d) Metritis.

Correct Answer: c) Pseudocyesis.
Explanation: Pseudocyesis, or false pregnancy, results from hormonal imbalances, often presenting with physical and behavioral signs of pregnancy without embryo development.

Question 94: _____ provides a means to measure the expired dioxide concentration of expired air, whereas _____ indicates a noninvasive measurement of the hemoglobin-oxygen saturation.

a) Blood gas analysis; capnography
b) Capnography; pulse oximetry
c) Pulse oximetry; capnography
d) Capnography; blood gas analysis

Correct Answer: b) Capnography; pulse oximetry
Explanation: Capnography measures the concentration of carbon dioxide in expired air, while pulse oximetry assesses oxygen saturation in the blood, crucial for monitoring respiratory and circulatory efficiency.

Question 95: The classic signs of gastric dilation volvulus (GDV) include all of the following except:

a) Bloating.
b) Vomiting.
c) Straining to defecate.
d) Retching.

Correct Answer: c) Straining to defecate.
Explanation: GDV is characterized by bloating, retching, and vomiting due to stomach rotation, while straining to defecate is not a typical sign of this condition.

Question 96: _____ result from antibody binding to the RBC surface and removal of a portion of the membrane by macrophages; this occurs in immune hemolytic anemia (IHA), which is most commonly recognized in dogs.

a) Echinocytes
b) Acanthocytes
c) Spherocytes
d) Leptocytes

Correct Answer: c) Spherocytes
Explanation: Spherocytes are red blood cells that become sphere-shaped due to membrane loss, typically seen in immune hemolytic anemia, especially in dogs.

Question 97: Postoperative incision infections and cellulitis can both be treated with:

a) Bandaging.
b) Drainage.

c) Aspiration.
d) Warm compresses and systemic antibiotics.

Correct Answer: d) Warm compresses and systemic antibiotics.
Explanation: Warm compresses and systemic antibiotics are effective in treating postoperative infections, promoting healing and reducing inflammation.

Question 98: Cestodes are:

a) Larval tapeworms.
b) Adult roundworms.
c) Larval roundworms.
d) Adult tapeworms.

Correct Answer: d) Adult tapeworms.
Explanation: Cestodes refer to adult tapeworms, parasitic flatworms that inhabit the intestines of their hosts, requiring specific antiparasitic treatments.

Question 99: The placenta in a bovine patient is considered retained if not expelled by _____ hours.

a) 6
b) 12
c) 2
d) 24

Correct Answer: b) 12
Explanation: In cattle, the placenta should be expelled within 2 to 4 hours post-calving; if retained beyond 12 hours, it necessitates veterinary intervention to prevent complications.

Question 100: Bob the dog has trouble walking at home and moves around as little as possible, which is not normal for him. On palpating the joints in Bob's hind leg, the veterinary assistant detects the following symptoms: pain, swelling, crepitus, decreased range of motion, and joint laxity. These are consistent with a diagnosis of:

a) OA.
b) MG.
c) FLUTD.
d) IMHA.

Correct Answer: a) OA.
Explanation: Osteoarthritis (OA) is characterized by joint pain, swelling, and restricted movement, evident in Bob's symptoms, typically confirmed through radiographic examination.

Question 101: Which antiseptic and disinfectant is bactericidal but does not kill spores or fungi; it has no residual effects; and it is both painful and cytotoxic when used in open wounds?

a) Quaternary ammonium
b) Chlorhexidine
c) Povidone-iodine
d) Alcohol

Correct Answer: d) Alcohol
Explanation: Alcohol acts as a bactericidal agent with no efficacy against spores or fungi, unsuitable for open wounds due to its painful and cytotoxic nature.

Question 102: A new horse owner calls to say her 6-year-old quarter horse gelding is sweating, kicking at his abdomen, pawing, and rolling. This horse is exhibiting signs of:

a) Abdominal pain (colic).
b) Neck pain.

c) A headache.
d) Lameness (leg pain).

Correct Answer: a) Abdominal pain (colic).
Explanation: The horse displays classic signs of colic, a common equine condition involving abdominal pain, requiring prompt veterinary assessment and management.

Question 103: Therapeutic drug monitoring is:

a) Recommended when a drug has a narrow therapeutic range.
b) The periodic measurement of the amount of drug in the blood.
c) Recommended when the pharmacokinetics of a drug varies greatly between recipients.
d) All of the above.

Correct Answer: d) All of the above.
Explanation: Therapeutic drug monitoring ensures optimal drug efficacy and safety by measuring blood drug levels, especially crucial for drugs with narrow therapeutic windows or variable kinetics.

Question 104: The "flash" sterilization setting on the autoclave is used for:

a) Cleaning the autoclave.
b) Motorized equipment such as orthopedic drills.
c) Items sensitive to heat, such as rubber and some plastics.
d) Emergency (very rapid) sterilization of instruments.

Correct Answer: d) Emergency (very rapid) sterilization of instruments.
Explanation: Flash sterilization rapidly sterilizes instruments in emergencies, utilizing high temperatures for quick decontamination in urgent surgical scenarios.

Question 105: As a complication of celiotomy, your patient experiences ____, a temporary loss of intestinal motility.

a) Evisceration
b) Megaesophagus
c) Ileus
d) Diarrhea

Correct Answer: c) Ileus
Explanation: Ileus involves temporary intestinal motility loss, often post-surgery, requiring medical management to restore normal gastrointestinal function.

Question 106: _____ refers to an increased response to a stimulus that is normally painful so that less and less stimulation is required to produce pain, whereas _____ refers to the production of pain in response to a stimulus that does not normally provoke pain.

a) Allodynia; hyperalgesia
b) Nociception; analgesia
c) Analgesia; hyperalgesia
d) Hyperalgesia; allodynia

Correct Answer: d) Hyperalgesia; allodynia
Explanation: Hyperalgesia and allodynia describe abnormal pain responses, with hyperalgesia increasing pain sensitivity and allodynia causing pain from non-painful stimuli.

Question 107: Which of the following is a common cause of feline idiopathic cystitis?

a) Viral infection
b) High-fat diet
c) Stress
d) Excessive exercise

Correct Answer: c) Stress
Explanation: Stress is a significant factor in feline idiopathic cystitis, causing bladder inflammation without infection, often managed through environmental enrichment and stress reduction.

Question 108: Which of the following is a characteristic of a malignant tumor?

a) Slow growth
b) Well-defined borders
c) Ability to metastasize
d) Uniform cell size

Correct Answer: c) Ability to metastasize
Explanation: Malignant tumors possess aggressive traits such as rapid growth, invasion, and metastasis, necessitating thorough diagnostic and therapeutic approaches.

Question 109: Which of the following is used to measure blood glucose levels?

a) Hematocrit
b) Glucometer
c) Sphygmomanometer
d) Thermometer

Correct Answer: b) Glucometer
Explanation: A glucometer is employed to measure blood glucose levels, crucial for managing conditions like diabetes mellitus in both humans and animals.

Question 110: What is the primary function of erythrocytes in the blood?

a) Oxygen transport
b) Immune response
c) Blood clotting
d) Hormone transport

Correct Answer: a) Oxygen transport
Explanation: Erythrocytes, or red blood cells, primarily transport oxygen from the lungs to tissues and facilitate carbon dioxide removal, vital for cellular respiration.

Question 111: Which of the following is a common cause of feline upper respiratory infections?

a) Fungal infection
b) Bacterial infection
c) Viral infection
d) Parasitic infection

Correct Answer: c) Viral infection
Explanation: Viral infections, primarily caused by feline herpesvirus and calicivirus, are leading causes of upper respiratory infections in cats, requiring supportive care and vaccination.

Question 112: Which of the following is a common symptom of canine hypothyroidism?

a) Hyperactivity
b) Weight loss
c) Lethargy
d) Increased appetite

Correct Answer: c) Lethargy
Explanation: Canine hypothyroidism often results in lethargy, weight gain, and skin changes due to reduced metabolic activity, managed with hormone replacement therapy.

Question 113: What is the main purpose of administering a pre-anesthetic medication?

a) To induce vomiting
b) To stimulate appetite
c) To reduce anxiety and provide analgesia
d) To increase heart rate

Correct Answer: c) To reduce anxiety and provide analgesia
Explanation: Pre-anesthetic medications calm the patient and provide pain relief, enhancing anesthesia safety and efficacy by minimizing stress and discomfort.

Question 114: Which of the following is a common method for diagnosing canine heartworm disease?

a) Urinalysis
b) Fecal flotation
c) Blood antigen test
d) Skin biopsy

Correct Answer: c) Blood antigen test
Explanation: Canine heartworm disease is diagnosed using blood antigen tests, detecting heartworm proteins, crucial for initiating appropriate treatment and control measures.

Question 115: Which of the following is a common cause of hypercalcemia in dogs?

a) Vitamin D deficiency
b) Renal failure
c) Hypoparathyroidism
d) Cancer

Correct Answer: d) Cancer
Explanation: Cancer, particularly lymphoma and anal gland adenocarcinoma, is a common cause of hypercalcemia in dogs, necessitating thorough evaluation and management.

Question 116: Which of the following is a common symptom of feline diabetes mellitus?

a) Weight gain
b) Increased thirst
c) Hyperactivity
d) Decreased appetite

Correct Answer: b) Increased thirst
Explanation: Feline diabetes mellitus often presents with increased thirst and urination, weight loss, and increased appetite due to insulin deficiency, requiring insulin therapy and dietary management.

Question 117: Which of the following is a common method for diagnosing canine Addison's disease?

a) Skin biopsy
b) ACTH stimulation test
c) Fecal analysis
d) Urinalysis

Correct Answer: b) ACTH stimulation test
Explanation: Addison's disease in dogs is diagnosed using the ACTH stimulation test, assessing adrenal gland response and cortisol production, guiding hormone replacement therapy.

Question 118: Which of the following is a common cause of anemia in dogs?

a) Obesity
b) Parasitic infection
c) Excessive exercise
d) High-fiber diet

Correct Answer: b) Parasitic infection
Explanation: Parasitic infections, such as hookworms and fleas, are common causes of anemia in dogs by consuming blood, emphasizing regular parasite control and treatment.

Question 119: Which of the following is a common symptom of canine leptospirosis?

a) Increased appetite
b) Vomiting
c) Weight gain
d) Hyperactivity

Correct Answer: b) Vomiting
Explanation: Canine leptospirosis often causes vomiting, fever, and renal or hepatic damage, requiring antibiotic treatment and supportive care to prevent severe outcomes.

Question 120: Which of the following is a common method for diagnosing feline hyperthyroidism?

a) Urinalysis
b) Blood test for thyroid hormones
c) Fecal analysis
d) Skin biopsy

Correct Answer: b) Blood test for thyroid hormones
Explanation: Feline hyperthyroidism is diagnosed by measuring elevated thyroid hormone levels in the blood, guiding treatment to manage excess hormone production.

Question 121: Which of the following is a common cause of pancreatitis in cats?

a) High-fiber diet
b) Obesity
c) Viral infection
d) Excessive exercise

Correct Answer: b) Obesity
Explanation: Obesity is a significant risk factor for pancreatitis in cats, leading to inflammation of the pancreas, managed through dietary changes and supportive care.

Question 122: Which of the following is a common symptom of canine parvovirus infection?

a) Increased appetite
b) Vomiting
c) Weight gain
d) Hyperactivity

Correct Answer: b) Vomiting
Explanation: Canine parvovirus infection causes severe vomiting and diarrhea, leading to dehydration and requiring intensive supportive care and isolation to prevent spread.

Question 123: Which of the following is a common method for diagnosing feline leukemia virus (FeLV)?

a) Urinalysis
b) Blood smear
c) ELISA test
d) Skin biopsy

Correct Answer: c) ELISA test
Explanation: Feline leukemia virus is diagnosed using ELISA tests to detect viral antigens in the blood, important for managing this contagious disease.

Question 124: Which of the following is a common cause of hypothyroidism in dogs?

a) Viral infection
b) Immune-mediated destruction of thyroid gland
c) Excessive exercise
d) High-carbohydrate diet

Correct Answer: b) Immune-mediated destruction of thyroid gland

Explanation: Hypothyroidism in dogs commonly arises from immune-mediated thyroid gland destruction, leading to reduced hormone production and requiring hormone replacement therapy.

Question 125: Which of the following is a common symptom of feline panleukopenia?

a) Increased appetite
b) Vomiting
c) Weight gain
d) Hyperactivity

Correct Answer: b) Vomiting

Explanation: Feline panleukopenia, caused by feline parvovirus, presents with vomiting, diarrhea, and severe immunosuppression, requiring supportive care and vaccination.

Question 126: Which of the following is a common method for diagnosing canine Lyme disease?

a) Fecal flotation
b) Blood test for antibodies
c) Skin biopsy
d) Urinalysis

Correct Answer: b) Blood test for antibodies

Explanation: Lyme disease in dogs is diagnosed through blood tests detecting antibodies to Borrelia burgdorferi, guiding appropriate antibiotic treatment.

Question 127: Which of the following is a common cause of liver disease in cats?

a) Hypothyroidism
b) Obesity
c) High-protein diet
d) Excessive exercise

Correct Answer: b) Obesity

Explanation: Obesity can lead to hepatic lipidosis in cats, a severe liver condition requiring nutritional support and weight management for recovery.

Question 128: Which of the following is a common symptom of canine distemper?

a) Increased thirst
b) Nasal discharge
c) Weight gain
d) Hyperactivity

Correct Answer: b) Nasal discharge

Explanation: Canine distemper presents with respiratory symptoms like nasal discharge, alongside gastrointestinal and neurological signs, necessitating vaccination for prevention.

Question 129: Which of the following is a common method for diagnosing feline immunodeficiency virus (FIV)?

a) Urinalysis
b) Blood test for antibodies
c) Fecal analysis
d) Skin biopsy

Correct Answer: b) Blood test for antibodies
Explanation: FIV infection in cats is diagnosed through blood tests detecting antibodies, essential for managing this immunosuppressive viral disease.

Question 130: Which of the following is a common cause of arthritis in cats?

a) High-carbohydrate diet
b) Excessive exercise
c) Obesity
d) Hypothyroidism

Correct Answer: c) Obesity
Explanation: Obesity exacerbates arthritis in cats by increasing joint stress, highlighting the need for weight management and joint support measures.

Question 131: Which of the following is a common symptom of feline calicivirus infection?

a) Increased appetite
b) Oral ulcers
c) Weight gain
d) Hyperactivity

Correct Answer: b) Oral ulcers
Explanation: Feline calicivirus infection often results in oral ulcers and respiratory symptoms, necessitating supportive care and vaccination for prevention.

Question 132: In situations in which the veterinary staff is having difficulty stimulating a calf to breathe, _____ can be injected under the animal's _____.

a) Doxapram hydrochloride; upper eyelid
b) Epinephrine; tongue
c) Doxapram hydrochloride; tongue
d) Epinephrine; upper eyelid

Correct Answer: c) Doxapram hydrochloride; tongue
Explanation: Doxapram hydrochloride is a respiratory stimulant injected under the tongue to stimulate breathing in calves, especially when natural respiration is impaired.

Question 133: Syncope is:

a) Breathing deeply.
b) A sympathomimetic agent.
c) A tranquilizer commonly used in show horses to help them cope with the stress in the judging arena.
d) Fainting.

Correct Answer: d) Fainting.
Explanation: Syncope refers to fainting or a temporary loss of consciousness due to a sudden drop in blood flow to the brain, often requiring a medical assessment to identify underlying causes.

Question 134: Serum enzymes cannot be used to detect:

a) Cholestasis.
b) Muscle damage.
c) Hepatocellular injury.
d) Drug overdose.

Correct Answer: d) Drug overdose.
Explanation: Serum enzymes are effective in diagnosing conditions like cholestasis and muscle damage but are not suitable for detecting drug overdoses, which require different diagnostic methods.

Question 135: Which of the following terms describes the presence of an opening in a surgical drape to allow exposure to a specific area while covering a broader area?

a) Cut-out
b) Surgical stage slit
c) Fenestration
d) Window

Correct Answer: c) Fenestration
Explanation: Fenestration in surgical drapes allows targeted exposure of the surgical field while maintaining sterility of the surrounding area, facilitating efficient surgical procedures.

Question 136: When selecting a cuff to use to indirectly measure a cat's or dog's blood pressure, the _____ of the cuff should be approximately _____ of the circumference of the limb at the site of cuff placement.

a) Circumference; 30%
b) Width; 40%
c) Length; 40%
d) Diameter; 30%

Correct Answer: b) Width; 40%
Explanation: Proper blood pressure measurement requires that the cuff width be approximately 40% of the limb's circumference, ensuring accurate readings and patient comfort.

Question 137: A test for gastrointestinal parasites, _____ requires that the solution used in the test must have a higher specific gravity than that of the parasitic material.

a) Fecal flotation
b) Fecal suspension
c) Fecal sedimentation
d) Direct smear of fecal matter

Correct Answer: a) Fecal flotation
Explanation: Fecal flotation tests rely on solutions with higher specific gravity than parasitic eggs, allowing them to float for easier identification and diagnosis of parasitic infections.

Question 138: Which of the following tests is essential for the evaluation of primary renal disease?

a) Urinalysis
b) Serum chemistry panel
c) WBC
d) CBC

Correct Answer: a) Urinalysis
Explanation: Urinalysis is crucial for assessing renal function, identifying abnormalities like proteinuria or hematuria, and guiding the diagnosis and management of kidney disease.

Question 139: Fluid collected from thoracic and abdominal effusions can be put in EDTA tubes to:

a) Prevent clotting (in case the sample is contaminated with blood).
b) Keep it sterile.
c) Prevent cloudiness during centrifugation.
d) Preserve clarity and color.

Correct Answer: a) Prevent clotting (in case the sample is contaminated with blood).
Explanation: EDTA tubes prevent clotting in effusion samples potentially contaminated with blood, ensuring the sample remains suitable for accurate laboratory analysis.

Question 140: Arterial blood samples should be drawn from the _____ or femoral artery.

a) Dorsal metatarsal
b) Saphenous
c) Cephalic
d) Caudal

Correct Answer: a) Dorsal metatarsal
Explanation: The dorsal metatarsal and femoral arteries are common sites for arterial blood sampling, providing access to arterial blood for gas analysis and other diagnostics.

Question 141: An abnormal P wave likely indicates:

a) Ventricular chamber enlargement.
b) An electrical impulse of supraventricular origin.
c) Right or left atrial enlargement.
d) Bundle branch block.

Correct Answer: c) Right or left atrial enlargement.
Explanation: Abnormal P waves suggest atrial enlargement, indicating changes in atrial size or function, often associated with specific cardiovascular conditions.

Question 142: When passing sharp instruments or scalpel blades, the sharp components should be passed:

a) Only after asking the surgeon to verify that the instrument or blade is the right one.
b) Slowly.
c) In such a way that the surgeon's open palm is avoided (i.e., pass the instrument or blade from your pen-hold grasp to the surgeon's pen-hold grasp).
d) Away from the surgeon's hand.

Correct Answer: d) Away from the surgeon's hand.
Explanation: Passing sharp instruments with the blade away from the surgeon's hand prevents accidental injury, ensuring safety in the operating room.

Question 143: At high doses, narcotics can cause excitement in:

a) Cats.
b) Horses.
c) Collie breeds or mixes.
d) Goats.

Correct Answer: b) Horses.
Explanation: In horses, high doses of narcotics like opioids can lead to excitement, necessitating careful dosing and often co-administration with sedatives to manage this reaction.

Question 144: Amino acids are made up of carbon, oxygen, _____, and _____.

a) Phosphorus; potassium
b) Nitrogen; sulfur
c) Calcium; phosphorus
d) Protein; nitrogen

Correct Answer: b) Nitrogen; sulfur
Explanation: Amino acids, the building blocks of proteins, consist of carbon, oxygen, nitrogen, and sulfur, playing a crucial role in various physiological processes.

Question 145: When a large section of intestine has become necrotic, it is necessary to perform _____ and _____.

a) Resection; intussusception
b) Resection; anastomosis

c) Intussusception; resection
d) Intussusception; anastomosis

Correct Answer: b) Resection; anastomosis
Explanation: Surgical intervention involving resection and anastomosis is required to remove necrotic intestine and restore gastrointestinal continuity.

Question 146: Tail docking and dewclaw removal in a puppy should occur between days:

a) 3 and 5.
b) 15 and 20.
c) 7 and 10.
d) 10 and 14.

Correct Answer: a) 3 and 5.
Explanation: Tail docking and dewclaw removal are ideally performed between 3 to 5 days of age to minimize discomfort and promote optimal healing in puppies.

Question 147: What is the first thing a technician should ascertain from a telephone triage with an owner who is worried about his or her pet?

a) Whether the animal is having difficulty breathing
b) A name and phone number where the caller can be contacted if disconnected
c) Whether the animal is experiencing life-threatening breathing
d) None of the above

Correct Answer: b) A name and phone number where the caller can be contacted if disconnected
Explanation: Gathering contact information ensures communication continuity in emergencies, enabling the technician to assist the pet owner effectively.

Question 148: What certification identifies to the public those online pharmacy sites that are appropriately licensed and legitimately operating over the Internet?

a) NABP
b) VIPPS
c) USP
d) FDA

Correct Answer: b) VIPPS
Explanation: The Verified Internet Pharmacy Practice Sites (VIPPS) certification indicates legitimate online pharmacies, ensuring consumer safety and regulatory compliance.

Question 149: Which of the following drugs is used to treat ventricular tachycardia?

a) Dopamine
b) Lidocaine
c) Sodium bicarbonate
d) Glucocorticoids

Correct Answer: b) Lidocaine
Explanation: Lidocaine is an antiarrhythmic drug that stabilizes the cardiac membrane, effectively treating ventricular tachycardia and preventing life-threatening arrhythmias.

Question 150: What is the primary function of neutrophils in the immune system?

a) Produce antibodies
b) Phagocytize bacteria
c) Release histamine
d) Transport oxygen

Correct Answer: b) Phagocytize bacteria
Explanation: Neutrophils play a critical role in the immune system by engulfing and destroying bacteria, forming the first line of defense against infections.

Question 151: Which of the following vaccines is typically administered annually to dogs?

a) Rabies
b) Distemper
c) Bordetella
d) Parvovirus

Correct Answer: c) Bordetella
Explanation: The Bordetella vaccine is often given annually to dogs, particularly those in high-risk environments like kennels, to prevent respiratory infections.

Question 152: In cats, which condition is characterized by the presence of stones in the kidney or bladder?

a) Cystitis
b) Nephritis
c) Urolithiasis
d) Pyelonephritis

Correct Answer: c) Urolithiasis
Explanation: Urolithiasis refers to the formation of stones in the urinary tract, causing potential blockages and requiring dietary management or surgical intervention.

Question 153: Which of the following is a common cause of feline hyperthyroidism?

a) Iodine deficiency
b) Benign thyroid tumor
c) Obesity
d) Diabetes mellitus

Correct Answer: b) Benign thyroid tumor
Explanation: Feline hyperthyroidism is often due to benign thyroid tumors, leading to excess thyroid hormone production and requiring medical or surgical treatment.

Question 154: Which of the following is a common sign of canine Cushing's disease?

a) Hyperactivity
b) Hair loss
c) Weight gain
d) Increased thirst

Correct Answer: b) Hair loss
Explanation: Canine Cushing's disease often presents with hair loss, along with increased thirst, appetite, and abdominal enlargement, requiring diagnostic testing and management.

Question 155: Which of the following is a common diagnostic tool for assessing heart function in dogs?

a) X-ray
b) Electrocardiogram (ECG)
c) Ultrasound
d) MRI

Correct Answer: b) Electrocardiogram (ECG)
Explanation: An ECG records the heart's electrical activity, helping diagnose arrhythmias and other cardiac issues in dogs, guiding treatment decisions.

Question 156: Which of the following conditions is associated with an enlarged heart in cats?

a) Hyperthyroidism
b) Hypertrophic cardiomyopathy
c) Diabetes mellitus
d) Chronic renal failure

Correct Answer: b) Hypertrophic cardiomyopathy
Explanation: Hypertrophic cardiomyopathy causes heart muscle thickening and enlargement, affecting cardiac function and requiring medical management in cats.

Question 157: What is the main purpose of administering a prophylactic antibiotic?

a) To treat an existing infection
b) To prevent a potential infection
c) To reduce inflammation
d) To stimulate appetite

Correct Answer: b) To prevent a potential infection
Explanation: Prophylactic antibiotics are given to prevent infections, especially in surgical settings, reducing the risk of postoperative complications.

Question 158: Which of the following is a common cause of canine hypothyroidism?

a) Autoimmune thyroiditis
b) Iodine deficiency
c) Adrenal tumor
d) Diabetes mellitus

Correct Answer: a) Autoimmune thyroiditis
Explanation: Autoimmune thyroiditis is a leading cause of hypothyroidism in dogs, where the immune system attacks the thyroid gland, reducing hormone production.

Question 159: Which of the following is a common method for evaluating renal function in cats?

a) Fecal analysis
b) Blood urea nitrogen (BUN) test
c) Skin biopsy
d) Urinalysis

Correct Answer: b) Blood urea nitrogen (BUN) test
Explanation: The BUN test assesses kidney function by measuring urea levels in the blood, helping diagnose renal insufficiency or failure in cats.

Question 160: Which of the following is a common sign of feline diabetes mellitus?

a) Weight loss
b) Increased appetite
c) Lethargy
d) All of the above

Correct Answer: d) All of the above
Explanation: Feline diabetes presents with weight loss, increased appetite, and lethargy, resulting from insulin deficiency and requiring insulin therapy and dietary management.

Question 161: Which of the following is a common diagnostic test for detecting feline leukemia virus (FeLV)?

a) ELISA test
b) Fecal flotation

c) Skin biopsy
d) Urinalysis

Correct Answer: a) ELISA test
Explanation: The ELISA test detects FeLV antigens in the blood, aiding in the diagnosis and management of this viral infection in cats.

Question 162: Which of the following conditions is characterized by the presence of crystals in the urine?

a) Urolithiasis
b) Crystalluria
c) Pyelonephritis
d) Cystitis

Correct Answer: b) Crystalluria
Explanation: Crystalluria involves the presence of crystals in the urine, often associated with urinary tract disorders and requiring dietary or medical interventions.

Question 163: Which of the following is a common treatment for canine osteoarthritis?

a) Antibiotics
b) Joint supplements
c) Insulin therapy
d) Antidepressants

Correct Answer: b) Joint supplements
Explanation: Joint supplements, alongside pain management strategies, help alleviate symptoms of osteoarthritis in dogs, improving mobility and quality of life.

Question 164: Which of the following is a common cause of feline chronic kidney disease?

a) Hypertension
b) Protein-rich diet
c) Diabetes mellitus
d) Age-related degeneration

Correct Answer: d) Age-related degeneration
Explanation: Age-related degeneration is a leading cause of chronic kidney disease in cats, requiring dietary management and supportive therapies to slow progression.

Question 165: Which of the following is a common sign of canine Lyme disease?

a) Increased appetite
b) Joint pain
c) Weight gain
d) Hyperactivity

Correct Answer: b) Joint pain
Explanation: Lyme disease in dogs often presents with joint pain, fever, and lethargy, caused by Borrelia burgdorferi infection and requiring antibiotic treatment.

Question 166: Which of the following is a common method for diagnosing canine heartworm disease?

a) Urinalysis
b) Blood antigen test
c) Fecal flotation
d) Skin biopsy

Correct Answer: b) Blood antigen test
Explanation: The blood antigen test detects heartworm proteins in dogs, essential for diagnosing and managing heartworm disease to prevent severe cardiovascular complications.

Question 167: Which of the following is a common cause of hypercalcemia in cats?

a) Renal failure
b) Hyperparathyroidism
c) Obesity
d) Vitamin D deficiency

Correct Answer: b) Hyperparathyroidism
Explanation: Hyperparathyroidism can lead to elevated calcium levels in cats, necessitating diagnostic evaluation and appropriate treatment to prevent complications.

Question 168: Which of the following is a common sign of feline pancreatitis?

a) Increased appetite
b) Vomiting
c) Weight gain
d) Hyperactivity

Correct Answer: b) Vomiting
Explanation: Feline pancreatitis often presents with vomiting and abdominal pain, requiring supportive care and dietary adjustments for recovery.

Question 169: Which of the following is a common method for diagnosing canine Addison's disease?

a) Skin biopsy
b) ACTH stimulation test
c) Fecal analysis
d) Urinalysis

Correct Answer: b) ACTH stimulation test
Explanation: The ACTH stimulation test assesses adrenal gland function, diagnosing Addison's disease in dogs and guiding hormone replacement therapy.

Question 170: Which of the following is a common cause of anemia in cats?

a) High-fiber diet
b) Parasitic infection
c) Excessive exercise
d) Obesity

Correct Answer: b) Parasitic infection
Explanation: Parasitic infections, such as fleas or intestinal worms, commonly cause anemia in cats by consuming blood, emphasizing the need for effective parasite control.

Full Test 4 with Detailed Explanations

Question 1: The most common late postoperative complication of _____ is stricture, generally manifested as stranguria.

a) Urethrostomy
b) Ovariohysterectomy
c) Anastomosis
d) Onychectomy

Correct Answer: a) Urethrostomy
Explanation: Stricture formation is a common complication after urethrostomy, leading to narrowing from

scar tissue and resulting in difficulty urinating, known as stranguria. This can be exacerbated by self-mutilation of the surgical site.

Question 2: A veterinarian who has a patient with congestive heart failure (CHF) administers _____ in hopes of improving the heart's ability to pump blood by increasing the calcium concentration.

a) Enrofloxacin
b) Digoxin
c) Prednisone
d) Furosemide

Correct Answer: b) Digoxin
Explanation: Digoxin is used in CHF treatment to increase intracellular calcium, enhancing cardiac muscle contraction strength and improving heart function.

Question 3: An accumulation of purulent secretions and fluid within the lining of the uterus is termed:

a) Pyometra
b) Metritis
c) Endometriosis
d) Pyoderma

Correct Answer: a) Pyometra
Explanation: Pyometra is a serious uterine condition characterized by pus accumulation due to infection and endometrial changes, often requiring surgical intervention.

Question 4: After ethylene oxide sterilization, materials should be:

a) Quarantined in a well-ventilated area for at least 7 days.
b) Packed closely in an air-tight cabinet.
c) Rinsed well in sterile, distilled water.

Correct Answer: a) Quarantined in a well-ventilated area for at least 7 days.
Explanation: Proper aeration post-ethylene oxide sterilization is crucial to remove residual toxic gases, ensuring safety for subsequent use.

Question 5: Feeding inadequate forages with little or no grain can create a deficiency of usable _____ during the last trimester of pregnancy in ewes carrying twins or triplets and can lead to _____ and ____ in the mother.

a) Carbohydrates; paralysis; coma
b) Protein; abortion; paralysis
c) Protein; paralysis; coma
d) Carbohydrates; abortion; paralysis

Correct Answer: a) Carbohydrates; paralysis; coma
Explanation: Lack of carbohydrates in late pregnancy leads to energy deficits, causing paralysis and coma in ewes, especially those with multiple fetuses.

Question 6: Bovine respiratory disease syndrome (BRDS), commonly called _____, is caused by a combination of respiratory bacteria, viruses, and _____.

a) Hardware disease; stress
b) Founder; poor nutrition
c) Shipping fever; stress
d) Lumpy jaw; enterotoxins

Correct Answer: c) Shipping fever; stress
Explanation: Shipping fever arises from stress and pathogen exposure, leading to respiratory illnesses in cattle, often exacerbated by transportation and confinement.

Question 7: Swelling and infection along tissue planes in a postoperative incision that may be red, warm, and associated with elevated body temperature may be a sign of:

a) Decubital ulcer
b) Cellulitis
c) Dermal edema
d) Ascites

Correct Answer: b) Cellulitis
Explanation: Postoperative cellulitis involves redness, warmth, and fever, indicating an infection that requires prompt treatment to prevent further complications.

Question 8: _____ can result from the rupture of retropharyngeal lymph nodes occurring secondary to infectious strangles in horses.

a) Maxillary sinusitis
b) Allergic airway disease
c) Pleuritis
d) Guttural pouch empyema

Correct Answer: d) Guttural pouch empyema
Explanation: Strangles can lead to guttural pouch empyema when lymph node abscesses rupture, filling the pouches with pus and necessitating drainage.

Question 9: Measuring the hematocrit, hemoglobin concentration, and _____ can be used to determine the oxygen-carrying capacity of blood.

a) RBC count
b) Cell volume of reticulocytes
c) WBC count
d) Platelet volume distribution width

Correct Answer: a) RBC count
Explanation: RBC count, along with hematocrit and hemoglobin, provides a full picture of blood's ability to transport oxygen, vital for diagnosing conditions like anemia.

Question 10: As you review the nursing care plan for Sparky, a rabbit, the data you encounter will contain:

a) The veterinarian's list of orders related to his or her diagnosis.
b) Information about implementation of the patient's actual assessment or examination needs.
c) Information about interventions specific to your own evaluation of Sparky.
d) The SOAP format.

Correct Answer: c) Information about interventions specific to your own evaluation of Sparky.
Explanation: The nursing care plan involves tailored interventions based on specific evaluations, ensuring a personalized approach to Sparky's care.

Question 11: Which of the following bacteria is most likely associated with the gangrenous form of mastitis in sheep and goats?

a) Staphylococcus aureus
b) Streptococcus
c) Pasteurella haemolytica
d) Pseudomonas

Correct Answer: a) Staphylococcus aureus
Explanation: Staphylococcus aureus is a common pathogen in gangrenous mastitis, causing severe tissue damage and potential systemic effects in affected animals.

Question 12: You discover that your patient is unable to breathe unless the patient is upright, a sign referred to as:

a) Orthopnea
b) Dyspnea
c) Hypoxemia
d) Hypoxia

Correct Answer: a) Orthopnea
Explanation: Orthopnea is a respiratory condition where patients can only breathe comfortably in an upright position, often associated with heart or lung issues.

Question 13: Which method of helping a downed cow stand is the best option for supporting an animal for long periods of time?

a) Pulley system
b) Hydroflotation
c) Sling
d) Hip lifter

Correct Answer: b) Hydroflotation
Explanation: Hydroflotation supports down cows with minimal trauma, allowing for prolonged support and improving the chances of recovery compared to other methods.

Question 14: An echogram of your patient, a cat, shows an increased thickness of the left ventricle wall and a small ventricular lumen, which confirms a diagnosis of:

a) Hypertrophic cardiomyopathy (HCM)
b) Degenerative atrioventricular valve disease
c) Dilated cardiomyopathy (DCM)
d) Aortic thromboembolism (ATE)

Correct Answer: a) Hypertrophic cardiomyopathy (HCM)
Explanation: HCM in cats is characterized by thickened ventricular walls and reduced chamber size, affecting heart function and requiring careful management.

Question 15: When you add liquid reagent to a serum sample:

a) The chemical reaction produces a colored chemical product.
b) It preserves that sample for shipment to a laboratory.
c) It clots and solidifies the sample.
d) It causes evaporation and a desiccated product that can be viewed microscopically.

Correct Answer: a) The chemical reaction produces a colored chemical product.
Explanation: Adding liquid reagent to serum initiates a chemical reaction, resulting in a color change that can be measured to determine various blood parameters.

Question 16: Which of the following drugs promotes diuresis and decreases cerebral edema in a patient following cardiac arrest by drawing water from the interstitial space between cells?

a) Mannitol
b) Dobutamine
c) Glucocorticoids
d) Lidocaine

Correct Answer: a) Mannitol
Explanation: Mannitol is an osmotic diuretic that draws fluid from tissues into the bloodstream, reducing cerebral edema and promoting diuresis, particularly important post-cardiac arrest.

Question 17: Bloody diarrhea and pale mucous membranes in very young puppies are signs of:

a) Ancylostoma caninum
b) Trichuris vulpis
c) Strongylus vulgaris
d) Ascarids

Correct Answer: a) Ancylostoma caninum
Explanation: Ancylostoma caninum, or canine hookworms, are blood-feeding parasites causing anemia and bloody diarrhea in puppies due to their voracious feeding habits.

Question 18: Which of the following conditions can cause hypoxia?

a) Reduced blood flow
b) Hypoventilation
c) Decreased oxygen-carrying capacity
d) All of the above

Correct Answer: d) All of the above
Explanation: Hypoxia arises from reduced blood flow, hypoventilation, or decreased oxygen-carrying capacity, each affecting oxygen delivery to tissues.

Question 19: As a general rule of thumb, the PaO2 should be approximately _____ times the FiO2.

a) 5
b) 3
c) 250
d) 10

Correct Answer: a) 5
Explanation: PaO2, the partial pressure of oxygen in arterial blood, is typically about five times the FiO2 (fraction of inspired oxygen), indicating efficient oxygen exchange.

Question 20: All horses in the United States should be vaccinated against:

a) Eastern and Western equine and West Nile encephalomyelitis
b) Eastern and Western encephalitis and strangles
c) Tetanus and influenza
d) Heaves and tetanus

Correct Answer: a) Eastern and Western equine and West Nile encephalomyelitis
Explanation: Vaccination against these viruses is crucial for horses in the U.S. due to their prevalence and mosquito-borne transmission, preventing severe neurological diseases.

Question 21: Which of the following may fall under the role of a surgical assistant in the postoperative management of a patient?

a) Participate in writing the medical report
b) Assure that any biopsy samples collected during the surgery are properly identified and submitted
c) Clean the wound and surrounding skin immediately after surgery before the animal becomes fully conscious
d) All of the above are correct

Correct Answer: d) All of the above are correct
Explanation: A surgical assistant's role includes comprehensive postoperative responsibilities such as documentation, sample management, and wound care, ensuring optimal patient recovery.

Question 22: It is your first day of work, and you are checking on a hospitalized patient. You see the phrase "Monitor for strangulation" in the medical report. Strangulation refers to:

a) Ileus
b) A large umbilical hernia
c) Intussusception
d) Loss of the intestinal blood supply with devitalization and possible intestinal perforation, which is seen in conjunction with some hernias

Correct Answer: d) Loss of the intestinal blood supply with devitalization and possible intestinal perforation, which is seen in conjunction with some hernias
Explanation: Strangulation involves compromised blood supply leading to tissue death, often linked with hernias, necessitating urgent surgical intervention.

Question 23: Guttural pouch mycosis is caused by a:

a) Bacteria
b) Fungus
c) Virus
d) Prion

Correct Answer: b) Fungus
Explanation: Guttural pouch mycosis, commonly caused by Aspergillus spp., leads to fungal infection in horses, potentially causing severe bleeding or nerve damage.

Question 24: High reticulocyte counts of more than 60,000/ml in dogs and more than 50,000/ml in cats are compatible with:

a) Ingestion of wilted maple leaves or onions
b) Lead toxicity
c) Ingestion of zinc-containing objects
d) Regenerative anemia

Correct Answer: d) Regenerative anemia
Explanation: High reticulocyte counts indicate active red blood cell production, often seen in regenerative anemia, where the body responds to blood loss or hemolysis.

Question 25: Highly irritating drugs can severely damage blood vessels and surrounding tissue if:

a) Injected outside the vein
b) Given with epinephrine
c) Given in combination with dimethyl sulfoxide (DMSO)
d) Not given with corticosteroids

Correct Answer: a) Injected outside the vein
Explanation: Extravasation, or leakage of drugs outside the vein, can lead to severe tissue damage, highlighting the importance of proper intravenous administration.

Question 26: The total hip prosthesis consists of a long stem that fits inside the proximal _____; a special cup replaces the _____.

a) Humerus; acetabulum
b) Femur; greater trochanter
c) Femur; acetabulum
d) Femur; femoral head

Correct Answer: c) Femur; acetabulum
Explanation: A total hip prosthesis involves replacing the femoral head with a prosthetic stem and the acetabulum with a cup, restoring joint function in hip dysplasia cases.

Question 27: You are examining a fecal specimen microscopically. The initial plane of focus should be that of air bubbles because:

a) Most helminth eggs are found in this plane
b) Segments are most easily identified in this plane
c) It is the most powerful setting
d) This is the plane most useful in detecting the helminthic mouth (the most immediate identifying factor)

Correct Answer: a) Most helminth eggs are found in this plane
Explanation: Helminth eggs typically float to the plane of air bubbles in fecal specimens, making this the ideal focus point for parasitological examinations.

Question 28: A trematode is commonly referred to as:

a) Any flatworm
b) Any roundworm
c) A tapeworm
d) A fluke

Correct Answer: d) A fluke
Explanation: Trematodes, or flukes, are parasitic flatworms infecting various animals, distinguished by their leaf-like shape and complex life cycles.

Question 29: Medications dispensed that are considered unsafe for laypersons to administer without monitoring by a licensed veterinarian are called _____ drugs and bear the "caution" sign, which restricts the use of the drug.

a) Counterfeit
b) Compounded
c) Legend
d) Controlled

Correct Answer: c) Legend
Explanation: Legend drugs, requiring a prescription, are regulated to prevent misuse due to their potential for harm if improperly administered.

Question 30: Every time you enter a ward that holds infectious patients, you wash your hands and don shoe covers, a gown, and examination gloves before entering. This is referred to as _____ nursing.

a) Barrier
b) Zoonotic
c) Nosocomic
d) Isolation

Correct Answer: a) Barrier
Explanation: Barrier nursing involves protective measures to prevent the spread of infection, crucial in managing contagious patients and ensuring healthcare safety.

Question 31: Which disinfectant is effective against bacteria, but not against spores or some viruses and is very bland and nontoxic?

a) Povidone-iodine
b) Alcohol
c) Quaternary ammonium
d) Chlorhexidine

Correct Answer: c) Quaternary ammonium
Explanation: Quaternary ammonium compounds are effective against bacteria and are safe for use, but they lack efficacy against spores and certain viruses.

Question 32: Low-pressure bleeding from small vessels can be controlled by:

a) Gently wiping the area with sterile gauze
b) Doing nothing; low-pressure bleeding should be allowed to stop on its own
c) Sustained pressure with a dry surgical glove
d) Sustained pressure through a gauze sponge

Correct Answer: d) Sustained pressure through a gauze sponge
Explanation: Applying pressure with gauze is a standard method for controlling low-pressure bleeding, promoting clot formation and hemostasis.

Question 33: Trocar, sleeve, blunt obturator, triangulation, and light cable are all terms used in _____ surgery.

a) Orthopedic
b) Emergency
c) Ophthalmologic
d) Arthroscopic

Correct Answer: d) Arthroscopic
Explanation: Arthroscopic surgery involves minimally invasive techniques using tools like the trocar and light cable, offering precise joint visualization and treatment.

Question 34: Taper needles are most commonly used to pierce _____ tissue.

a) Muscle, tendon, and ligament
b) Skin, sinus, and cartilage
c) Intestinal, subcutaneous, and fascia
d) Brain, liver, and kidney

Correct Answer: c) Intestinal, subcutaneous, and fascia
Explanation: Taper needles are designed to pierce delicate tissues like intestines and fascia without tearing, ensuring minimal trauma during suturing.

Question 35: For tracheostomy in a calf, you will use a _____ mm ID tube.

a) 15- to 20-
b) 10- to 15-
c) 5- to 10-
d) 10- to 12-

Correct Answer: c) 5- to 10-
Explanation: A 5- to 10-mm ID tube is appropriate for tracheostomy in calves, ensuring adequate airway support in cases of upper airway obstruction.

Question 36: It is imperative to a calf's survival to receive colostrum within the first _____ of life.

a) Week
b) 2 hours
c) Day
d) 6 hours

Correct Answer: d) 6 hours
Explanation: Colostrum provides essential antibodies and nutrients, and its timely intake within 6 hours postpartum is critical for neonatal health and immunity.

Question 37: Which diagnostic test is most useful for detecting heartworm infection in dogs?

a) Fecal flotation
b) Thoracic radiographs

c) ELISA antigen test
d) Complete blood count (CBC)

Correct Answer: c) ELISA antigen test
Explanation: The ELISA antigen test is highly specific and sensitive for detecting heartworm in dogs, identifying the presence of adult female heartworm antigens in the bloodstream.

Question 38: Which type of fracture is characterized by a bone breaking into several pieces?

a) Greenstick
b) Comminuted
c) Transverse
d) Oblique

Correct Answer: b) Comminuted
Explanation: A comminuted fracture involves the bone shattering into multiple fragments, often requiring surgical intervention for stabilization and healing.

Question 39: Which of the following is a zoonotic disease?

a) Canine parvovirus
b) Feline leukemia
c) Rabies
d) Distemper

Correct Answer: c) Rabies
Explanation: Rabies is a zoonotic viral disease that affects the nervous system of mammals, including humans, and is transmitted through saliva, often via bites.

Question 40: Which vitamin is essential for proper blood clotting?

a) Vitamin A
b) Vitamin D
c) Vitamin E
d) Vitamin K

Correct Answer: d) Vitamin K
Explanation: Vitamin K is crucial for synthesizing clotting factors, playing a key role in the coagulation process to prevent excessive bleeding.

Question 41: Which of the following is a common sign of feline hyperthyroidism?

a) Weight gain
b) Lethargy
c) Increased appetite
d) Hair loss

Correct Answer: c) Increased appetite
Explanation: Feline hyperthyroidism typically results in increased appetite due to heightened metabolism, often accompanied by weight loss and hyperactivity.

Question 42: Which part of the central nervous system is primarily responsible for coordinating movement and balance?

a) Cerebrum
b) Cerebellum
c) Brainstem
d) Thalamus

Correct Answer: b) Cerebellum

Explanation: The cerebellum is integral to motor control, coordinating movements, maintaining posture, and ensuring balance, essential for smooth physical activity.

Question 43: The term for difficulty swallowing is:

a) Dysphagia
b) Dysphonia
c) Dysuria
d) Dyspnea

Correct Answer: a) Dysphagia

Explanation: Dysphagia refers to difficulty in swallowing, which can result from neurological, muscular, or anatomical issues affecting the swallowing mechanism.

Question 44: Which electrolyte imbalance is most likely to cause cardiac arrhythmias?

a) Hypocalcemia
b) Hyperkalemia
c) Hypophosphatemia
d) Hypermagnesemia

Correct Answer: b) Hyperkalemia

Explanation: Hyperkalemia, characterized by elevated potassium levels, can disrupt cardiac electrical activity, leading to dangerous arrhythmias.

Question 45: Which organ is primarily responsible for detoxifying drugs and toxins in the body?

a) Kidneys
b) Spleen
c) Liver
d) Pancreas

Correct Answer: c) Liver

Explanation: The liver plays a central role in detoxification, metabolizing drugs and toxins to ensure they are safely eliminated from the body.

Question 46: Which blood cell type is primarily responsible for oxygen transport?

a) Platelets
b) White blood cells
c) Red blood cells
d) Lymphocytes

Correct Answer: c) Red blood cells

Explanation: Red blood cells contain hemoglobin, a protein essential for oxygen transport from the lungs to tissues throughout the body.

Question 47: Which hormone is responsible for regulating blood sugar levels by facilitating glucose uptake into cells?

a) Insulin
b) Glucagon
c) Cortisol
d) Thyroxine

Correct Answer: a) Insulin

Explanation: Insulin, produced by the pancreas, lowers blood sugar levels by promoting cellular glucose uptake, crucial for energy production and homeostasis.

Question 48: Which condition is characterized by the inflammation of the lining of the heart and its valves?

a) Pericarditis
b) Endocarditis
c) Myocarditis
d) Cardiomyopathy

Correct Answer: b) Endocarditis
Explanation: Endocarditis involves inflammation of the endocardium, often due to infection, affecting heart valves and potentially leading to severe cardiac dysfunction.

Question 49: Which species is most susceptible to copper toxicity?

a) Horses
b) Sheep
c) Cattle
d) Goats

Correct Answer: b) Sheep
Explanation: Sheep are particularly sensitive to copper, with excessive intake leading to toxicity characterized by liver damage and hemolytic anemia.

Question 50: Which of the following is the primary function of the nephron in the kidney?

a) Produce hormones
b) Filter blood
c) Store urine
d) Regulate body temperature

Correct Answer: b) Filter blood
Explanation: Nephrons filter blood, removing waste products and excess substances to form urine, crucial for maintaining fluid and electrolyte balance.

Question 51: Which of the following is an example of a long bone?

a) Femur
b) Skull
c) Vertebra
d) Pelvis

Correct Answer: a) Femur
Explanation: The femur is a long bone, characterized by a shaft and two ends, crucial for support, movement, and hematopoiesis (blood cell production).

Question 52: Which condition is characterized by the accumulation of pus in a body cavity?

a) Hemothorax
b) Empyema
c) Ascites
d) Hematoma

Correct Answer: b) Empyema
Explanation: Empyema refers to pus accumulation, typically in the pleural space, often due to infection, requiring drainage and antibiotic treatment.

Question 53: Which type of immunity is acquired through vaccination?

a) Passive natural immunity
b) Passive artificial immunity

c) Active natural immunity
d) Active artificial immunity

Correct Answer: d) Active artificial immunity
Explanation: Vaccination induces active artificial immunity by stimulating the immune system to produce a protective response without causing disease.

Question 54: What is the primary function of platelets in the blood?

a) Transport oxygen
b) Fight infections
c) Clot blood
d) Regulate blood pressure

Correct Answer: c) Clot blood
Explanation: Platelets are essential for hemostasis, forming clots to prevent bleeding and facilitating wound healing processes.

Question 55: Which of the following parasites is known for causing "creeping eruption" in humans?

a) Hookworm
b) Tapeworm
c) Roundworm
d) Whipworm

Correct Answer: a) Hookworm
Explanation: Hookworms cause creeping eruption, or cutaneous larva migrans, when larvae penetrate human skin, causing itchy, serpiginous tracks.

Question 56: Which structure in the eye is responsible for focusing light onto the retina?

a) Cornea
b) Lens
c) Iris
d) Sclera

Correct Answer: b) Lens
Explanation: The lens focuses light onto the retina, enabling clear vision by adjusting its shape to accommodate near and distant objects.

Question 57: Which nutrient is essential for the production of thyroid hormones?

a) Iron
b) Calcium
c) Iodine
d) Magnesium

Correct Answer: c) Iodine
Explanation: Iodine is crucial for synthesizing thyroid hormones, which regulate metabolism and are vital for growth and development.

Question 58: Which type of muscle is under voluntary control?

a) Cardiac muscle
b) Smooth muscle
c) Skeletal muscle
d) Involuntary muscle

Correct Answer: c) Skeletal muscle
Explanation: Skeletal muscle is under voluntary control, allowing conscious movement and coordination of the body.

Question 60: The placenta in a bovine patient is considered retained if not expelled by _____ hours.

a) 24
b) 12
c) 6
d) 2

Correct Answer: b) 12
Explanation: In cattle, the placenta is typically expelled within 2 to 4 hours after birth. If not expelled by 12 hours, it is considered retained, necessitating veterinary intervention to prevent complications like infection.

Question 61: RBCs from _____ have the largest diameter and the least anisocytosis.

a) Cats
b) Horses
c) Sheep
d) Dogs

Correct Answer: d) Dogs
Explanation: Among domestic animals, canine red blood cells have the largest diameter and exhibit minimal anisocytosis, indicating uniformity in size, which is useful for diagnosing various blood disorders.

Question 62: _____, you give the operating room a thorough cleaning that includes all permanent structures, floors, and cabinets, as well as removing, cleaning, and disinfecting all movable equipment.

a) Once a week
b) At the end of the surgery day
c) At the beginning of the surgery day
d) Once a month

Correct Answer: a) Once a week
Explanation: Weekly deep cleaning of the operating room is essential to prevent infection, encompassing all surfaces and equipment, ensuring a sterile environment for surgical procedures.

Question 63: Which nutritional myodegenerative disease may be caused by a deficiency of gestational vitamin E and/or selenium?

a) Caseous lymphadenitis
b) Johne disease
c) Caprine arthritis-encephalitis
d) White muscle disease

Correct Answer: d) White muscle disease
Explanation: White muscle disease results from selenium and vitamin E deficiency during gestation, affecting muscle function in young animals, especially lambs and calves, often requiring supplementation.

Question 64: What is the last step in draping a patient before equine orthopedic surgery?

a) An adhesive, impervious plastic, iodine-impregnated drape is wrapped over the incision site.
b) The limb is fed through a fenestration up to the sterile hand towels.
c) An impervious orthopedic stockinet is placed over the limb.
d) A large drape is fenestrated by cutting a 'cross' in the center of the drape to accommodate the limb.

Correct Answer: a) An adhesive, impervious plastic, iodine-impregnated drape is wrapped over the incision site.
Explanation: The adhesive, iodine-impregnated drape provides an additional sterile barrier over the incision site, crucial for preventing contamination during orthopedic procedures.

Question 65: In arthroscopic surgery, burs (or burrs) are:

a) Removed from the animal's coat before the procedure.
b) A type of forceps used to grasp and remove osteochondral chip fragments.
c) The pumps used to deliver fluids to the surgical site.
d) Often referred to as a motorized arthroplasty system.

Correct Answer: d) Often referred to as a motorized arthroplasty system.
Explanation: Motorized burs in arthroscopic surgery are used for precise bone shaping and removal, enhancing surgical accuracy and reducing damage to surrounding tissues.

Question 66: Sarcomas can arise from _____, whereas carcinomas can arise from _____.

a) Organs; cartilage
b) Mucous membranes; bone
c) Skin; connective tissue
d) Cartilage; lymph nodes

Correct Answer: d) Cartilage; lymph nodes
Explanation: Sarcomas originate from mesenchymal tissues like cartilage, whereas carcinomas derive from epithelial tissues, often spreading to lymph nodes and other organs.

Question 67: All horses in the United States should be vaccinated against:

a) Tetanus and influenza.
b) Eastern and Western equine and West Nile encephalomyelitis.
c) Heaves and tetanus.
d) Eastern and Western encephalitis and strangles.

Correct Answer: b) Eastern and Western equine and West Nile encephalomyelitis.
Explanation: Vaccination against these viruses is vital for equine health in the U.S., protecting against mosquito-borne diseases common in spring and summer months.

Question 68: Which of the following is not one of the three physical sterilization methods?

a) Heat
b) Radiation
c) Filtration
d) Water

Correct Answer: d) Water
Explanation: Physical sterilization methods include heat, radiation, and filtration, each effectively eliminating microorganisms without using chemical agents.

Question 69: Which of the following statements regarding automated hematology analyzers is not true?

a) Hematology analyzers use light scatter, impedance technology, and various staining methods to count and evaluate cells.
b) Special stains can be used to differentiate various cell populations.
c) Instrument settings for the size of each cell type are universal to all species.
d) Results are generally accurate, reproducible, and ready in a short period of time.

Correct Answer: c) Instrument settings for the size of each cell type are universal to all species.
Explanation: Hematology analyzers require species-specific settings to accurately measure cell sizes and types, as variations exist between different animal species.

Question 70: What covers the feet of horses to help decrease contamination in the surgical suite?

a) Obstetric sleeves
b) Sterile surgical tape

c) Paper booties
d) Fluid bags

Correct Answer: a) Obstetric sleeves
Explanation: Obstetric sleeves are used to cover horse hooves during surgery, minimizing the risk of contaminating the sterile field with dirt and bacteria.

Question 71: In some species, neutrophils are called _____ because of the intense staining of the granules.

a) Heterophils
b) Acanthocytes
c) Eccentrocytes
d) Metarubricytes

Correct Answer: a) Heterophils
Explanation: Heterophils, found in species like rabbits and birds, are similar to neutrophils but have intensely staining granules that help identify them under a microscope.

Question 72: Which of the following must always be supplemented to beef cattle feeding with pasture grasses?

a) Minerals
b) Energy in the form of grain
c) Fat
d) Protein

Correct Answer: a) Minerals
Explanation: Minerals are essential for cattle health, especially when grazing on pasture grasses, which may lack sufficient mineral content, requiring supplementation.

Question 73: Polydioxanone is a _____ suture material.

a) Synthetic nonabsorbable
b) Natural absorbable
c) Synthetic absorbable
d) Natural nonabsorbable

Correct Answer: c) Synthetic absorbable
Explanation: Polydioxanone is a commonly used synthetic absorbable suture known for its strength and gradual absorption, suitable for internal tissue repair.

Question 74: Which of the following is an example of a temporary surgical implant?

a) Drains
b) Wires
c) Ingesta
d) Screws

Correct Answer: a) Drains
Explanation: Drains are temporary surgical implants used to remove excess fluid from surgical sites, preventing infection and promoting healing.

Question 75: The position of a recumbent horse should be changed every ____ hours to help prevent the formation of decubital ulcers.

a) 2
b) 6
c) 4
d) 8

Correct Answer: b) 6
Explanation: Changing the position of a recumbent horse every 6 hours helps prevent pressure sores, ensuring blood flow and reducing the risk of tissue necrosis.

Question 76: Which part of the bovine reproductive tract is responsible for producing progesterone during pregnancy?

a) Ovaries
b) Uterus
c) Placenta
d) Corpus luteum

Correct Answer: d) Corpus luteum
Explanation: The corpus luteum forms on the ovary after ovulation and secretes progesterone, a hormone essential for maintaining pregnancy in cattle.

Question 77: Which of the following is a major cause of bloat in ruminants?

a) Excessive water intake
b) High-fat diets
c) Rapid fermentation of carbohydrates
d) Protein deficiency

Correct Answer: c) Rapid fermentation of carbohydrates
Explanation: Rapid fermentation of carbohydrates, especially from lush pastures or grain, produces excessive gas, leading to bloat, a life-threatening condition in ruminants.

Question 78: Which type of vaccine contains a virus that has been weakened so it cannot cause disease?

a) Killed vaccine
b) Recombinant vaccine
c) Toxoid vaccine
d) Modified live vaccine

Correct Answer: d) Modified live vaccine
Explanation: Modified live vaccines contain attenuated viruses that stimulate a strong immune response without causing the disease, providing effective protection.

Question 79: Which of the following is a zoonotic disease transmitted by ticks?

a) Canine distemper
b) Lyme disease
c) Feline leukemia
d) Parvovirus

Correct Answer: b) Lyme disease
Explanation: Lyme disease, caused by the bacterium Borrelia burgdorferi, is transmitted by ticks and can affect both animals and humans, necessitating tick control measures.

Question 80: Which type of suture pattern is best for closing skin incisions in a manner that allows for excellent apposition and minimal tension?

a) Interrupted horizontal mattress
b) Interrupted cruciate
c) Continuous subcuticular
d) Simple interrupted

Correct Answer: c) Continuous subcuticular

Explanation: Continuous subcuticular sutures provide excellent skin apposition, minimize tension, and result in a cosmetically pleasing incision closure, commonly used in various surgeries.

Question 81: Which method is commonly used for euthanizing small animals in a humane manner?

a) Drowning
b) Asphyxiation
c) Barbiturate overdose
d) Blunt force trauma

Correct Answer: c) Barbiturate overdose

Explanation: Barbiturate overdose, typically with intravenous pentobarbital, is a humane and rapid method for euthanizing small animals, ensuring minimal distress and pain.

Question 82: What is the primary purpose of the rumen in ruminants?

a) Digesting proteins
b) Absorbing water
c) Fermenting fibrous plant material
d) Producing bile

Correct Answer: c) Fermenting fibrous plant material

Explanation: The rumen houses microbes that ferment fibrous plant material, breaking down cellulose and providing ruminants with energy and essential nutrients.

Question 83: Which of the following is a common sign of metabolic acidosis in animals?

a) Hypoventilation
b) Bradycardia
c) Hyperventilation
d) Hypertension

Correct Answer: c) Hyperventilation

Explanation: Animals with metabolic acidosis often hyperventilate to compensate for increased acidity by expelling carbon dioxide, a volatile acid, from the bloodstream.

Question 84: Which of the following is a common cause of dystocia in cattle?

a) Uterine torsion
b) Anemia
c) Lameness
d) Hypocalcemia

Correct Answer: a) Uterine torsion

Explanation: Uterine torsion, a rotation of the uterus, can obstruct the birth canal, leading to dystocia, requiring prompt veterinary intervention to resolve.

Question 85: Which of the following is the most common nutritional deficiency in swine worldwide?

a) Vitamin C
b) Calcium
c) Iron
d) Vitamin D

Correct Answer: c) Iron

Explanation: Iron deficiency is common in piglets as they lack sufficient iron reserves and must be supplemented to prevent anemia and promote healthy growth.

Question 86: Which of the following is a clinical sign of hypothyroidism in dogs?

a) Weight loss
b) Increased appetite
c) Hyperactivity
d) Weight gain

Correct Answer: d) Weight gain
Explanation: Hypothyroidism in dogs often leads to weight gain due to a slow metabolism, along with lethargy and hair loss, requiring hormonal supplementation.

Question 87: Which of the following is a primary component of a balanced diet for adult dogs?

a) High fat content
b) Excessive carbohydrates
c) Adequate protein
d) Low fiber

Correct Answer: c) Adequate protein
Explanation: Adequate protein is essential for maintaining muscle mass and overall health in adult dogs, playing a key role in a balanced diet.

Question 88: Which disease is characterized by inflammation of the gums and supporting structures of the teeth in dogs and cats?

a) Gingivitis
b) Periodontal disease
c) Halitosis
d) Stomatitis

Correct Answer: b) Periodontal disease
Explanation: Periodontal disease involves inflammation of the gums and supporting tooth structures, leading to tooth loss if untreated, common in dogs and cats.

Question 89: Which of the following is a common cause of anemia in young puppies?

a) Parasitic infection
b) Excessive exercise
c) Overfeeding
d) Vitamin D deficiency

Correct Answer: a) Parasitic infection
Explanation: Parasitic infections, such as hookworms, can cause significant blood loss in young puppies, leading to anemia and requiring prompt treatment.

Question 90: Which of the following is a common sign of liver disease in cats?

a) Vomiting
b) Increased thirst
c) Jaundice
d) Seizures

Correct Answer: c) Jaundice
Explanation: Jaundice, or yellowing of the skin and eyes, is a common sign of liver disease in cats, indicative of bile accumulation due to liver dysfunction.

Question 91: Which of the following is a common cause of laminitis in horses?

a) Dehydration
b) High grain intake
c) Excessive salt intake
d) Protein deficiency

Correct Answer: b) High grain intake

Explanation: High grain intake can lead to laminitis in horses due to rapid fermentation and endotoxin release, causing inflammation and damage to the hoof structures.

Question 92: Which type of cell is primarily responsible for the immune response in animals?

a) Red blood cells
b) Platelets
c) Lymphocytes
d) Neurons

Correct Answer: c) Lymphocytes

Explanation: Lymphocytes, including B and T cells, are crucial for the adaptive immune response, identifying and neutralizing pathogens in the body.

Question 93: Which of the following is a common sign of dehydration in animals?

a) Increased appetite
b) Lethargy
c) Hyperactivity
d) Excessive urination

Correct Answer: b) Lethargy

Explanation: Lethargy, along with sunken eyes and dry mucous membranes, is a common indicator of dehydration, requiring prompt fluid replenishment.

Question 94: Which of the following is a common cause of colic in horses?

a) Excessive exercise
b) Sand ingestion
c) Protein deficiency
d) Vitamin overdose

Correct Answer: b) Sand ingestion

Explanation: Sand ingestion can lead to colic in horses by causing irritation and blockage in the gastrointestinal tract, necessitating careful management and prevention.

Question 95: Which of the following is a zoonotic disease transmitted by mosquitoes?

a) Lyme disease
b) West Nile virus
c) Feline leukemia
d) Distemper

Correct Answer: b) West Nile virus

Explanation: West Nile virus is a zoonotic disease spread by mosquitoes, capable of infecting birds, horses, and humans, emphasizing the need for vector control.

Question 96: Which of the following is a common cause of hypocalcemia in lactating dairy cows?

a) Excessive grain intake
b) Lack of exercise
c) Low dietary calcium
d) High fiber diet

Correct Answer: c) Low dietary calcium

Explanation: Lactating dairy cows with insufficient calcium intake can develop hypocalcemia, impacting milk production and cow health, often addressed with calcium supplementation.

Question 97: Which of the following is a common sign of heart failure in dogs?

a) Weight gain
b) Increased appetite
c) Coughing
d) Seizures

Correct Answer: c) Coughing
Explanation: Coughing, particularly at night, is a common sign of heart failure in dogs, resulting from fluid accumulation in the lungs due to poor heart function.

Question 98: Which of the following is a common cause of urinary tract infections in cats?

a) High grain diet
b) Obesity
c) Dehydration
d) High protein diet

Correct Answer: c) Dehydration
Explanation: Dehydration can lead to concentrated urine, increasing the risk of urinary tract infections in cats, underscoring the importance of adequate water intake.

Question 99: Which of the following is a common cause of hypothyroidism in dogs?

a) Autoimmune disease
b) Trauma
c) High-fat diet
d) Excessive exercise

Correct Answer: a) Autoimmune disease
Explanation: Autoimmune thyroiditis is a leading cause of hypothyroidism in dogs, where the immune system attacks the thyroid gland, reducing hormone production.

Question 100: Which of the following is a common sign of diabetes mellitus in cats?

a) Weight gain
b) Increased thirst
c) Lethargy
d) Hair loss

Correct Answer: b) Increased thirst
Explanation: Increased thirst, along with frequent urination and weight loss, is a hallmark of diabetes mellitus in cats, resulting from elevated blood glucose levels.

Question 101: Which of the following is a common cause of anemia in cats?

a) Kidney disease
b) Excessive exercise
c) Overfeeding
d) Vitamin C deficiency

Correct Answer: a) Kidney disease
Explanation: Kidney disease can lead to anemia in cats due to reduced erythropoietin production, a hormone necessary for red blood cell production.

Question 103: As you review the nursing care plan for Sparky, a rabbit, the data you encounter will contain:

a) Information about implementation of the patient's actual assessment or examination needs.
b) The veterinarian's list of orders related to his or her diagnosis.
c) Information about interventions specific to your own evaluation of Sparky.
d) The SOAP format.

Correct Answer: c) Information about interventions specific to your own evaluation of Sparky.
Explanation: A nursing care plan is a personalized document that outlines specific interventions based on the technician's evaluation of the patient, ensuring tailored care and treatment.

Question 104: The ST segment indicates the _____ repolarization.

a) Time interval from ventricular depolarization to
b) Positive ventricular
c) Negative ventricular
d) Biphasic ventricular

Correct Answer: a) Time interval from ventricular depolarization to
Explanation: The ST segment on an ECG represents the time from ventricular depolarization to repolarization, crucial for diagnosing heart conditions like ischemia or infarction.

Question 105: A modified Wright or Wright-Giemsa stain:

a) Is of lower quality than most commercially available quick stains.
b) Has the advantage that the stain itself is not permanent.
c) Is very expensive but essential for detection of cutaneous mast cell tumors.
d) Will stain mast cell granules and granules in some lymphocytes purple.

Correct Answer: d) Will stain mast cell granules and granules in some lymphocytes purple.
Explanation: Modified Wright or Wright-Giemsa stain is essential in veterinary cytology for identifying mast cell tumors and certain lymphocytes by staining granules purple.

Question 106: All of the following can contribute to wound dehiscence and evisceration except:

a) Drug therapy.
b) Tension on the incision line.
c) Surgical débridement.
d) Using inappropriate suture material to close the wound.

Correct Answer: c) Surgical débridement.
Explanation: Surgical débridement is a controlled process of removing necrotic tissue to promote healing, unlike factors such as tension and inappropriate sutures that can cause wound complications.

Question 107: Cerebrospinal (CSF) fluid from a horse is collected at the:

a) Cervical thoracic junction.
b) Sacrococcygeal junction.
c) Lumbosacral space.
d) Atlantooccipital space.

Correct Answer: c) Lumbosacral space
Explanation: Collecting CSF from the lumbosacral space is preferred in horses for diagnosing spinal cord diseases, offering a safe approach under sedation.

Question 108: A small dog is brought into the clinic by his owner because he is exhibiting _____, a symptom identified as stridor.

a) Excessive, continual sneezing
b) High-pitched inspiratory wheezing
c) Loud snorting sounds
d) Loud snoring with apnea

Correct Answer: b) High-pitched inspiratory wheezing
Explanation: Stridor is characterized by a high-pitched wheezing sound during inspiration, often indicating an upper airway obstruction requiring prompt evaluation.

Question 109: Surgical catgut is a _____ suture material.

a) Natural absorbable
b) Synthetic nonabsorbable
c) Synthetic absorbable
d) Natural nonabsorbable

Correct Answer: a) Natural absorbable
Explanation: Catgut, derived from animal intestines, is a natural absorbable suture material commonly used for internal suturing due to its biodegradability.

Question 110: Which of the following practices helps ensure adequate steam penetration in the autoclave?

a) Stacking packs on top of each other
b) Leaving less than 2 cm of space between packs and between the packs and autoclave walls
c) Keeping the pack size smaller than 30 cm by 30 cm by 50 cm
d) Keeping the pack weight below 5 kg

Correct Answer: c) Keeping the pack size smaller than 30 cm by 30 cm by 50 cm
Explanation: Limiting the size of packs helps ensure even steam penetration during autoclaving, critical for achieving effective sterilization.

Question 111: Because the power equipment you need to sterilize cannot tolerate the high temperatures or steam associated with autoclaving, you are choosing to use gas sterilization with:

a) Glutaraldehyde.
b) Iodine.
c) Phenolic.
d) Ethylene oxide.

Correct Answer: d) Ethylene oxide.
Explanation: Ethylene oxide is a gaseous sterilant used for heat-sensitive equipment, ensuring sterilization without damaging delicate instruments.

Question 112: Gloved hands may be rested on a sterile drape or clasped in front of the body in the zone between the _____ and _____.

a) Armpits; waist
b) Shoulders; waist
c) Shoulders; hips
d) Chin; waist

Correct Answer: b) Shoulders; waist
Explanation: Maintaining gloved hands between the shoulders and waist prevents contamination, preserving the sterile field essential in surgical environments.

Question 113: Guttural pouch mycosis is caused by a:

a) Virus.
b) Bacteria.
c) Fungus.
d) Prion.

Correct Answer: c) Fungus
Explanation: Guttural pouch mycosis in horses is typically caused by Aspergillus species, a fungal infection that can result in severe complications if untreated.

Question 114: Trichuris vulpis of the dog, fox, and coyote can be found in the:

a) Small intestine.
b) Stomach.

c) Cecum.
d) Right ventricle and pulmonary arteries.

Correct Answer: c) Cecum.
Explanation: Trichuris vulpis, the whipworm, resides in the cecum and colon, where it can cause gastrointestinal disturbances and requires appropriate antiparasitic treatment.

Question 115: _____ are the predominant type of circulating cell in cattle, sheep, and goats.

a) Monocytes
b) Basophils
c) Lymphocytes
d) Mast cells

Correct Answer: c) Lymphocytes
Explanation: Lymphocytes dominate the circulating leukocyte population in ruminants, playing a key role in adaptive immunity and infection response.

Question 116: Which of the following is true regarding the impact of disease on pharmacokinetics?

a) Geriatric patients commonly have an increased hepatic metabolism.
b) Cardiovascular disease increases the risk of toxicity to the heart and brain due to increased blood distribution to those organs.
c) Kidney disease or failure interferes with the pharmacokinetics of a drug when frequent urination rapidly expels the drug from the body.
d) The gastrointestinal tract of a geriatric patient absorbs drugs more quickly than that of a young patient.

Correct Answer: b) Cardiovascular disease increases the risk of toxicity to the heart and brain due to increased blood distribution to those organs.
Explanation: In cardiovascular disease, altered blood flow can enhance drug delivery to vital organs, potentially increasing toxicity risks, requiring dose adjustments.

Question 117: Which of the following is an example of an isotonic crystalloid solution used in veterinary medicine?

a) 5% Dextrose in water
b) Lactated Ringer's solution
c) Hypertonic saline
d) 3% Dextrose in saline

Correct Answer: b) Lactated Ringer's solution
Explanation: Lactated Ringer's solution is an isotonic crystalloid commonly used for rehydration and electrolyte balance in veterinary patients, mimicking plasma composition.

Question 118: Which of the following is a zoonotic disease caused by a protozoan parasite?

a) Canine distemper
b) Toxoplasmosis
c) Feline leukemia
d) Parvovirus

Correct Answer: b) Toxoplasmosis
Explanation: Toxoplasmosis, caused by Toxoplasma gondii, is a zoonotic protozoan infection, often transmitted through undercooked meat or cat feces, posing risks to humans.

Question 119: Which of the following is a common cause of regurgitation in dogs?

a) Gastric ulcer
b) Esophageal obstruction

c) Intestinal blockage
d) Pancreatitis

Correct Answer: b) Esophageal obstruction
Explanation: Esophageal obstruction, due to foreign bodies or strictures, can lead to regurgitation, requiring diagnostic imaging and intervention for resolution.

Question 120: Which of the following is a common sign of hyperthyroidism in cats?

a) Weight gain
b) Increased appetite
c) Lethargy
d) Hair loss

Correct Answer: b) Increased appetite
Explanation: Hyperthyroidism in cats often presents with increased appetite and weight loss due to elevated metabolic rates from excessive thyroid hormone production.

Question 121: Which of the following is a common cause of cough in horses?

a) Lungworm infestation
b) Laminitis
c) Colic
d) Navicular disease

Correct Answer: a) Lungworm infestation
Explanation: Lungworm infestation in horses can cause respiratory symptoms including coughing, necessitating antiparasitic treatment and environmental management.

Question 122: Which of the following is a common cause of hypoglycemia in dogs?

a) Obesity
b) Excessive carbohydrate intake
c) Insulin overdose
d) High protein diet

Correct Answer: c) Insulin overdose
Explanation: Insulin overdose in diabetic dogs can lead to hypoglycemia, characterized by weakness and seizures, requiring immediate glucose administration.

Question 123: Which of the following is a common cause of pruritus in cats?

a) Hypercalcemia
b) Flea allergy dermatitis
c) Hypothyroidism
d) Hypernatremia

Correct Answer: b) Flea allergy dermatitis
Explanation: Flea allergy dermatitis is a prevalent cause of pruritus in cats, resulting from hypersensitivity to flea saliva, necessitating flea control measures.

Question 124: Which of the following is a common cause of seizures in dogs?

a) Hypothyroidism
b) Epilepsy
c) Hyperkalemia
d) Hyperglycemia

Correct Answer: b) Epilepsy
Explanation: Epilepsy is a frequent cause of seizures in dogs, requiring medical management to control seizure activity and improve quality of life.

Question 125: Which of the following is a common sign of kidney disease in cats?

a) Increased appetite
b) Decreased thirst
c) Increased urination
d) Weight gain

Correct Answer: c) Increased urination
Explanation: Increased urination and thirst are indicative of kidney disease in cats due to impaired kidney function, necessitating dietary and medical management.

Question 126: Which of the following is a common cause of pancreatitis in dogs?

a) Low-fat diet
b) High protein intake
c) High-fat diet
d) High fiber intake

Correct Answer: c) High-fat diet
Explanation: A high-fat diet can trigger pancreatitis in dogs, characterized by inflammation of the pancreas and requiring dietary modification and supportive care.

Question 127: Which of the following is a common sign of anemia in dogs?

a) Jaundice
b) Hyperactivity
c) Pale mucous membranes
d) Weight gain

Correct Answer: c) Pale mucous membranes
Explanation: Pale mucous membranes in dogs suggest anemia, due to reduced red blood cells or hemoglobin, necessitating diagnostic evaluation and treatment.

Question 128: Which of the following is a common cause of feline lower urinary tract disease (FLUTD)?

a) Hyperthyroidism
b) Obesity
c) Urinary crystals
d) Hepatic lipidosis

Correct Answer: c) Urinary crystals
Explanation: Urinary crystals contribute to FLUTD, causing irritation and blockage in cats, requiring dietary management and increased water intake.

Question 129: Which of the following is a common sign of respiratory distress in horses?

a) Weight gain
b) Lethargy
c) Nasal flaring
d) Increased appetite

Correct Answer: c) Nasal flaring
Explanation: Nasal flaring in horses indicates respiratory distress, often accompanied by labored breathing, necessitating prompt veterinary assessment.

Question 130: Which of the following is a common cause of hypercalcemia in dogs?

a) Hyperparathyroidism
b) Hypothyroidism

c) Diabetes mellitus
d) Anemia

Correct Answer: a) Hyperparathyroidism
Explanation: Hyperparathyroidism leads to elevated calcium levels in dogs, often due to parathyroid gland tumors, requiring surgical intervention or medical management.

Question 131: Which of the following is a common cause of vomiting in cats?

a) Dental disease
b) Hairballs
c) Hyperthyroidism
d) Diabetes mellitus

Correct Answer: b) Hairballs
Explanation: Hairballs, resulting from grooming, are a frequent cause of vomiting in cats, often managed with dietary adjustments and grooming.

Question 132: Which of the following is a common sign of congestive heart failure in dogs?

a) Hyperactivity
b) Coughing
c) Increased appetite
d) Weight loss

Correct Answer: b) Coughing
Explanation: Coughing, especially at night, is a common sign of congestive heart failure in dogs, due to fluid accumulation in the lungs, requiring medical intervention.

Question 133: Which of the following is a common cause of diarrhea in adult horses?

a) Sand colic
b) Obesity
c) Laminitis
d) Navicular disease

Correct Answer: a) Sand colic
Explanation: Sand colic, caused by ingestion of sand, leads to diarrhea and colic in horses, necessitating management strategies to reduce sand intake.

Question 134: Which of the following is a common cause of dermatitis in dogs?

a) Hypocalcemia
b) Atopic dermatitis
c) Hyperglycemia
d) Hyperthyroidism

Correct Answer: b) Atopic dermatitis
Explanation: Atopic dermatitis, an allergic skin condition, is a frequent cause of itching and inflammation in dogs, requiring allergy testing and management.

Question 135: Which of the following is a common sign of liver disease in dogs?

a) Increased energy
b) Jaundice
c) Hyperactivity
d) Weight gain

Correct Answer: b) Jaundice
Explanation: Jaundice, or yellowing of the skin and eyes, indicates liver dysfunction in dogs, requiring diagnostic evaluation and supportive care.

Question 136: Which of the following is a common cause of lameness in horses?

a) Dental disease
b) Laminitis
c) Colic
d) Hyperthyroidism

Correct Answer: b) Laminitis
Explanation: Laminitis, inflammation of the hoof tissues, is a common cause of lameness in horses, often linked to dietary factors and requiring prompt treatment.

Question 137: Which of the following is a common cause of ear infections in dogs?

a) Excessive bathing
b) Hypothyroidism
c) Hyperactivity
d) Allergies

Correct Answer: d) Allergies
Explanation: Allergies often lead to ear infections in dogs, causing inflammation and discharge, necessitating allergy identification and management.

Question 138: Which of the following is a common sign of feline infectious peritonitis (FIP)?

a) Increased appetite
b) Weight gain
c) Fluid accumulation in the abdomen
d) Hyperactivity

Correct Answer: c) Fluid accumulation in the abdomen
Explanation: FIP in cats is characterized by fluid buildup in the abdomen or chest, often with fever and lethargy, requiring supportive care.

Question 139: Which of the following is a common cause of obesity in cats?

a) High protein diet
b) Lack of exercise
c) Hyperthyroidism
d) Diabetes mellitus

Correct Answer: b) Lack of exercise
Explanation: Sedentary lifestyles and excessive calorie intake contribute to obesity in cats, necessitating dietary management and increased physical activity.

Question 140: Which of the following is a common cause of abscesses in cats?

a) Dental disease
b) Flea bites
c) Feline leukemia
d) Bite wounds

Correct Answer: d) Bite wounds
Explanation: Bite wounds from fights often lead to abscess formation in cats, requiring drainage and antibiotic treatment to prevent infection.

Question 141: Which of the following is a common sign of hyperadrenocorticism (Cushing's disease) in dogs?

a) Weight loss
b) Increased thirst

c) Hyperactivity
d) Lethargy

Correct Answer: b) Increased thirst
Explanation: Cushing's disease in dogs often presents with increased thirst and urination, due to excessive cortisol production, necessitating medical management.

Question 142: Which of the following is a common cause of constipation in cats?

a) Dehydration
b) Hyperactivity
c) Dental disease
d) Hyperthyroidism

Correct Answer: a) Dehydration
Explanation: Dehydration leads to constipation in cats by causing dry, hard stools, requiring increased fluid intake and dietary adjustments.

Question 143: Which of the following is a common sign of pyometra in dogs?

a) Increased energy
b) Decreased thirst
c) Vaginal discharge
d) Weight gain

Correct Answer: c) Vaginal discharge
Explanation: Pyometra, a uterine infection, often presents with purulent vaginal discharge in dogs, requiring surgical intervention for resolution.

Question 144: Which of the following is a common cause of respiratory distress in birds?

a) Feather plucking
b) Aspergillosis
c) Egg binding
d) Obesity

Correct Answer: b) Aspergillosis
Explanation: Aspergillosis, a fungal infection, causes respiratory distress in birds, necessitating antifungal treatment and environmental management.

Question 146: When selecting a cuff to measure a cat's or dog's blood pressure indirectly, the _____ of the cuff should be approximately _____ of the circumference of the limb at the site of cuff placement.

a) length; 40%
b) diameter; 30%
c) width; 40%
d) circumference; 30%

Correct Answer: c) width; 40%
Explanation: The width of a blood pressure cuff should be about 40% of the limb circumference where it is placed. This ensures accurate blood pressure readings by providing proper fit and occlusion.

Question 147: As a general rule of thumb, the PaO2 should be approximately _____ times the FiO2.

a) 250
b) 10
c) 3
d) 5

Correct Answer: d) 5

Explanation: PaO2 (partial pressure of oxygen in arterial blood) is typically five times the FiO2 (fraction of inspired oxygen) under normal physiological conditions, aiding in assessing a patient's oxygenation status.

Question 148: The veterinarian suspects a horse has a Salmonella infection. To detect this, you collect a total of _____ fecal samples for culture at least _____ hours between samplings.

a) three; 12
b) three; 24
c) six; 24
d) five; 12

Correct Answer: d) five; 12

Explanation: To accurately diagnose Salmonella, five fecal samples are collected at 12-hour intervals, as intermittent shedding can make detection challenging.

Question 149: In preparation for a vaginal examination on a cow with dystocia, which of the following is not true?

a) Some veterinarians prefer to begin by cleaning out the rectum.
b) It is imperative to clean the perineal area before the rectal portion of the examination.
c) The perineal scrub will decrease uterine and vaginal contamination.
d) The perineal scrub is not intended to achieve asepsis.

Correct Answer: b) It is imperative to clean the perineal area before the rectal portion of the examination.

Explanation: In practice, the perineal area should ideally be cleaned after a rectal exam to avoid contamination. The scrub reduces contamination but does not achieve full asepsis.

Question 150: The average heart rate (HR) (in beats per minute) can be calculated by counting the number of:

a) P waves in a predetermined time period and multiplying by the number of QRS complexes.
b) Millimeters between two R waves and dividing into 3000 at 50 mm/sec paper speed.
c) Millimeters between two R waves and dividing into 1500 at 25 mm/sec paper speed.
d) QRS complexes in a predetermined time period and multiplying by a specific factor.

Correct Answer: d) QRS complexes in a predetermined time period and multiplying by a specific factor.

Explanation: Calculating heart rate involves counting QRS complexes over a set time, then multiplying by a factor to extrapolate beats per minute, ensuring accurate cardiac assessment.

Question 151: Variation in the PR interval may occur with:

a) Left atrial enlargement.
b) Right atrial enlargement.
c) Right ventricular enlargement.
d) Atrioventricular dissociation.

Correct Answer: d) Atrioventricular dissociation.

Explanation: Atrioventricular dissociation can cause PR interval variation, indicating asynchronous atrial and ventricular contractions, which requires further cardiac evaluation.

Question 152: A Rouleaux formulation:

a) Is normal in horses and often shows RBCs appearing like stacked coins.
b) Indicates anemia in cats and shows RBCs clumped together irregularly.
c) Most commonly occurs in dogs with immune-mediated hemolytic anemia.
d) Is a false platelet count.

Correct Answer: a) Is normal in horses and often shows RBCs appearing like stacked coins.
Explanation: Rouleaux formation, where RBCs stack like coins, is physiologically normal in horses and some other species, aiding in hematological assessments.

Question 153: As you monitor your postsurgical patient, you are aware that packed cell volume (PCV) and total protein (TP) values can drop up to _____ due to anesthesia and surgery, even if no blood loss occurs.

a) 20%
b) 10%
c) 15%
d) 35%

Correct Answer: b) 10%
Explanation: Post-surgery, a 10% drop in PCV and TP is expected due to fluid shifts and dilution, even without blood loss, aiding in postoperative monitoring.

Question 154: Increased serum _____ is a normal physiologic response in the fasted horse.

a) Gamma-glutamyl transferase
b) Sorbitol dehydrogenase
c) Bilirubin
d) Creatine phosphokinase

Correct Answer: c) Bilirubin
Explanation: Fasting increases serum bilirubin in horses, a normal physiological response, not indicative of liver disease, essential in interpreting lab results.

Question 155: In the process known as malignant transformation, an initiated cell undergoes mutations caused by an agent or event that stimulate proliferation of the cell to grow into a neoplasm. This stage is called:

a) Promotion.
b) Progression.
c) Initiation.
d) Proliferation.

Correct Answer: a) Promotion.
Explanation: Promotion is the stage where an initiated cell proliferates due to external stimuli, critical in cancer development, emphasizing the need for preventive measures.

Question 156: The classic signs of gastric dilation volvulus (GDV) include all of the following except:

a) Retching.
b) Straining to defecate.
c) Bloating.
d) Vomiting.

Correct Answer: b) Straining to defecate.
Explanation: GDV is marked by bloating, retching, and vomiting due to stomach torsion, but not straining to defecate, aiding in differential diagnosis.

Question 157: Hypoalbuminemia may develop from loss through:

a) The gastrointestinal tract.
b) Decreased production due to liver failure.
c) The kidney.
d) All of the above.

Correct Answer: d) All of the above.
Explanation: Hypoalbuminemia results from losses via the GI tract or kidneys, or decreased hepatic production, crucial for diagnosing underlying conditions.

Question 158: Which of the following bacteria is most likely associated with the gangrenous form of mastitis in sheep and goats?

a) Pasteurella haemolytica
b) Pseudomonas
c) Streptococcus
d) Staphylococcus aureus

Correct Answer: d) Staphylococcus aureus
Explanation: Staphylococcus aureus causes gangrenous mastitis in small ruminants, a severe condition requiring prompt veterinary intervention.

Question 159: Anisocytosis can be determined using _____ as a mathematical index.

a) MCH
b) Hgb
c) MCV
d) RDW

Correct Answer: d) RDW
Explanation: RDW, the red cell distribution width, quantifies anisocytosis, reflecting RBC size variability, useful in diagnosing anemia types.

Question 160: Acute laminitis may be due to sudden excess ingestion of _____, or secondary to other diseases, which occur during the _____ period.

a) Mycotoxins; neonatal
b) Grain; postparturient
c) Salt; postparturient
d) Calcium; neonatal

Correct Answer: b) Grain; postparturient
Explanation: Acute laminitis often follows excessive grain intake or diseases in the postparturient period, emphasizing dietary management in prevention.

Question 161: Feeding inadequate forages with little or no grain can create a deficiency of usable _____ during the last trimester of pregnancy in ewes carrying twins or triplets and can lead to _____ and _____ in the mother.

a) Protein; paralysis; coma
b) Carbohydrates; abortion; paralysis
c) Carbohydrates; paralysis; coma
d) Protein; abortion; paralysis

Correct Answer: c) Carbohydrates; paralysis; coma
Explanation: Lack of carbohydrates during late pregnancy in ewes can cause metabolic disorders, resulting in paralysis and coma, highlighting nutritional needs.

Question 162: After performing CPCR on a dog, the animal develops opisthotonus with rigidity in all four limbs. Where is the lesion, and what is the prognosis?

a) Intervertebral disk; fair
b) Brainstem; grave
c) Brainstem; fair
d) Cerebrum; poor

Correct Answer: b) Brainstem; grave
Explanation: Opisthotonus post-CPCR suggests a brainstem lesion with a grave prognosis, indicating severe neurological damage requiring immediate attention.

Question 163: You and your colleagues attend a lecture on the _____ of a disease to which animals in your patient's farming community have been exposed recently. This particular lecture, then, gives you increased understanding of the mechanism for the development of this particular disease.

a) Pathology
b) Histopathology
c) Etiology
d) Pathogenesis

Correct Answer: d) Pathogenesis
Explanation: Understanding pathogenesis provides insight into the disease development process, essential for effective intervention and treatment planning.

Question 164: Pregnant broodmares should be vaccinated for _____ to prevent abortion caused by this disease.

a) Botulism
b) Potomac horse fever
c) Rabies
d) Equine herpesvirus infection

Correct Answer: d) Equine herpesvirus infection
Explanation: Vaccination against equine herpesvirus prevents abortion in broodmares, a vital measure in reproductive health management.

Question 165: You are in charge of training personnel for the new isolation ward of your veterinary hospital. Your coverage of diseases will most likely include a thorough discussion of:

a) Heaves, strangles, and colitis.
b) Heaves, EHV-1, and influenza.
c) Colitis, neurologic EHV-1, and strangles.
d) Strangles, heaves, and colitis.

Correct Answer: c) Colitis, neurologic EHV-1, and strangles.
Explanation: Isolation protocols in veterinary hospitals focus on highly contagious diseases like colitis, neurologic EHV-1, and strangles to prevent outbreaks.

Question 166: You are attempting to calibrate a microscope. Starting on low power (10´ magnification), you focus on the 2-mm line on the stage micrometer and then rotate the eyepiece so that the hash-mark scale is parallel to the stage micrometer scale, aligning the zero point on both scales. Now you notice that the 0.125-mm mark aligns with the "10" hash mark on the eyepiece. What is the distance between each hash mark on the eyepiece?

a) 0.125 μm
b) 1.25 μm
c) 0.0125 μm
d) 12.5 μm

Correct Answer: d) 12.5 μm
Explanation: Aligning the micrometer scales reveals each hash on the eyepiece is 12.5 μm, aiding precise measurements, crucial in microscopic analysis.

Question 167: Adult pentastomes are always associated with infecting the _____ of the host.

a) Respiratory system
b) Cardiovascular system

c) Mesenchymal tissues
d) Digestive system

Correct Answer: a) Respiratory system
Explanation: Adult pentastomes primarily infect the respiratory system, including snakes and reptiles, necessitating specific management strategies for affected hosts.

Question 168: In the QRS complex, a tall R wave indicates:

a) Ectopic atrial activation.
b) Left ventricular enlargement.
c) Right ventricular enlargement.
d) Myocardial ischemia.

Correct Answer: b) Left ventricular enlargement.
Explanation: A tall R wave in the QRS complex suggests left ventricular enlargement, important in diagnosing cardiac conditions in veterinary patients.

Question 169: Serum enzymes cannot be used to detect:

a) Drug overdose.
b) Muscle damage.
c) Cholestasis.
d) Hepatocellular injury.

Correct Answer: a) Drug overdose.
Explanation: Serum enzymes reflect liver and muscle conditions but do not indicate drug overdose, requiring alternative diagnostic approaches.

Question 170: _____ result from antibody binding to the RBC surface and removal of a portion of the membrane by macrophages; this occurs in immune hemolytic anemia (IHA), which is most commonly recognized in dogs.

a) Acanthocytes
b) Leptocytes
c) Spherocytes
d) Echinocytes

Correct Answer: c) Spherocytes
Explanation: Spherocytes, altered RBCs from antibody action in IHA, are key in diagnosing hemolytic anemias, especially in dogs, guiding treatment plans.

Full Test 5 with Detailed Explanations

Question 1: Joint supplements are used more commonly in _____ than in any other species.

a) horses
b) dogs
c) camelids
d) cattle

Correct Answer: a) horses
Explanation: Horses frequently experience joint stress due to their size and activity levels, making joint supplements and chondroprotective agents popular for maintaining joint health.

Question 2: Normal serum from horses should be:

a) reddish colored
b) pink and milky
c) clear and colorless
d) light yellow

Correct Answer: d) light yellow
Explanation: The light yellow color of horse serum is due to the presence of bilirubin, which is normal, as opposed to the clearer serum found in dogs and cats.

Question 3: Which of the following is a pair of heavy operating scissors with a straight or curved blade used to cut tough tissue?

a) Lister scissors
b) Metzenbaum scissors
c) Bard-Parker scissors
d) Mayo scissors

Correct Answer: d) Mayo scissors
Explanation: Mayo scissors are robust instruments designed for cutting dense tissues like fascia, making them essential in surgical procedures.

Question 4: Another name for nucleated RBCs is:

a) eccentrocytes
b) Heinz bodies
c) metarubricytes
d) Howell Jolly bodies

Correct Answer: c) metarubricytes
Explanation: Metarubricytes, or nucleated RBCs, are immature red blood cells seen in certain conditions, indicating bone marrow response or stress.

Question 5: Taper needles are most commonly used to pierce _____ tissue.

a) muscle, tendon, and ligament
b) skin, sinus, and cartilage
c) intestinal, subcutaneous, and fascia
d) brain, liver, and kidney

Correct Answer: c) intestinal, subcutaneous, and fascia
Explanation: Taper needles are preferred for soft tissues like intestines and fascia to minimize trauma, spreading tissue rather than cutting.

Question 6: Which of the following statements concerning transduction is most accurate?

a) Transduction is the conversion of energy into electrical impulses in specialized nerve endings in response to pain that exceeds the nociceptor's threshold.
b) Transduction is the conduction of nerve impulses from the nociceptor to the thalamus.
c) Transduction involves the conduction of a painful sensation to a nerve cell located entirely within the central nervous system (CNS) that activates sympathetic reflexes.
d) Transduction is the process of carrying a pain nerve impulse along peripheral nerves to the spinal cord.

Correct Answer: a) Transduction is the conversion of energy into electrical impulses in specialized nerve endings in response to pain that exceeds the nociceptor's threshold.
Explanation: Transduction involves converting noxious stimuli into nerve impulses, a critical first step in the pain pathway.

Question 7: _____ is a CNS disease that results from an underlying defect in thiamine metabolism.

a) Polioencephalomalacia
b) Gangrenous mastitis
c) Agammaglobulinemia
d) Keratoconjunctivitis

Correct Answer: a) Polioencephalomalacia
Explanation: Polioencephalomalacia is caused by thiamine deficiency, leading to neurological symptoms, and requires prompt treatment with thiamine supplementation.

Question 8: How many major canine blood groups have been identified?

Correct Answer: 8
Explanation: Canine blood groups, such as DEA 1.1 and others, are crucial for transfusion compatibility to prevent adverse reactions.

Question 9: Optimal temperature for housing most mammals and birds is?

Correct Answer: 65-84 degrees F
Explanation: Maintaining an ambient temperature between 65-84°F ensures comfort and health in mammals and birds, preventing temperature-related stress.

Question 10: In dogs and cats, the blood chemistry tests most commonly used to evaluate liver function are?

Correct Answer: alanine transaminase and aspartate aminotransferase
Explanation: ALT and AST are key liver enzymes measured to assess liver health and function in small animals, indicating liver cell damage.

Question 11: Potentiated penicillins?

Correct Answer: are active against B-lactamase-producing bacteria
Explanation: Potentiated penicillins, combined with B-lactamase inhibitors, enhance antibiotic efficacy against resistant bacterial strains.

Question 12: Correct term for an increased leukocyte count not due to cancer?

Correct Answer: leukocytosis
Explanation: Leukocytosis refers to elevated white blood cell count, often indicative of infection or inflammation, distinct from leukemic processes.

Question 13: Cholinergic agents do all of the following except?

a) Cause peripheral vasodilation
b) Increase gastrointestinal motility
c) Induce salivation
d) Cause miosis

Correct Answer: a) Cause peripheral vasodilation
Explanation: Cholinergic agents enhance parasympathetic activity, increasing secretions and motility, but do not cause vasodilation, a sympathetic response.

Question 14: Not a sign of fluid volume overload?

a) Edema
b) Hypertension
c) Tachycardia
d) Dry mucous membranes

Correct Answer: d) Dry mucous membranes
Explanation: Dry mucous membranes indicate dehydration, whereas fluid overload presents with edema, hypertension, and possible tachycardia.

Question 15: You regularly order 6 10-ml vials per month of a drug that has a concentration of 50mg/ml. Now that same drug is available in only 20ml vials of 10mg/ml. How many vials should you order this month to get the same total amount of drug?

Correct Answer: 15 vials
Explanation: Previously, 3000mg were obtained monthly (6 vials x 10ml x 50mg/ml). With the new concentration (20ml x 10mg/ml = 200mg/vial), 15 vials are needed to match the 3000mg.

Question 16: Causative agent of Tyzzer disease?

Correct Answer: Clostridium piliforme
Explanation: Clostridium piliforme causes Tyzzer's disease, primarily affecting rodents, and requires specific diagnosis and management strategies.

Question 17: Which situation would the vet definitely not be held liable for damages?

a) An animal dies due to a surgical error.
b) An animal contracts an infection from unsterile equipment.
c) A medication error leads to adverse effects.
d) An animal dies as a result of the client's not following written directions relating to treatment.

Correct Answer: d) An animal dies as a result of the client's not following written directions relating to treatment.
Explanation: Veterinarians are not liable when clients fail to follow prescribed care instructions, highlighting the importance of client compliance.

Question 18: How many muscle heads are in the canine triceps brachii group?

Correct Answer: 3
Explanation: The canine triceps brachii comprises three heads: the long, lateral, and medial, essential for forelimb extension.

Question 19: In goats, night blindness, poor appetite, weight loss, unthrifty appearance with a poor hair coat, and a thick nasal discharge have resulted from a lack of vitamin?

Correct Answer: A
Explanation: Vitamin A deficiency in goats leads to night blindness and poor health, emphasizing the need for balanced nutrition.

Question 20: When clients are instructed to bring in a fecal sample, how much are they told to collect?

Correct Answer: 1-2 teaspoons
Explanation: A small fecal amount (1-2 teaspoons) suffices for diagnostic testing, ensuring accuracy without overwhelming laboratory processes.

Question 21: In radiography, the term "mAs" refers to?

a) Milliampere-seconds, which control the quantity of X-ray photons produced.
b) Maximum allowable seconds for exposure.
c) Minimum acceptable sensitivity of the film.
d) Measurement of absorbed scatter.

Correct Answer: a) Milliampere-seconds, which control the quantity of X-ray photons produced.
Explanation: "mAs" in radiography refers to milliampere-seconds, determining the number of X-ray photons, crucial for image quality and exposure.

Question 22: The primary function of the cerebellum is?

a) Regulating emotions.
b) Coordination of voluntary movements.
c) Processing auditory information.
d) Controlling cardiovascular function.

Correct Answer: b) Coordination of voluntary movements.

Explanation: The cerebellum coordinates voluntary movements, ensuring smooth, balanced motor activity, vital for normal physical function.

Question 23: Which of the following is not a common symptom of hyperthyroidism in cats?

a) Weight gain
b) Increased appetite
c) Hyperactivity
d) Increased thirst

Correct Answer: a) Weight gain

Explanation: Hyperthyroid cats usually experience weight loss despite increased appetite and hyperactivity, contrasting with hypothyroid weight gain.

Question 24: A dog presents with a sudden onset of paralysis in the hind limbs. Which condition is most likely?

a) Intervertebral disc disease
b) Hip dysplasia
c) Osteoarthritis
d) Patellar luxation

Correct Answer: a) Intervertebral disc disease

Explanation: Sudden hind limb paralysis in dogs often indicates intervertebral disc disease, requiring urgent veterinary intervention.

Question 25: What is the normal gestation period for a domestic cat?

a) 58-65 days
b) 70-75 days
c) 40-50 days
d) 80-85 days

Correct Answer: a) 58-65 days

Explanation: The normal gestation period for cats is 58-65 days, essential for planning breeding and anticipating kitten births.

Question 26: Which parasite is known for causing "walking dandruff" in animals?

a) Sarcoptes scabiei
b) Cheyletiella spp.
c) Demodex canis
d) Otodectes cynotis

Correct Answer: b) Cheyletiella spp.

Explanation: Cheyletiella mites, causing "walking dandruff," are visible moving flakes on the skin surface, requiring specific treatment.

Question 27: Which of the following is a zoonotic disease?

a) Canine parvovirus
b) Feline leukemia
c) Rabies
d) Canine distemper

Correct Answer: c) Rabies

Explanation: Rabies is zoonotic, transmissible between animals and humans, necessitating stringent vaccination and control measures.

Question 28: What is the primary role of platelets in the body?

a) Oxygen transport
b) Immune response
c) Blood clotting
d) Hormone regulation

Correct Answer: c) Blood clotting
Explanation: Platelets are crucial for hemostasis, forming clots to prevent bleeding, thus playing a vital role in wound healing.

Question 29: Which structure in the eye is responsible for focusing light onto the retina?

a) Cornea
b) Lens
c) Iris
d) Pupil

Correct Answer: b) Lens
Explanation: The lens focuses light onto the retina, adjusting for distance to provide clear vision, critical for visual acuity.

Question 30: In which part of the digestive system does most nutrient absorption occur?

a) Stomach
b) Large intestine
c) Small intestine
d) Esophagus

Correct Answer: c) Small intestine
Explanation: The small intestine is the primary site for nutrient absorption, with villi and microvilli increasing surface area for efficient uptake.

Question 31: Which of the following conditions is characterized by inflammation of the uveal tract of the eye?

a) Cataract
b) Glaucoma
c) Uveitis
d) Conjunctivitis

Correct Answer: c) Uveitis
Explanation: Uveitis involves inflammation of the uveal tract, causing eye pain, redness, and potential vision loss, requiring prompt treatment.

Question 32: Which of the following is a common cause of otitis externa in dogs?

a) Bacterial infection
b) Fungal infection
c) Parasitic infection
d) All of the above

Correct Answer: d) All of the above
Explanation: Otitis externa in dogs can result from bacterial, fungal, or parasitic infections, necessitating comprehensive diagnostic and treatment approaches.

Question 33: Which hormone is primarily responsible for regulating metabolism?

a) Insulin
b) Thyroxine
c) Cortisol
d) Estrogen

Correct Answer: b) Thyroxine

Explanation: Thyroxine, produced by the thyroid gland, regulates metabolism, influencing energy expenditure and metabolic rate.

Question 34: What is the main function of bile in the digestive system?

a) Break down carbohydrates
b) Emulsify fats
c) Absorb proteins
d) Neutralize stomach acid

Correct Answer: b) Emulsify fats

Explanation: Bile emulsifies fats in the small intestine, increasing surface area for lipase action, crucial for fat digestion and absorption.

Question 35: Which of the following is a common sign of dehydration in animals?

a) Shiny coat
b) Bright eyes
c) Elastic skin
d) Sunken eyes

Correct Answer: d) Sunken eyes

Explanation: Sunken eyes, along with dry mucous membranes and decreased skin elasticity, indicate dehydration, necessitating rehydration treatment.

Question 36: Which of the following is not a component of the axial skeleton?

a) Skull
b) Vertebrae
c) Ribs
d) Femur

Correct Answer: d) Femur

Explanation: The axial skeleton includes the skull, vertebrae, and ribs, while the femur is part of the appendicular skeleton.

Question 37: What is the primary function of the spleen?

a) Produce insulin
b) Filter blood and recycle iron
c) Store bile
d) Absorb nutrients

Correct Answer: b) Filter blood and recycle iron

Explanation: The spleen filters blood, recycles iron from old red blood cells, and plays a role in immune response.

Question 38: Which of the following is a fungal infection that affects the skin?

a) Ringworm
b) Demodicosis
c) Scabies
d) Flea allergy dermatitis

Correct Answer: a) Ringworm

Explanation: Ringworm is a contagious fungal infection affecting the skin, requiring antifungal treatment to resolve.

Question 39: Which is the largest organ in the body?

a) Liver
b) Heart
c) Skin
d) Lungs

Correct Answer: c) Skin
Explanation: The skin is the body's largest organ, serving as a protective barrier and playing roles in sensation and temperature regulation.

Question 40: Which of the following is a common cause of diarrhea in puppies?

a) Overeating
b) Parvovirus
c) Stress
d) All of the above

Correct Answer: d) All of the above
Explanation: Diarrhea in puppies can result from overeating, infections like parvovirus, and stress, each requiring different management strategies.

Question 41: What is the primary purpose of vaccinations?

a) Treat infections
b) Prevent diseases
c) Relieve symptoms
d) Diagnose conditions

Correct Answer: b) Prevent diseases
Explanation: Vaccinations stimulate the immune system to develop immunity against specific diseases, crucial for disease prevention.

Question 42: Which vitamin is essential for blood clotting?

a) Vitamin A
b) Vitamin D
c) Vitamin E
d) Vitamin K

Correct Answer: d) Vitamin K
Explanation: Vitamin K is essential for synthesizing clotting factors, playing a vital role in the blood coagulation process.

Question 43: Which is the primary site of protein digestion?

a) Mouth
b) Stomach
c) Small intestine
d) Large intestine

Correct Answer: b) Stomach
Explanation: Protein digestion begins in the stomach, where pepsin breaks down proteins into smaller peptides for further digestion.

Question 44: Which condition is characterized by the dilation and twisting of the stomach, common in large breed dogs?

a) Bloat
b) Gastritis
c) Colitis
d) Enteritis

Correct Answer: a) Bloat

Explanation: Bloat, or gastric dilatation-volvulus (GDV), involves stomach dilation and twisting, requiring emergency treatment to prevent life-threatening complications.

Question 45: Which of the following is a non-steroidal anti-inflammatory drug (NSAID) used in veterinary medicine?

a) Prednisone
b) Meloxicam
c) Enalapril
d) Metoclopramide

Correct Answer: b) Meloxicam

Explanation: Meloxicam is an NSAID used to manage pain and inflammation in animals, commonly prescribed for joint issues and post-surgery.

Question 46: Which part of the brain controls balance and coordination?

a) Cerebrum
b) Medulla oblongata
c) Cerebellum
d) Hypothalamus

Correct Answer: c) Cerebellum

Explanation: The cerebellum controls balance and coordination, ensuring smooth, coordinated muscle movements for physical activity.

Question 47: Which of the following is an ectoparasite?

a) Tapeworm
b) Roundworm
c) Flea
d) Hookworm

Correct Answer: c) Flea

Explanation: Fleas are ectoparasites, living on the host's skin, causing itching and potentially transmitting diseases, requiring control measures.

Question 48: Which is the largest artery in the body?

a) Carotid artery
b) Femoral artery
c) Aorta
d) Pulmonary artery

Correct Answer: c) Aorta

Explanation: The aorta is the largest artery, distributing oxygenated blood from the heart to the rest of the body, essential for circulation.

Question 49: Which of the following is not a function of the liver?

a) Produce bile
b) Store glycogen
c) Filter toxins
d) Produce insulin

Correct Answer: d) Produce insulin

Explanation: The liver is responsible for producing bile, storing glycogen, and filtering toxins, but insulin production is a function of the pancreas.

Question 50: A free-roaming dog is brought to your clinic for listlessness and dyspnea. When performing venipuncture, you notice that the animal seems to have a prolonged clotting time. You suspect that the patient may have ingested?

Correct Answer: anticoagulant rodent poison
Explanation: Anticoagulant rodent poisons, like warfarin, inhibit the vitamin K cycle, leading to prolonged clotting times and bleeding disorders in animals.

Question 51: The primary ovarian structure responsible for the release of estrogen is?

Correct Answer: follicle
Explanation: The follicle, specifically the Graafian follicle, releases estrogen, a hormone critical for regulating the estrous cycle and reproductive function.

Question 52: The higher the hematocrit and total protein values, the greater the degree of?

Correct Answer: dehydration
Explanation: Elevated hematocrit and total protein values often indicate dehydration, as fluid loss concentrates blood components, increasing their apparent levels.

Question 53: The minimum relative humidity in a neonatal puppy housing unit should be?

Correct Answer: 50%
Explanation: Maintaining a minimum relative humidity of 50% is crucial for neonatal puppies to prevent dehydration and support healthy respiratory function.

Question 54: Cardiac arrhythmias that occur during anesthesia are commonly associated with all of the following except?

a) Hypoxia
b) Hypercapnia
c) Acidosis
d) Normocapnia

Correct Answer: d) Normocapnia
Explanation: Cardiac arrhythmias during anesthesia are linked to hypoxia, hypercapnia, and acidosis, but not normocapnia, which indicates normal CO2 levels.

Question 55: Two tooth buds that grow together to form one larger tooth is referred to as?

Correct Answer: fusion
Explanation: Fusion occurs when two developing tooth buds join, resulting in a single, larger tooth, often with a shared root system.

Question 56: Anterior drawer movement detects a problem with the?

Correct Answer: stifle
Explanation: Anterior drawer movement is a diagnostic test for stifle joint instability, particularly indicative of cranial cruciate ligament rupture.

Question 57: The underlying disease for most cases of feline aortic thromboembolism is?

Correct Answer: myocardial disease
Explanation: Myocardial disease, especially hypertrophic cardiomyopathy, is a common precursor to feline aortic thromboembolism, causing clot formation.

Question 58: Local anesthetics?

Correct Answer: prevent nerve cell depolarization
Explanation: Local anesthetics block sodium channels, preventing nerve cell depolarization and interrupting pain signal transmission.

Question 59: A male guinea pig is called a?

Correct Answer: boar
Explanation: In guinea pigs, the male is referred to as a boar, while the female is known as a sow, similar to some farm animals.

Question 60: False about the eruption of permanent teeth?

a) Permanent incisors erupt lingual to deciduous ones
b) Permanent lower canines erupt buccal to the deciduous canines
c) Permanent premolars replace deciduous ones
d) Permanent molars do not have deciduous precursors

Correct Answer: b) Permanent lower canines erupt buccal to the deciduous canines
Explanation: Permanent lower canines actually erupt lingual to the deciduous canines, not buccal, ensuring alignment in the dental arch.

Question 61: Failure of an organ or a part of an organ to grow to its full size is an example of?

Correct Answer: hypoplasia
Explanation: Hypoplasia refers to the underdevelopment or incomplete development of an organ or tissue, resulting in reduced size or function.

Question 62: Steatorrhea refers to?

Correct Answer: fat in the stool
Explanation: Steatorrhea is the presence of excess fat in feces, indicating malabsorption or pancreatic insufficiency, often requiring dietary adjustments.

Question 63: To supply nearly adequate nutrition via the IV route, solutions used must be?

Correct Answer: hypertonic
Explanation: Hypertonic solutions provide concentrated nutrients and electrolytes for parenteral nutrition, essential when oral intake is insufficient.

Question 64: Which drug is the most potent sedative?

a) Diazepam
b) Acepromazine
c) Detomidine
d) Xylazine

Correct Answer: c) Detomidine
Explanation: Detomidine is a potent sedative with strong analgesic properties, primarily used in horses for its rapid onset and reliable effects.

Question 65: To flash sterilize an instrument, the autoclave settings should be?

Correct Answer: 270 degrees F, 30 lb pressure, 4 min, fast exhaust
Explanation: Flash sterilization at 270°F for 4 minutes under 30 lb pressure with a fast exhaust is used for urgent sterilization needs.

Question 66: Which agent, method, or device is most appropriate for sterilizing a pair of dissecting scissors to be used in a surgical procedure?

a) Dry heat sterilization
b) Ethylene oxide gas
c) Liquid chemical disinfectant
d) Gamma radiation

Correct Answer: c) Liquid chemical disinfectant
Explanation: Liquid chemical disinfectants are effective for sterilizing instruments like dissecting scissors, particularly when heat sterilization is unsuitable.

Question 67: On a CBC, all of the following findings could be expected in a patient with an infection, except?

a) Leukocytosis
b) Left shift
c) Narrow buffy coat
d) Anemia

Correct Answer: c) Narrow buffy coat
Explanation: A narrow buffy coat is not typical in infections, which usually cause leukocytosis and a left shift, indicating increased white blood cells.

Question 68: What species has multiple forms of reticulocytes?

Correct Answer: cat
Explanation: Cats have two forms of reticulocytes: aggregate and punctate, with aggregate forms indicating more recent bone marrow activity.

Question 69: An expectorant is a drug that acts to?

Correct Answer: liquefy and dilute viscous secretions in the respiratory tract
Explanation: Expectorants help clear mucus from the airways by liquefying and diluting thick secretions, aiding in their expulsion.

Question 70: The extent to which measurements agree with the true value of the quantity measured is?

Correct Answer: accuracy
Explanation: Accuracy denotes how close a measurement is to the actual or true value, crucial for reliable and valid data collection.

Question 71: The most common mistake made in treating periodontal disease is?

Correct Answer: inadequate root planing
Explanation: Inadequate root planing leaves bacterial plaque and calculus on tooth roots, perpetuating periodontal disease progression.

Question 72: In pigs, how long can a stress neutrophilia last?

Correct Answer: 8 hours
Explanation: Stress neutrophilia, characterized by increased neutrophils due to stress, can persist for up to 8 hours in pigs, impacting diagnostic interpretations.

Question 73: What type of dressing best helps debride a wound with extensive tissue damage?

Correct Answer: wet saline dressing
Explanation: Wet saline dressings aid in wound debridement by maintaining moisture, softening necrotic tissue, and facilitating its removal.

Question 74: Fresh frozen plasma can be stored up to___ and still contain clotting factors.

Correct Answer: 12 months
Explanation: Fresh frozen plasma retains clotting factors for up to 12 months when stored properly, critical for managing coagulopathies.

Question 75: A cat diagnosed with hyperthyroidism may be offered a number of treatment options, including all but which of the following?

a) Radioactive iodine therapy
b) Surgical thyroidectomy
c) Methimazole
d) Fenbendazole medical management

Correct Answer: d) Fenbendazole medical management
Explanation: Fenbendazole is an antiparasitic, not used for hyperthyroidism; treatments include medication, surgery, or radioactive iodine.

Question 76: Sialoschesis is the?

Correct Answer: suppression of the flow of saliva
Explanation: Sialoschesis refers to decreased or suppressed saliva flow, potentially caused by medication or disease, affecting oral health.

Question 77: The principal cation in extracellular fluid is?

Correct Answer: Na^+
Explanation: Sodium (Na^+) is the primary cation in extracellular fluid, crucial for maintaining fluid balance and nerve function.

Question 78: Which cranial nerve provides parasympathetic innervation to the heart, lungs, stomach, and small intestine?

Correct Answer: vagus (X)
Explanation: The vagus nerve (CN X) supplies parasympathetic fibers to various organs, influencing heart rate, digestion, and respiratory function.

Question 79: Dry matter refers to the?

Correct Answer: analysis of nutrient after moisture has been removed
Explanation: Dry matter analysis calculates nutritional content without water, providing insights into food quality and nutrient density.

Question 80: Which unit of measure is most commonly used for serum potassium?

Correct Answer: mEq
Explanation: Milliequivalents (mEq) are used to express serum potassium concentration, reflecting its ionic activity in biological systems.

Question 81: Which of the following is not part of the gastrointestinal (GI) tract?

a) Esophagus
b) Liver
c) Stomach
d) Small intestine

Correct Answer: b) Liver
Explanation: The liver is an accessory organ, not part of the GI tract itself, which includes the esophagus, stomach, and intestines.

Question 82: Which enzyme is responsible for breaking down proteins in the stomach?

a) Amylase
b) Pepsin
c) Lipase
d) Trypsin

Correct Answer: b) Pepsin
Explanation: Pepsin, activated in the acidic environment of the stomach, is the primary enzyme for protein digestion, breaking them into peptides.

Question 83: Which of the following is a symptom of hypoglycemia in animals?

a) Hyperactivity
b) Seizures

c) Increased thirst
d) Weight gain

Correct Answer: b) Seizures
Explanation: Hypoglycemia, low blood sugar, can cause seizures due to insufficient glucose for brain function, requiring immediate intervention.

Question 84: What is the function of the epiglottis?

a) Protect the heart
b) Aid in digestion
c) Prevent food from entering the trachea
d) Regulate body temperature

Correct Answer: c) Prevent food from entering the trachea
Explanation: The epiglottis closes over the trachea during swallowing, preventing food or liquid from entering the airway, ensuring safe ingestion.

Question 85: Which of the following is not a characteristic of a malignant tumor?

a) Invasive
b) Encapsulated
c) Rapid growth
d) Metastatic potential

Correct Answer: b) Encapsulated
Explanation: Malignant tumors are invasive and can metastasize, while benign tumors are often encapsulated, limiting their spread.

Question 86: Which hormone is responsible for milk production in mammals?

a) Oxytocin
b) Prolactin
c) Estrogen
d) Testosterone

Correct Answer: b) Prolactin
Explanation: Prolactin stimulates milk production in the mammary glands, essential for lactation and nurturing offspring.

Question 87: Which of the following is a characteristic of heartworm disease in dogs?

a) Increased urination
b) Coughing
c) Vomiting
d) Diarrhea

Correct Answer: b) Coughing
Explanation: Heartworm disease causes coughing due to pulmonary artery and lung involvement, often leading to respiratory distress in affected dogs.

Question 88: What is the primary function of red blood cells?

a) Fight infections
b) Clot blood
c) Transport oxygen
d) Store nutrients

Correct Answer: c) Transport oxygen
Explanation: Red blood cells transport oxygen from the lungs to tissues and return carbon dioxide for exhalation, vital for cellular respiration.

Question 89: Which structure separates the thoracic cavity from the abdominal cavity?

a) Liver
b) Diaphragm
c) Lungs
d) Stomach

Correct Answer: b) Diaphragm
Explanation: The diaphragm, a muscular structure, separates the thoracic and abdominal cavities, playing a crucial role in respiration.

Question 90: Which vitamin is necessary for calcium absorption?

a) Vitamin A
b) Vitamin B12
c) Vitamin C
d) Vitamin D

Correct Answer: d) Vitamin D
Explanation: Vitamin D enhances calcium absorption in the gut, crucial for bone health and maintaining proper calcium levels in the body.

Question 91: Which of the following is a common cause of liver disease in dogs?

a) Overeating
b) Heartworm infection
c) Canine adenovirus type 1
d) Fungal infection

Correct Answer: c) Canine adenovirus type 1
Explanation: Canine adenovirus type 1 causes infectious canine hepatitis, a significant cause of liver disease, preventable by vaccination.

Question 92: What is the main function of the kidneys?

a) Produce bile
b) Filter blood and produce urine
c) Synthesize vitamin D
d) Store glycogen

Correct Answer: b) Filter blood and produce urine
Explanation: The kidneys filter waste from the blood, regulating fluid and electrolyte balance, and produce urine for excretion.

Question 93: Which of the following is not a type of white blood cell?

a) Neutrophil
b) Erythrocyte
c) Lymphocyte
d) Monocyte

Correct Answer: b) Erythrocyte
Explanation: Erythrocytes are red blood cells, while neutrophils, lymphocytes, and monocytes are types of white blood cells involved in the immune response.

Question 94: Which of the following is a common sign of anemia in animals?

a) Jaundice
b) Lethargy
c) Hyperactivity
d) Increased appetite

Correct Answer: b) Lethargy
Explanation: Anemia causes lethargy due to reduced oxygen delivery to tissues, leading to fatigue and decreased activity levels.

Question 95: What is the role of the pancreas in digestion?

a) Produce bile
b) Secrete digestive enzymes and insulin
c) Absorb nutrients
d) Store vitamins

Correct Answer: b) Secrete digestive enzymes and insulin
Explanation: The pancreas secretes enzymes for digestion and insulin for blood sugar regulation, playing dual roles in metabolism and digestion.

Question 96: Which of the following is an example of a zoonotic disease?

a) Tetanus
b) Tuberculosis
c) Canine distemper
d) Feline leukemia

Correct Answer: b) Tuberculosis
Explanation: Tuberculosis is a zoonotic disease, transmissible between animals and humans, emphasizing the need for public health vigilance.

Question 97: Which of the following conditions is characterized by high blood sugar levels?

a) Hypothyroidism
b) Hyperthyroidism
c) Diabetes mellitus
d) Addison's disease

Correct Answer: c) Diabetes mellitus
Explanation: Diabetes mellitus involves high blood sugar due to insulin deficiency or resistance, requiring dietary and medical management.

Question 98: Which of the following is a function of the lymphatic system?

a) Produce red blood cells
b) Transport oxygen
c) Maintain fluid balance and defend against infections
d) Store fat

Correct Answer: c) Maintain fluid balance and defend against infections
Explanation: The lymphatic system regulates fluid balance and provides immune defense, filtering lymph and housing lymphocytes.

Question 99: Which part of the ear is responsible for balance?

a) Cochlea
b) Tympanic membrane
c) Semicircular canals
d) Eustachian tube

Correct Answer: c) Semicircular canals
Explanation: The semicircular canals in the inner ear detect head movements, playing a crucial role in maintaining balance and equilibrium.

Question 100: Which of the following is not a function of the skin?

a) Protection
b) Sensation
c) Hormone production
d) Temperature regulation

Correct Answer: c) Hormone production
Explanation: The skin protects, senses environmental changes, and regulates temperature, but does not produce hormones, primarily the function of glands.

Question 101: What is the primary function of the large intestine in the digestive system?

a) Digest carbohydrates
b) Absorb nutrients
c) Absorb water and electrolytes
d) Produce enzymes

Correct Answer: c) Absorb water and electrolytes
Explanation: The large intestine absorbs water and electrolytes from indigestible food residues, forming and storing feces for excretion.

Question 102: Which of the following is a sign of an upper respiratory infection in cats?

a) Diarrhea
b) Sneezing
c) Vomiting
d) Itching

Correct Answer: b) Sneezing
Explanation: Sneezing is a common symptom of upper respiratory infections in cats, often accompanied by nasal discharge and ocular signs.

Question 103: Which of the following is a characteristic of a benign tumor?

a) Invasive
b) Slow-growing
c) Metastatic potential
d) Unencapsulated

Correct Answer: b) Slow-growing
Explanation: Benign tumors are typically slow-growing and encapsulated, lacking the invasive and metastatic characteristics of malignant tumors.

Question 104: What medical record format takes more time to compile?

Correct Answer: problem-oriented medical records
Explanation: Problem-oriented medical records (POMR) require detailed documentation of each patient issue separately, making the process more time-consuming compared to source-oriented formats.

Question 105: What measure would be of no use in monitoring patients given succinylcholine?

Correct Answer: jaw muscle tone
Explanation: Succinylcholine, a muscle relaxant, causes muscle paralysis including that of the jaw, making jaw muscle tone an unreliable monitoring measure.

Question 106: In the equine, what term describes a drainage tract resulting from a crack in the white line?

Correct Answer: gravel
Explanation: "Gravel" refers to an infection or abscess that drains through a tract formed from a crack in the white line of a horse's hoof.

Question 107: A small filament produces an image of?

Correct Answer: greater detail than a large filament
Explanation: A small filament in x-ray machines provides finer detail due to reduced focal spot size, enhancing image sharpness and resolution.

Question 108: Pin indexing on an inhalant anesthetic machine is used to?

Correct Answer: prevent oxygen and nitrous oxide cylinders from being exchanged
Explanation: The pin index safety system ensures correct gas cylinder connections, avoiding potentially dangerous mix-ups between oxygen and nitrous oxide.

Question 109: A rabbit with a purulent nasal discharge and conjunctivitis would most likely be affected by?

Correct Answer: snuffles
Explanation: "Snuffles" is a common term for Pasteurellosis in rabbits, characterized by purulent nasal discharge and conjunctivitis caused by Pasteurella multocida.

Question 110: Which structure is not part of the large intestine?

Correct Answer: ileum
Explanation: The ileum is part of the small intestine, while the large intestine includes the cecum, colon, rectum, and anal canal.

Question 111: Why are intensifying screens added to an x-ray cassette?

Correct Answer: to cause light exposure of the film
Explanation: Intensifying screens convert x-ray photons to visible light, reducing exposure needed to produce an image and minimizing radiation dose.

Question 112: What effect do procaine and benzathine have on penicillin G?

Correct Answer: they prolong absorption of penicillin G from the injection site
Explanation: Procaine and benzathine slow penicillin G absorption, providing longer-lasting therapeutic levels and reducing dosing frequency.

Question 113: According to the Punnett square, in a cross of Bb x Bb, the F1 generations will be made up of?

Correct Answer: 25%, 50%, and 25%, or 1:2:1
Explanation: In a Bb x Bb cross, the F1 generation's genotype ratio is 1 BB: 2 Bb: 1 bb, or phenotypically, 3 dominant: 1 recessive trait.

Question 114: The PCV of the abdominal fluid of an animal with a urologic injury is?

Correct Answer: lower than the peripheral PCV
Explanation: Abdominal fluid in urologic injuries often has lower PCV than peripheral blood due to dilution by urine leakage.

Question 115: When autoclaving, the minimum temperature and exposure time for the center of the surgical packs is?

Correct Answer: 250 degrees F for 15 minutes
Explanation: Adequate sterilization in an autoclave requires maintaining 250°F for at least 15 minutes to ensure all microorganisms are destroyed.

Question 116: A new in-house test has been developed with 80% sensitivity and 100% specificity. What does this mean?

Correct Answer: 20% will be false negative
Explanation: An 80% sensitivity indicates 20% of true positives may be missed (false negatives), while 100% specificity confirms no false positives.

Question 117: The adrenal cortex is made up of all of the following except?

Correct Answer: zona medullata

Explanation: The adrenal cortex includes the zona glomerulosa, zona fasciculata, and zona reticularis; the medulla is a separate inner region.

Question 118: When using hand instruments to clean teeth?

Correct Answer: use a modified pen grasp with overlapping pull strokes that are directed away from the gingival margin

Explanation: A modified pen grasp offers precision and control, and strokes away from the gingival margin prevent tissue damage during scaling.

Question 119: Mus musculus is the scientific name of the?

Correct Answer: mouse

Explanation: Mus musculus is the scientific name for the common house mouse, widely used in medical and genetic research.

Question 120: Neuromuscular blocking agents?

Correct Answer: do not cross the blood-brain barrier

Explanation: Neuromuscular blockers act peripherally, causing muscle paralysis without affecting central nervous system function, as they don't cross the blood-brain barrier.

Question 121: The term that refers to making an incision through the abdominal wall is?

Correct Answer: laparotomy

Explanation: A laparotomy involves surgical incision into the abdominal wall, allowing access to the abdominal organs for diagnostic or therapeutic purposes.

Question 122: What disease is most dangerous in a herd of breeding horses?

Correct Answer: rhinopneumonitis

Explanation: Equine rhinopneumonitis, caused by Equine Herpesvirus, poses significant risks including respiratory disease, abortion, and neurological disorders in breeding horses.

Question 123: If a film is too dark and the image appears overpenetrated, you should?

Correct Answer: decrease kVp 10-15%

Explanation: Reducing kVp by 10-15% decreases x-ray penetration, lightening the film to achieve appropriate contrast and detail.

Question 124: Tyzzer's disease is most commonly seen in what animal?

Correct Answer: rodent

Explanation: Caused by Clostridium piliforme, Tyzzer's disease primarily affects rodents, resulting in liver necrosis, diarrhea, and high mortality rates.

Question 125: Spasmodic muscular contractions that produce heat to help maintain normal body temperature are called?

Correct Answer: shivering

Explanation: Shivering involves involuntary muscle contractions generating heat to raise body temperature, a natural response to cold exposure.

Question 126: The opening at the distal end of the simple stomach that allows for emptying of its contents into the duodenum is called the?

Correct Answer: pylorus

Explanation: The pylorus is the stomach's distal opening into the duodenum, controlling the passage of gastric contents into the small intestine.

Question 127: Digoxin has a narrow therapeutic index. What does this mean?

Correct Answer: plasma drug concentrations that produce toxicity are very close to the minimum concentration at which a beneficial effect occurs

Explanation: The narrow therapeutic index of digoxin means careful monitoring is essential, as small dosing errors can lead to toxicity.

Question 128: In radiographs, an apical abscess appears as a?

Correct Answer: radiolucent area around the apex of the tooth

Explanation: An apical abscess manifests as a radiolucent area on x-rays, indicating bone destruction around the tooth's root apex due to infection.

Question 129: What is the appropriate time to soak an instrument in a cold sterilization solution before adequate sterilization is achieved?

Correct Answer: 10 minutes

Explanation: Cold sterilization typically requires at least 10 minutes of immersion for effective microbial reduction, though longer times may be recommended.

Question 130: What species is not a social animal and should be housed alone?

Correct Answer: hamster

Explanation: Hamsters are solitary by nature and can become stressed or aggressive when housed with others, making solitary housing preferable.

Question 131: What is the primary role of platelets in the body?

a) Transport oxygen
b) Produce antibodies
c) Facilitate blood clotting
d) Regulate blood pressure

Correct Answer: c) Facilitate blood clotting

Explanation: Platelets are essential for hemostasis, aggregating at injury sites to form clots, preventing excessive bleeding and promoting healing.

Question 132: What is the most common cause of hyperthyroidism in cats?

a) Iodine deficiency
b) Thyroid adenoma
c) Parathyroid hyperplasia
d) Pituitary tumor

Correct Answer: b) Thyroid adenoma

Explanation: Hyperthyroidism in cats is most often caused by a benign thyroid adenoma, leading to excess thyroid hormone production and metabolic acceleration.

Question 133: Which vitamin is essential for blood clotting?

a) Vitamin A
b) Vitamin C
c) Vitamin D
d) Vitamin K

Correct Answer: d) Vitamin K

Explanation: Vitamin K is vital for synthesizing clotting factors in the liver, facilitating normal coagulation and preventing excessive bleeding.

Question 134: Which part of the brain regulates heart rate and blood pressure?

a) Cerebellum
b) Medulla oblongata
c) Thalamus
d) Hippocampus

Correct Answer: b) Medulla oblongata
Explanation: The medulla oblongata controls autonomic functions such as heart rate and blood pressure, essential for maintaining homeostasis.

Question 135: Which of the following is a symptom of Cushing's disease in dogs?

a) Increased appetite
b) Weight loss
c) Hair growth
d) Decreased thirst

Correct Answer: a) Increased appetite
Explanation: Dogs with Cushing's disease, or hyperadrenocorticism, often exhibit increased appetite, weight gain, and hair loss due to elevated cortisol levels.

Question 136: What is the main function of the spleen?

a) Produce bile
b) Filter blood and store red blood cells
c) Secrete insulin
d) Absorb nutrients

Correct Answer: b) Filter blood and store red blood cells
Explanation: The spleen filters blood, removing old or damaged red blood cells, and stores blood components, playing a key role in immune response.

Question 137: Which condition results from a deficiency of insulin in the body?

a) Addison's disease
b) Hyperthyroidism
c) Diabetes insipidus
d) Diabetes mellitus

Correct Answer: d) Diabetes mellitus
Explanation: Diabetes mellitus results from insufficient insulin or insulin resistance, leading to elevated blood glucose levels and metabolic disturbances.

Question 138: Which of the following is not a component of the central nervous system?

a) Brain
b) Spinal cord
c) Peripheral nerves
d) Cerebellum

Correct Answer: c) Peripheral nerves
Explanation: Peripheral nerves are part of the peripheral nervous system, while the brain, spinal cord, and cerebellum make up the central nervous system.

Question 139: What is the primary purpose of the lymph nodes in the body?

a) Produce hormones
b) Filter lymph and house immune cells
c) Store calcium
d) Regulate temperature

Correct Answer: b) Filter lymph and house immune cells
Explanation: Lymph nodes filter pathogens from lymph and provide a site for immune cell activation, crucial for defending against infections.

Question 140: Which of the following is a characteristic of a viral infection?

a) Antibiotic sensitivity
b) High fever
c) Presence of pus
d) Lymphocyte predominance in the bloodstream

Correct Answer: d) Lymphocyte predominance in the bloodstream
Explanation: Viral infections often lead to increased lymphocytes, as they target viruses, unlike bacterial infections which respond to antibiotics.

Question 141: Which organ is primarily responsible for detoxifying chemicals and metabolizing drugs in the body?

a) Kidneys
b) Liver
c) Pancreas
d) Spleen

Correct Answer: b) Liver
Explanation: The liver detoxifies chemicals and metabolizes drugs, converting them into safer compounds for elimination or processing.

Question 142: Which hormone regulates the body's water balance and is stored in the posterior pituitary gland?

a) Oxytocin
b) Vasopressin (ADH)
c) Prolactin
d) Thyroxine

Correct Answer: b) Vasopressin (ADH)
Explanation: Vasopressin, or antidiuretic hormone (ADH), regulates water retention by the kidneys, maintaining fluid balance and blood pressure.

Question 143: Which of the following is a function of the alveoli in the lungs?

a) Filter air
b) Produce surfactant
c) Exchange gases between air and blood
d) Trap dust particles

Correct Answer: c) Exchange gases between air and blood
Explanation: Alveoli facilitate gas exchange, allowing oxygen to enter the blood and carbon dioxide to be expelled during respiration.

Question 144: Which of the following is a common sign of dehydration in animals?

a) Increased salivation
b) Tacky mucous membranes
c) Hyperactive behavior
d) Decreased heart rate

Correct Answer: b) Tacky mucous membranes
Explanation: Dehydration leads to tacky or dry mucous membranes, indicating insufficient fluid levels, often accompanied by skin tenting and sunken eyes.

Question 145: Which structure in the eye is responsible for detecting light and converting it into neural signals?

a) Cornea
b) Lens
c) Retina
d) Iris

Correct Answer: c) Retina
Explanation: The retina contains photoreceptor cells that detect light and convert it into electrical signals, which are sent to the brain for visual processing.

Question 146: Which of the following is a non-steroidal anti-inflammatory drug (NSAID) commonly used in veterinary medicine?

a) Prednisone
b) Furosemide
c) Meloxicam
d) Enalapril

Correct Answer: c) Meloxicam
Explanation: Meloxicam is an NSAID used to treat pain and inflammation in animals, particularly effective in managing arthritis and postoperative discomfort.

Question 147: Which of the following is a symptom of feline lower urinary tract disease (FLUTD)?

a) Increased appetite
b) Frequent urination
c) Vomiting
d) Itchy skin

Correct Answer: b) Frequent urination
Explanation: FLUTD often presents with frequent urination, straining, and blood in the urine, indicating bladder or urethral irritation or obstruction.

Question 148: Which cell type is responsible for producing antibodies?

a) T-lymphocytes
b) B-lymphocytes
c) Erythrocytes
d) Neutrophils

Correct Answer: b) B-lymphocytes
Explanation: B-lymphocytes, or B-cells, differentiate into plasma cells that produce antibodies, key components of the adaptive immune response.

Question 149: Which of the following is a characteristic of a bacterial infection?

a) Lymphocyte predominance
b) Neutrophil predominance
c) Viral load increase
d) Fungal spore production

Correct Answer: b) Neutrophil predominance
Explanation: Bacterial infections typically cause an increase in neutrophils, the body's primary defense against bacterial pathogens.

Question 150: Which mineral is essential for the formation of hemoglobin in red blood cells?

a) Calcium
b) Iron

c) Sodium
d) Potassium

Correct Answer: b) Iron
Explanation: Iron is a critical component of hemoglobin, the molecule responsible for oxygen transport in red blood cells, and its deficiency leads to anemia.

Question 151: Which hormone is responsible for the development of secondary sexual characteristics in males?

a) Estrogen
b) Progesterone
c) Testosterone
d) Insulin

Correct Answer: c) Testosterone
Explanation: Testosterone drives the development of male secondary sexual characteristics, such as increased muscle mass and facial hair growth.

Question 152: Which of the following is a sign of heart failure in dogs?

a) Increased thirst
b) Coughing
c) Weight gain
d) Hyperactivity

Correct Answer: b) Coughing
Explanation: Coughing in dogs can indicate heart failure, as fluid buildup from poor heart function leads to pulmonary congestion and respiratory issues.

Question 153: Which part of the digestive system is primarily responsible for nutrient absorption?

a) Stomach
b) Small intestine
c) Large intestine
d) Esophagus

Correct Answer: b) Small intestine
Explanation: The small intestine, particularly the jejunum and ileum, is the main site for nutrient absorption, facilitated by its extensive surface area and villi.

Question 154: Which of the following is a common cause of ear infections in dogs?

a) Dry air
b) Fungal spores
c) Yeast overgrowth
d) Vitamin deficiency

Correct Answer: c) Yeast overgrowth
Explanation: Yeast overgrowth, often due to moisture and poor ventilation, is a frequent cause of ear infections in dogs, requiring antifungal treatment.

Question 155: Which structure in the heart prevents backflow of blood from the ventricles into the atria?

a) Aortic valve
b) Mitral valve
c) Pulmonary valve
d) Tricuspid valve

Correct Answer: b) Mitral valve

Explanation: The mitral valve, along with the tricuspid valve, prevents backflow from the ventricles to the atria, ensuring unidirectional blood flow during contraction.

Question 156: Which of the following is not a function of the liver?

a) Produce bile
b) Store glycogen
c) Filter toxins
d) Produce insulin

Correct Answer: d) Produce insulin

Explanation: The pancreas, not the liver, is responsible for insulin production; the liver's roles include detoxification, bile production, and glycogen storage.

Question 157: Which vitamin is essential for blood clotting?

a) Vitamin A
b) Vitamin C
c) Vitamin K
d) Vitamin D

Correct Answer: c) Vitamin K

Explanation: Vitamin K is crucial for synthesizing proteins required for blood coagulation. It plays an essential role in preventing excessive bleeding and ensuring proper wound healing. Deficiencies in vitamin K can lead to bleeding disorders due to impaired clot formation.

Question 158: What is the most common color of the safelight used in a darkroom for processing blue-light sensitive film?

a) Red
b) Green
c) Brown
d) Yellow

Correct Answer: c) Brown

Explanation: Brown safelights are used for blue-light sensitive films because they filter out blue and green light, which could otherwise expose the film and ruin the image quality.

Question 159: What is an example of a sexually dimorphic pet bird?

a) African Grey Parrot
b) Grey Cockatiel
c) Lovebird
d) Budgerigar

Correct Answer: b) Grey Cockatiel

Explanation: Grey cockatiels exhibit sexual dimorphism; males have a brighter orange cheek patch and less barring on the tail feathers, while females have more subdued coloration and barring.

Question 160: What is a common cause of gastric ulcers in ferrets?

a) Escherichia coli
b) Helicobacter mustelae
c) Streptococcus
d) Clostridium

Correct Answer: b) Helicobacter mustelae

Explanation: Helicobacter mustelae is a bacterium that can colonize the stomach lining of ferrets, leading to inflammation and ulceration, similar to H. pylori in humans.

Question 161: What rat is also known as the hooded rat?

a) Sprague-Dawley rat
b) Wistar rat
c) Long-Evans rat
d) Fischer rat

Correct Answer: c) Long-Evans rat
Explanation: The Long-Evans rat is known as the hooded rat due to its characteristic black or dark-colored "hood" covering the head and extending down the back.

Question 162: Prolapse of the lacrimal gland is described as?

a) Dacryocystitis
b) Dacryocystoptosis
c) Blepharitis
d) Conjunctivitis

Correct Answer: b) Dacryocystoptosis
Explanation: Dacryocystoptosis refers to the prolapse or displacement of the lacrimal gland, often seen in "cherry eye" conditions in dogs, where the gland protrudes from its normal position.

Question 163: Which surgical procedure is least likely to combat canine hip dysplasia's debilitating complications?

a) Femoral head ostectomy
b) Triple pelvic osteotomy
c) Total hip replacement
d) Intramedullary pinning

Correct Answer: d) Intramedullary pinning
Explanation: Intramedullary pinning stabilizes fractures but does not address the joint instability or degeneration associated with hip dysplasia, unlike procedures like total hip replacement.

Question 164: During the maintenance period of anesthesia in a cat or dog, respiratory rates lower than how many breaths/min may indicate excessive anesthetic depth that should be reported to the vet?

a) 12
b) 10
c) 8
d) 15

Correct Answer: c) 8
Explanation: Respiratory rates below 8 breaths per minute during anesthesia can suggest excessive anesthetic depth, requiring immediate adjustment to prevent respiratory depression.

Question 165: The parasite also known as a lung fluke is?

a) Fasciola hepatica
b) Paragonimus species
c) Dirofilaria immitis
d) Taenia saginata

Correct Answer: b) Paragonimus species
Explanation: Paragonimus species are lung flukes that infect the respiratory system, causing lung disease in various mammals, including humans and dogs, upon ingestion of contaminated water or food.

Question 166: What is micturition?

a) Urine production
b) Emptying the bladder
c) Kidney filtration
d) Ureter contraction

Correct Answer: b) Emptying the bladder

Explanation: Micturition is the process of expelling urine from the bladder through the urethra, controlled by neural and muscular mechanisms.

Question 167: Aspirin may be safely used in cats as an NSAID, but it should be noted that its half-life in this species approximates?

a) 6 hours
b) 12 hours
c) 24 hours
d) 30 hours

Correct Answer: d) 30 hours

Explanation: Cats metabolize aspirin slowly due to limited glucuronyl transferase enzyme activity, resulting in an extended half-life of approximately 30 hours, requiring careful dosing intervals.

Question 168: For a large dog receiving CPR, compressions and respirations should be administered at?

a) 80 compressions/minute, respirations every 1-2 seconds
b) 60 compressions/minute, respirations every 3-5 seconds
c) 100 compressions/minute, respirations every 5-10 seconds
d) 40 compressions/minute, respirations every 5-7 seconds

Correct Answer: b) 60 compressions/minute, respirations every 3-5 seconds

Explanation: During CPR on large dogs, consistent chest compressions at 60 per minute and respirations every 3-5 seconds help maintain circulation and oxygenation until spontaneous activity resumes.

Question 169: What causes diarrhea in dogs and humans?

a) Salmonella
b) Campylobacter
c) E. coli
d) Giardia

Correct Answer: b) Campylobacter

Explanation: Campylobacter bacteria are a common cause of diarrhea in both dogs and humans, often transmitted through contaminated food or water, requiring antimicrobial treatment if severe.

Question 170: An all-white breed of goat is the?

a) Nubian
b) Alpine
c) Saanen
d) Boer

Correct Answer: c) Saanen

Explanation: The Saanen goat is known for its all-white coat, high milk production, and docile temperament, making it a popular dairy breed worldwide.

Full Test 6 with Detailed Explanations

Question 1: What type of epithelial cell is capable of significant variation in shape, depending on changes in the size of the organ it lines?

a) Squamous epithelium
b) Cuboidal epithelium
c) Transitional epithelium
d) Columnar epithelium

Correct Answer: c) Transitional epithelium
Explanation: Transitional epithelium lines organs such as the bladder, allowing for stretch and contraction without damage, accommodating fluctuating volumes.

Question 2: What is the PCV of a normal adult dog?

a) 25-35%
b) 37-55%
c) 60-70%
d) 10-20%

Correct Answer: b) 37-55%
Explanation: Packed cell volume (PCV) indicates the proportion of blood volume occupied by red blood cells, with 37-55% being the normal range for adult dogs.

Question 3: Grid cutoff can be described as?

a) Incorrect grid placement leading to excessive radiation exposure
b) The grid absorbing more radiation than it should
c) Proper alignment between the x-ray beam and grid
d) The grid enhancing image quality

Correct Answer: b) The grid absorbing more radiation than it should
Explanation: Grid cutoff occurs when misalignment between the x-ray beam and grid leads to excessive radiation absorption, reducing image clarity.

Question 4: What nutrient is sometimes referred to as ash?

a) Carbohydrates
b) Proteins
c) Minerals
d) Fats

Correct Answer: c) Minerals
Explanation: "Ash" in nutritional analysis refers to the inorganic residue left after complete combustion, mainly consisting of essential minerals.

Question 5: Acetylcysteine (Mucomyst) is an antidote for what type of drug toxicity?

a) Ibuprofen
b) Aspirin
c) Acetaminophen
d) Morphine

Correct Answer: c) Acetaminophen
Explanation: Acetylcysteine replenishes glutathione, detoxifying harmful byproducts of acetaminophen metabolism, preventing liver damage following overdose.

Question 6: People may serve as the intermediate host of?

a) Taenia solium
b) Echinococcus granulosus
c) Dipylidium caninum
d) Toxoplasma gondii

Correct Answer: b) Echinococcus granulosus
Explanation: Humans can be intermediate hosts for Echinococcus granulosus, developing hydatid cysts when ingesting eggs from infected animal feces.

Question 7: Which species is prone to nasal dermatitis initiated by its burrowing activity?

a) Hamster
b) Rabbit
c) Gerbil
d) Rat

Correct Answer: c) Gerbil
Explanation: Gerbils often develop nasal dermatitis, or "sore nose," due to stress-induced burrowing behaviors and subsequent irritation.

Question 8: What heart rate is cause for concern if it falls below in an anesthetized cat?

a) 120 bpm
b) 150 bpm
c) 100 bpm
d) 90 bpm

Correct Answer: c) 100 bpm
Explanation: A heart rate below 100 bpm in anesthetized cats may indicate excessive anesthetic depth or cardiovascular distress, warranting immediate attention.

Question 9: Which organ has storage sinuses that hold blood and release it into circulation when the need for oxygen is increased?

a) Liver
b) Spleen
c) Kidneys
d) Heart

Correct Answer: b) Spleen
Explanation: The spleen stores blood in its sinuses, releasing it during hypoxia or increased demand, aiding in oxygen transport and immune response.

Question 10: Which breed of dog is particularly susceptible to heat stroke?

a) Labrador Retriever
b) English Bulldog
c) German Shepherd
d) Border Collie

Correct Answer: b) English Bulldog
Explanation: English Bulldogs are prone to heat stroke due to their brachycephalic (short-nosed) anatomy, impairing effective panting and heat dissipation.

Question 11: Diphenhydramine elixir is prescribed at 12.5 mg po q8h. The drug is available in 30ml bottles that contain 25mg/5ml. How long will one bottle last?

a) 8 days
b) 5 days
c) 4 days
d) 3 days

Correct Answer: c) 4 days
Explanation: A dose of 12.5 mg equals 2.5 ml per dose. At three doses per day (7.5 ml total), a 30 ml bottle will last 4 days.

Question 12: The armadillo is one of the few animal models of what human disease?

a) Tuberculosis
b) Leprosy
c) Malaria
d) Rabies

Correct Answer: b) Leprosy
Explanation: Armadillos can naturally contract Mycobacterium leprae, making them unique models for studying leprosy due to their low body temperature.

Question 13: In an isolation unit where sick animals are housed, the air pressure compared with that in quarters housing healthy animals must be?

a) Higher
b) Equal
c) Lower
d) Controlled

Correct Answer: c) Lower
Explanation: Lower air pressure in isolation prevents contaminated air from escaping the unit, reducing the spread of infectious agents to healthy animals.

Question 14: Which statement is true about anaerobic metabolism?

a) It produces more energy than aerobic metabolism
b) It requires oxygen to produce ATP
c) Glucose can be used
d) It results in the production of carbon dioxide and water

Correct Answer: c) Glucose can be used
Explanation: Anaerobic metabolism utilizes glucose to produce energy in the absence of oxygen, resulting in lactic acid as a byproduct.

Question 15: A focal-film distance that is too short causes the radiographed image to?

a) Appear too light
b) Appear too dark
c) Be distorted
d) Be blurred

Correct Answer: b) Appear too dark
Explanation: A short focal-film distance increases x-ray intensity at the film, making the image appear darker due to higher exposure.

Question 16: The lab animal species most likely to experience dystocia is a?

a) Rat
b) Rabbit
c) Guinea pig
d) Mouse

Correct Answer: c) Guinea pig
Explanation: Guinea pigs risk dystocia if bred after 6 months without previous litters, as pelvic fusion limits birth canal expansion.

Question 17: When taking a lateral thoracic radiograph, you should make sure the spine and sternum are?

a) Parallel to the table
b) Perpendicular to the table

c) Equidistant from the table
d) Angled at 45 degrees

Correct Answer: c) Equidistant from the table
Explanation: Ensuring the spine and sternum are equidistant prevents image distortion and ensures accurate representation of thoracic structures.

Question 18: What occurs in an animal with pregnancy toxemia?

a) Anemia
b) Hypocalcemia
c) Ketosis
d) Hypoglycemia

Correct Answer: c) Ketosis
Explanation: Pregnancy toxemia involves ketosis, where negative energy balance leads to fat breakdown and ketone production, causing metabolic complications.

Question 19: Vaporizers may be classified according to all of the following except the?

a) Type of anesthetic agent used
b) Temperature compensation
c) Precision of output
d) Type of breathing circuit with which they can be used

Correct Answer: d) Type of breathing circuit with which they can be used
Explanation: Vaporizers are classified by factors like precision, temperature compensation, and agent specificity, not by breathing circuit compatibility.

Question 20: What muscle is the main adductor of the shoulder?

a) Deltoid
b) Trapezius
c) Pectoralis
d) Latissimus dorsi

Correct Answer: c) Pectoralis
Explanation: The pectoralis major muscle adducts and medially rotates the shoulder, playing a key role in arm and shoulder movement.

Question 21: Ferret young are called?

a) Pups
b) Kits
c) Cubs
d) Fawns

Correct Answer: b) Kits
Explanation: Ferret offspring are known as kits, typically born in litters and requiring maternal care until weaning at about 6 weeks.

Question 22: When describing bone fractures, the two terms that mean the same thing are?

a) Comminuted and simple
b) Greenstick and transverse
c) Open and compound
d) Impacted and depressed

Correct Answer: c) Open and compound
Explanation: Open and compound fractures both refer to breaks where bone fragments penetrate the skin, posing infection risks.

Question 23: Protein that is not used by the body is converted to energy and the waste?

a) Is stored in the liver
b) Is excreted by the kidneys
c) Is converted into fat
d) Is exhaled as carbon dioxide

Correct Answer: b) Is excreted by the kidneys
Explanation: Unused protein is deaminated for energy, producing nitrogenous waste like urea, which is filtered and excreted by the kidneys.

Question 24: The recommended procedure for a dog that has just bitten a person is?

a) Euthanize the dog
b) Observe at home
c) Quarantine and observe for 10 days
d) Immediate vaccination

Correct Answer: c) Quarantine and observe for 10 days
Explanation: Quarantine and observation for rabies symptoms ensure safety, as rabies virus presence can manifest within this period post-exposure.

Question 25: The buccal surface of the mandibular molars in a dog refers to the?

a) Surface facing the tongue
b) Surface in contact with the cheek tissue
c) Surface near the gum line
d) Surface facing the palate

Correct Answer: b) Surface in contact with the cheek tissue
Explanation: The buccal surface faces the cheeks, important for dental assessments and procedures, especially in oral hygiene and disease evaluation.

Question 26: When a spinning-top test is performed on a full-wave rectified machine, how many dots should you see in 1/60 seconds?

a) 1
b) 2
c) 3
d) 4

Correct Answer: b) 2
Explanation: A full-wave rectified machine creates two pulses per cycle, so a 1/60 second exposure results in two dots, verifying exposure accuracy.

Question 27: Which vitamin is essential for blood clotting?

a) Vitamin A
b) Vitamin C
c) Vitamin K
d) Vitamin D

Correct Answer: c) Vitamin K
Explanation: Vitamin K is crucial for synthesizing clotting factors in the liver, ensuring proper hemostasis and preventing excessive bleeding.

Question 28: What is the role of hemoglobin in red blood cells?

a) Transport carbon dioxide
b) Transport oxygen

c) Fight infections
d) Regulate blood pressure

Correct Answer: b) Transport oxygen
Explanation: Hemoglobin binds oxygen in the lungs and releases it in tissues, facilitating cellular respiration and energy production.

Question 29: Which mineral is essential for the formation of hemoglobin?

a) Calcium
b) Iron
c) Magnesium
d) Potassium

Correct Answer: b) Iron
Explanation: Iron is integral to hemoglobin's structure, enabling it to bind and transport oxygen effectively; deficiency leads to anemia.

Question 30: Which organ is responsible for detoxifying chemicals and metabolizing drugs?

a) Kidney
b) Liver
c) Pancreas
d) Spleen

Correct Answer: b) Liver
Explanation: The liver processes toxins and drugs, converting them to less harmful substances for excretion, crucial for metabolic homeostasis.

Question 31: Which hormone regulates water balance and is stored in the posterior pituitary gland?

a) Oxytocin
b) Vasopressin (ADH)
c) Insulin
d) Glucagon

Correct Answer: b) Vasopressin (ADH)
Explanation: Vasopressin, or antidiuretic hormone (ADH), controls kidney water reabsorption, maintaining fluid balance and blood pressure.

Question 32: Which hormone is responsible for the development of secondary sexual characteristics in males?

a) Estrogen
b) Progesterone
c) Testosterone
d) Cortisol

Correct Answer: c) Testosterone
Explanation: Testosterone promotes male secondary sexual traits, such as increased muscle mass, facial hair, and deepening of the voice.

Question 33: What is the main function of the spleen?

a) Produce bile
b) Filter blood and store red blood cells
c) Produce insulin
d) Regulate calcium levels

Correct Answer: b) Filter blood and store red blood cells

Explanation: The spleen removes old or damaged red blood cells, stores blood, and facilitates immune responses, contributing to hematological and immune health.

Question 34: Which type of tissue is responsible for transmitting electrical signals in the body?

a) Connective tissue
b) Epithelial tissue
c) Muscle tissue
d) Nervous tissue

Correct Answer: d) Nervous tissue

Explanation: Nervous tissue, composed of neurons, transmits electrical impulses, coordinating sensory and motor functions throughout the body.

Question 35: Which part of the brain regulates heart rate and blood pressure?

a) Cerebellum
b) Hypothalamus
c) Medulla oblongata
d) Thalamus

Correct Answer: c) Medulla oblongata

Explanation: The medulla oblongata controls autonomic functions such as heart rate and blood pressure, essential for maintaining homeostasis.

Question 36: What is a common indicator of dehydration in animals?

a) Wet nose
b) Bright eyes
c) Tacky mucous membranes
d) Shiny coat

Correct Answer: c) Tacky mucous membranes

Explanation: Dehydration leads to tacky or dry mucous membranes, indicating insufficient fluid levels, often accompanied by skin tenting and sunken eyes.

Question 37: What structure in the eye is responsible for sensing light and converting it into neural signals?

a) Cornea
b) Lens
c) Retina
d) Iris

Correct Answer: c) Retina

Explanation: The retina contains photoreceptor cells that detect light and convert it into electrical signals, which are sent to the brain for visual processing.

Question 38: Which of these is a non-steroidal anti-inflammatory drug (NSAID) often used in veterinary practice?

a) Prednisone
b) Meloxicam
c) Acetaminophen
d) Amoxicillin

Correct Answer: b) Meloxicam

Explanation: Meloxicam is an NSAID used to treat pain and inflammation in animals, particularly effective in managing arthritis and postoperative discomfort.

Question 39: What is a typical symptom of feline lower urinary tract disease (FLUTD)?

a) Vomiting
b) Frequent urination
c) Hair loss
d) Increased appetite

Correct Answer: b) Frequent urination
Explanation: FLUTD often presents with frequent urination, straining, and blood in the urine, indicating bladder or urethral irritation or obstruction.

Question 40: Which type of cell is responsible for antibody production?

a) T-lymphocytes
b) Macrophages
c) B-lymphocytes
d) Neutrophils

Correct Answer: c) B-lymphocytes
Explanation: B-lymphocytes, or B-cells, differentiate into plasma cells that produce antibodies, key components of the adaptive immune response.

Question 41: What is a common characteristic of a bacterial infection?

a) Lymphopenia
b) Neutrophil predominance
c) Eosinophilia
d) Monocytosis

Correct Answer: b) Neutrophil predominance
Explanation: Bacterial infections typically cause an increase in neutrophils, the body's primary defense against bacterial pathogens.

Question 42: Which part of the digestive system is mainly responsible for absorbing nutrients?

a) Stomach
b) Large intestine
c) Small intestine
d) Esophagus

Correct Answer: c) Small intestine
Explanation: The small intestine, particularly the jejunum and ileum, is the main site for nutrient absorption, facilitated by its extensive surface area and villi.

Question 43: What structure in the heart prevents blood from flowing back into the atria from the ventricles?

a) Aortic valve
b) Pulmonary valve
c) Mitral valve
d) Semilunar valve

Correct Answer: c) Mitral valve
Explanation: The mitral valve, along with the tricuspid valve, prevents backflow from the ventricles to the atria, ensuring unidirectional blood flow during contraction.

Question 44: Which of the following is not a function of the liver?

a) Produce bile
b) Detoxify chemicals

c) Store glycogen
d) Produce insulin

Correct Answer: d) Produce insulin
Explanation: The pancreas, not the liver, is responsible for insulin production; the liver's roles include detoxification, bile production, and glycogen storage.

Question 45: What condition results from a lack of insulin in the body?

a) Hypoglycemia
b) Hyperthyroidism
c) Diabetes mellitus
d) Addison's disease

Correct Answer: c) Diabetes mellitus
Explanation: Diabetes mellitus results from insufficient insulin or insulin resistance, leading to elevated blood glucose levels and metabolic disturbances.

Question 46: Which organ is primarily responsible for detoxifying chemicals and metabolizing drugs?

a) Kidney
b) Liver
c) Pancreas
d) Spleen

Correct Answer: b) Liver
Explanation: The liver detoxifies chemicals and metabolizes drugs, converting them into safer compounds for elimination or processing.

Question 47: Which hormone regulates water balance and is stored in the posterior pituitary gland?

a) Oxytocin
b) Vasopressin (ADH)
c) Aldosterone
d) Cortisol

Correct Answer: b) Vasopressin (ADH)
Explanation: Vasopressin, or antidiuretic hormone (ADH), regulates water retention by the kidneys, maintaining fluid balance and blood pressure.

Question 48: What is the function of the alveoli in the lungs?

a) Produce surfactant
b) Exchange gases between air and blood
c) Filter dust and particles
d) Warm and humidify air

Correct Answer: b) Exchange gases between air and blood
Explanation: Alveoli facilitate gas exchange, allowing oxygen to enter the blood and carbon dioxide to be expelled during respiration.

Question 49: What is a common indicator of dehydration in animals?

a) Wet nose
b) Bright eyes
c) Tacky mucous membranes
d) Shiny coat

Correct Answer: c) Tacky mucous membranes
Explanation: Dehydration leads to tacky or dry mucous membranes, indicating insufficient fluid levels, often accompanied by skin tenting and sunken eyes.

Question 50: What structure in the eye is responsible for sensing light and converting it into neural signals?

a) Cornea
b) Lens
c) Retina
d) Iris

Correct Answer: c) Retina
Explanation: The retina contains photoreceptor cells that detect light and convert it into electrical signals, which are sent to the brain for visual processing.

Question 51: Which of these is a non-steroidal anti-inflammatory drug (NSAID) often used in veterinary practice?

a) Prednisone
b) Meloxicam
c) Acetaminophen
d) Amoxicillin

Correct Answer: b) Meloxicam
Explanation: Meloxicam is an NSAID used to treat pain and inflammation in animals, particularly effective in managing arthritis and postoperative discomfort.

Question 52: What is a typical symptom of feline lower urinary tract disease (FLUTD)?

a) Vomiting
b) Frequent urination
c) Hair loss
d) Increased appetite

Correct Answer: b) Frequent urination
Explanation: FLUTD often presents with frequent urination, straining, and blood in the urine, indicating bladder or urethral irritation or obstruction.

Question 53: Which type of cell is responsible for antibody production?

a) T-lymphocytes
b) Macrophages
c) B-lymphocytes
d) Neutrophils

Correct Answer: c) B-lymphocytes
Explanation: B-lymphocytes, or B-cells, differentiate into plasma cells that produce antibodies, key components of the adaptive immune response.

Question 54: What is a common characteristic of a bacterial infection?

a) Lymphopenia
b) Neutrophil predominance
c) Eosinophilia
d) Monocytosis

Correct Answer: b) Neutrophil predominance
Explanation: Bacterial infections typically cause an increase in neutrophils, the body's primary defense against bacterial pathogens.

Question 55: Which mineral is essential for forming hemoglobin in red blood cells?

a) Calcium
b) Iron
c) Magnesium
d) Potassium

Correct Answer: b) Iron
Explanation: Iron is a critical component of hemoglobin, the molecule responsible for oxygen transport in red blood cells, and its deficiency leads to anemia.

Question 56: Which hormone is responsible for the development of secondary sexual characteristics in males?

a) Estrogen
b) Progesterone
c) Testosterone
d) Cortisol

Correct Answer: c) Testosterone
Explanation: Testosterone drives the development of male secondary sexual characteristics, such as increased muscle mass and facial hair growth.

Question 57: Which of the following is a sign of heart failure in dogs?

a) Increased appetite
b) Coughing
c) Hair loss
d) Vomiting

Correct Answer: b) Coughing
Explanation: Coughing in dogs can indicate heart failure, as fluid buildup from poor heart function leads to pulmonary congestion and respiratory issues.

Question 58: Which part of the digestive system is mainly responsible for absorbing nutrients?

a) Stomach
b) Large intestine
c) Small intestine
d) Esophagus

Correct Answer: c) Small intestine
Explanation: The small intestine, particularly the jejunum and ileum, is the main site for nutrient absorption, facilitated by its extensive surface area and villi.

Question 59: What is a common cause of ear infections in dogs?

a) Bacterial infection
b) Yeast overgrowth
c) Mite infestation
d) Viral infection

Correct Answer: b) Yeast overgrowth
Explanation: Yeast overgrowth, often due to moisture and poor ventilation, is a frequent cause of ear infections in dogs, requiring antifungal treatment.

Question 60: What structure in the heart prevents blood from flowing back into the atria from the ventricles?

a) Aortic valve
b) Pulmonary valve

c) Mitral valve
d) Semilunar valve

Correct Answer: c) Mitral valve

Explanation: The mitral valve, along with the tricuspid valve, prevents backflow from the ventricles to the atria, ensuring unidirectional blood flow during contraction.

Question 61: Which of the following is not a function of the liver?

a) Produce bile
b) Detoxify chemicals
c) Store glycogen
d) Produce insulin

Correct Answer: d) Produce insulin

Explanation: The pancreas, not the liver, is responsible for insulin production; the liver's roles include detoxification, bile production, and glycogen storage.

Question 62: What type of epithelial cell is capable of significant shape variation based on the organ's size it lines?

a) Squamous epithelium
b) Cuboidal epithelium
c) Transitional epithelium
d) Columnar epithelium

Correct Answer: c) Transitional epithelium

Explanation: Transitional epithelium lines organs such as the bladder, allowing for stretch and contraction without damage, accommodating fluctuating volumes.

Question 63: What is the packed cell volume (PCV) for a normal adult dog?

a) 25-35%
b) 37-55%
c) 60-70%
d) 10-20%

Correct Answer: b) 37-55%

Explanation: Packed cell volume (PCV) indicates the proportion of blood volume occupied by red blood cells, with 37-55% being the normal range for adult dogs.

Question 64: How is grid cutoff described?

a) Incorrect grid placement leading to excessive radiation exposure
b) The grid absorbing more radiation than it should
c) Proper alignment between the x-ray beam and grid
d) The grid enhancing image quality

Correct Answer: b) The grid absorbing more radiation than it should

Explanation: Grid cutoff occurs when misalignment between the x-ray beam and grid leads to excessive radiation absorption, reducing image clarity.

Question 65: What nutrient is sometimes referred to as "ash" in nutritional analysis?

a) Carbohydrates
b) Proteins
c) Minerals
d) Fats

Correct Answer: c) Minerals
Explanation: "Ash" in nutritional analysis refers to the inorganic residue left after complete combustion, mainly consisting of essential minerals.

Question 66: What is a sarcolemma in muscle cells?

a) A protein that stores oxygen
b) The cell membrane enclosing a muscle fiber
c) The contractile unit of muscle fibers
d) A type of connective tissue

Correct Answer: b) The cell membrane enclosing a muscle fiber
Explanation: The sarcolemma is the specialized cell membrane surrounding muscle fibers, crucial for conducting electrical impulses and maintaining cell integrity.

Question 67: You make a 1:5 dilution of a serum sample and measure the urea nitrogen. The analyzer reads that the concentration of urea nitrogen is 30 mg/dl. What is the urea nitrogen level of the patient's serum?

a) 30 mg/dl
b) 60 mg/dl
c) 150 mg/dl
d) 120 mg/dl

Correct Answer: c) 150 mg/dl
Explanation: To find the actual concentration, multiply the measured value by the dilution factor. Here, 30 mg/dl x 5 = 150 mg/dl, reflecting the original serum concentration.

Question 68: The National Association of Veterinary Technicians in America adopting a code of ethics is an example of which branch of ethics?

a) Personal ethics
b) Social ethics
c) Official ethics
d) Descriptive ethics

Correct Answer: c) Official ethics
Explanation: Official ethics involve established codes or guidelines set by professional organizations, guiding behavior and decision-making within the field.

Question 69: Which drug is NOT useful in treating seizures?

a) Phenobarbital
b) Diazepam
c) Butorphanol
d) Levetiracetam

Correct Answer: c) Butorphanol
Explanation: Butorphanol, primarily a pain and cough suppressant, lacks efficacy in seizure management compared to other anticonvulsants like phenobarbital or diazepam.

Question 70: You are reading a cardiologist report discussing tricuspid valve insufficiency and a grade 3 murmur. The mitral valve is said to be normal. If you listened to this patient, where would you expect to hear the murmur the loudest?

a) Left side
b) Right side
c) Base of the heart
d) Apex of the heart

Correct Answer: b) Right side

Explanation: The tricuspid valve murmur is best auscultated on the right side of the thorax, as it is located between the right atrium and right ventricle.

Question 71: Which form of chocolate contains the highest level of theobromine?

a) Milk chocolate
b) Dark chocolate
c) White chocolate
d) Unsweetened baking chocolate

Correct Answer: d) Unsweetened baking chocolate

Explanation: Unsweetened baking chocolate has the highest theobromine content, posing significant toxicity risks to pets if ingested.

Question 72: How are different types of bladder stones identified?

a) Visual examination
b) Ultrasound imaging
c) Submit to lab for analysis
d) Chemical testing at home

Correct Answer: c) Submit to lab for analysis

Explanation: Laboratory analysis provides definitive identification of bladder stone composition, guiding appropriate treatment and dietary management.

Question 73: What type of vaccine is most commonly used for distemper-parvo in dogs?

a) Inactivated virus
b) Live attenuated virus
c) Recombinant virus
d) Subunit vaccine

Correct Answer: b) Modified live virus

Explanation: Modified live virus vaccines elicit strong immune responses, making them effective for preventing distemper and parvovirus in dogs.

Question 74: What is the term for a castration method in cattle that does not involve skin incision?

a) Open castration
b) Closed castration
c) Chemical castration
d) Surgical castration

Correct Answer: b) Closed castration

Explanation: Closed castration, using an emasculatome, avoids skin incisions, reducing infection risks and is referred to as bloodless castration.

Question 75: Which medication should be used cautiously in cats due to potential blindness risks?

a) Amoxicillin
b) Enrofloxacin
c) Prednisone
d) Metronidazole

Correct Answer: b) Enrofloxacin

Explanation: Enrofloxacin, at high doses, poses a risk of retinal damage in cats, leading to blindness, necessitating cautious use.

Question 76: How long does the estrus period typically last in dogs?

a) 1-3 days
b) 4-13 days
c) 14-21 days
d) 3-5 weeks

Correct Answer: b) 4-13 days
Explanation: Estrus in dogs generally spans 4 to 13 days, with ovulation and fertility peaks, crucial for breeding timing.

Question 77: The Tensilon test in dogs is used to diagnose which disease?

a) Epilepsy
b) Myasthenia gravis
c) Canine distemper
d) Lyme disease

Correct Answer: b) Myasthenia gravis
Explanation: The Tensilon test utilizes edrophonium chloride to temporarily improve muscle strength, diagnosing myasthenia gravis by inhibiting acetylcholinesterase.

Question 78: Which type of cell contains high levels of histamine and heparin?

a) Neutrophil
b) Eosinophil
c) Mast cell
d) Macrophage

Correct Answer: c) Mast cell
Explanation: Mast cells release histamine and heparin, mediating allergic reactions and inflammation, pivotal in immune responses.

Question 79: What is the primary role of platelets in the blood?

a) Oxygen transport
b) Blood clotting
c) Fighting infections
d) Hormone regulation

Correct Answer: b) To aid in blood clotting
Explanation: Platelets, or thrombocytes, aggregate at injury sites, releasing factors that form clots, preventing excessive bleeding.

Question 80: Which organ is often referred to as the "master gland" of the endocrine system?

a) Thyroid gland
b) Adrenal gland
c) Pituitary gland
d) Pancreas

Correct Answer: c) Pituitary gland
Explanation: The pituitary gland regulates various hormonal functions by secreting hormones that control other endocrine glands.

Question 81: What is the primary function of hemoglobin in red blood cells?

a) To transport oxygen
b) To fight infections
c) To store nutrients
d) To regulate pH

Correct Answer: a) To transport oxygen

Explanation: Hemoglobin binds oxygen in the lungs, transporting it to tissues, and facilitating cellular respiration and energy production.

Question 82: Which animal has a four-chambered stomach?

a) Horse
b) Pig
c) Cow
d) Rabbit

Correct Answer: c) Cow

Explanation: Cows, as ruminants, possess a four-chambered stomach (rumen, reticulum, omasum, abomasum) for efficient digestion of fibrous plant material.

Question 83: What vitamin is essential for vision and immune function?

a) Vitamin A
b) Vitamin B12
c) Vitamin C
d) Vitamin D

Correct Answer: a) Vitamin A

Explanation: Vitamin A supports vision by maintaining retinal health and bolsters immune defenses, preventing infections and maintaining epithelial tissues.

Question 84: What role do the kidneys play in the excretory system?

a) Produce red blood cells
b) Filter waste from the blood and form urine
c) Regulate body temperature
d) Store glycogen

Correct Answer: b) To filter waste from the blood and form urine

Explanation: Kidneys filter blood, removing waste products and excess substances, which are then excreted as urine, maintaining fluid and electrolyte balance.

Question 85: Which vitamin is primarily synthesized by the skin when exposed to sunlight?

a) Vitamin A
b) Vitamin B6
c) Vitamin C
d) Vitamin D

Correct Answer: d) Vitamin D

Explanation: Vitamin D synthesis in the skin is triggered by UV exposure, essential for calcium absorption and bone health.

Question 86: Which animal is the natural host for the parasite Toxoplasma gondii?

a) Dog
b) Bird
c) Cat
d) Rabbit

Correct Answer: c) Cat

Explanation: Cats are the definitive hosts for Toxoplasma gondii, where the parasite completes its life cycle, shedding oocysts into the environment.

Question 87: Which part of the brain processes visual information?

a) Frontal lobe
b) Parietal lobe
c) Temporal lobe
d) Occipital lobe

Correct Answer: d) Occipital lobe
Explanation: The occipital lobe, located at the back of the brain, is primarily involved in interpreting visual stimuli received from the eyes.

Question 88: Where does most nutrient absorption occur in the digestive system?

a) Stomach
b) Large intestine
c) Small intestine
d) Esophagus

Correct Answer: c) Small intestine
Explanation: The small intestine, with its extensive surface area, is the primary site for nutrient absorption, utilizing villi and microvilli to maximize efficiency.

Question 89: Which hormone lowers blood sugar levels?

a) Glucagon
b) Cortisol
c) Insulin
d) Adrenaline

Correct Answer: c) Insulin
Explanation: Insulin, produced by the pancreas, facilitates cellular glucose uptake, lowering blood sugar levels and maintaining metabolic balance.

Question 90: Which blood type is known as the universal donor?

a) A positive
b) B negative
c) O positive
d) O negative

Correct Answer: d) O negative
Explanation: O negative blood lacks A, B, and Rh antigens, making it compatible with all other blood types for transfusions, hence "universal donor."

Question 91: What is the main structural protein in skin and connective tissues?

a) Keratin
b) Elastin
c) Collagen
d) Albumin

Correct Answer: c) Collagen
Explanation: Collagen provides tensile strength and structural support in skin, tendons, and ligaments, maintaining integrity and elasticity.

Question 92: Which part of the cell is responsible for energy production?

a) Nucleus
b) Ribosome
c) Mitochondria
d) Golgi apparatus

Correct Answer: c) Mitochondria

Explanation: Mitochondria generate ATP through cellular respiration, powering cellular activities and acting as the cell's energy powerhouse.

Question 93: What is the role of the lymphatic system?

a) Maintain body temperature
b) Transport lymph and support immune function
c) Produce insulin
d) Store vitamins

Correct Answer: b) To transport lymph and support immune function

Explanation: The lymphatic system circulates lymph, removes waste, and houses lymphocytes, crucial for immune responses and fluid balance.

Question 94: Which vitamin is essential for collagen synthesis?

a) Vitamin A
b) Vitamin B6
c) Vitamin C
d) Vitamin E

Correct Answer: c) Vitamin C

Explanation: Vitamin C is vital for collagen synthesis, promoting skin health and wound healing, and functioning as an antioxidant.

Question 95: What is the primary function of the large intestine?

a) Digestion of fats
b) Absorb water and electrolytes
c) Produce digestive enzymes
d) Store bile

Correct Answer: b) To absorb water and electrolytes

Explanation: The large intestine absorbs water and electrolytes from indigestible food, forming and storing feces for excretion.

Question 96: Which mineral is important for thyroid hormone production?

a) Calcium
b) Iron
c) Iodine
d) Zinc

Correct Answer: c) Iodine

Explanation: Iodine is essential for synthesizing thyroid hormones (T3 and T4), regulating metabolism and growth.

Question 97: What is the term for the process by which plants convert sunlight into chemical energy?

a) Respiration
b) Fermentation
c) Photosynthesis
d) Transpiration

Correct Answer: c) Photosynthesis

Explanation: Photosynthesis enables plants to convert sunlight into glucose and oxygen, sustaining life on Earth by providing food and oxygen.

Question 98: Which part of the nervous system controls involuntary actions?

a) Central nervous system
b) Peripheral nervous system
c) Autonomic nervous system
d) Somatic nervous system

Correct Answer: c) Autonomic nervous system
Explanation: The autonomic nervous system regulates involuntary functions, like heart rate and digestion, maintaining homeostasis.

Question 99: What is the primary function of white blood cells?

a) To transport oxygen
b) To defend against infections
c) To clot blood
d) To balance electrolytes

Correct Answer: b) To defend against infections
Explanation: White blood cells, or leukocytes, identify and neutralize pathogens, playing a central role in the immune response.

Question 100: Which hormone triggers ovulation in females?

a) Follicle-stimulating hormone (FSH)
b) Luteinizing hormone (LH)
c) Estrogen
d) Progesterone

Correct Answer: b) Luteinizing hormone (LH)
Explanation: Luteinizing hormone surges mid-cycle, prompting ovulation and enabling potential fertilization and conception.

Question 101: A deficiency in which vitamin can lead to scurvy?

a) Vitamin A
b) Vitamin B12
c) Vitamin C
d) Vitamin D

Correct Answer: c) Vitamin C
Explanation: Vitamin C deficiency causes scurvy, characterized by bleeding gums, anemia, and connective tissue breakdown.

Question 102: Which part of the brain coordinates voluntary movements?

a) Cerebrum
b) Medulla oblongata
c) Cerebellum
d) Hypothalamus

Correct Answer: c) Cerebellum
Explanation: The cerebellum coordinates voluntary movements, ensuring balance, posture, and precise motor control.

Question 103: What is the main function of the respiratory system?

a) To circulate blood
b) To filter waste products
c) To facilitate gas exchange
d) To produce hormones

Correct Answer: c) To facilitate gas exchange
Explanation: The respiratory system exchanges oxygen and carbon dioxide between the air and bloodstream, essential for cellular respiration.

Question 104: Which gland produces melatonin to regulate sleep-wake cycles?

a) Thyroid gland
b) Pituitary gland
c) Pineal gland
d) Adrenal gland

Correct Answer: c) Pineal gland
Explanation: The pineal gland secretes melatonin, modulating sleep patterns and circadian rhythms in response to light exposure.

Question 105: Which mineral is necessary for muscle contraction and nerve function?

a) Sodium
b) Potassium
c) Calcium
d) Magnesium

Correct Answer: c) Calcium
Explanation: Calcium ions are crucial for muscle contractions and neurotransmitter release, facilitating nerve impulse transmission.

Question 106: Which component of the eye regulates light entry?

a) Cornea
b) Iris
c) Lens
d) Pupil

Correct Answer: d) Pupil
Explanation: The pupil adjusts its size in response to light intensity, controlling the amount entering the eye for optimal vision.

Question 107: Which organ primarily regulates blood sugar levels?

a) Liver
b) Kidneys
c) Pancreas
d) Stomach

Correct Answer: c) Pancreas
Explanation: The pancreas produces insulin and glucagon, hormones that regulate blood glucose levels, maintaining metabolic balance.

Question 108: What is the main purpose of the skeletal system?

a) Produce hormones
b) Provide support and protection
c) Transport oxygen
d) Regulate body temperature

Correct Answer: b) To provide support and protection
Explanation: The skeletal system supports body structure, protects vital organs, and facilitates movement through attachment sites for muscles.

Question 109: Which vitamin aids in calcium absorption?

a) Vitamin A
b) Vitamin B12
c) Vitamin C
d) Vitamin D

Correct Answer: d) Vitamin D
Explanation: Vitamin D enhances intestinal calcium absorption, crucial for bone health and preventing disorders like osteoporosis.

Question 110: What is the main function of the circulatory system?

a) To digest food
b) To transport nutrients and oxygen
c) To filter waste
d) To produce hormones

Correct Answer: b) To transport nutrients and oxygen
Explanation: The circulatory system delivers oxygen, nutrients, and hormones to cells and removes waste, sustaining bodily functions.

Question 111: Which hormone is key in metabolism regulation?

a) Insulin
b) Cortisol
c) Thyroxine (T4)
d) Adrenaline

Correct Answer: c) Thyroxine (T4)
Explanation: Thyroxine, produced by the thyroid gland, regulates metabolism, influencing energy levels and growth.

Question 112: What is the primary role of the integumentary system?

a) To regulate temperature
b) To protect the body from external damage
c) To transport nutrients
d) To produce red blood cells

Correct Answer: b) To protect the body from external damage
Explanation: The integumentary system, including skin, hair, and nails, acts as a barrier against pathogens and physical damage.

Question 113: Which mineral is essential for oxygen transport in blood?

a) Calcium
b) Magnesium
c) Iron
d) Zinc

Correct Answer: c) Iron
Explanation: Iron, a component of hemoglobin, is vital for oxygen transport from the lungs to tissues and carbon dioxide removal.

Question 114: Which part of the ear helps maintain balance?

a) Cochlea
b) Eustachian tube
c) Vestibular system
d) Tympanic membrane

Correct Answer: c) Vestibular system

Explanation: The vestibular system, within the inner ear, detects head movements and position, aiding in balance and spatial orientation.

Question 115: Which vitamin is crucial for blood clotting?

a) Vitamin A
b) Vitamin B12
c) Vitamin C
d) Vitamin K

Correct Answer: d) Vitamin K

Explanation: Vitamin K is essential for synthesizing clotting factors, preventing excessive bleeding and ensuring proper hemostasis.

Question 116: What role do sweat glands play in the skin?

a) To store fat
b) To regulate body temperature
c) To produce hormones
d) To protect against UV rays

Correct Answer: b) To regulate body temperature

Explanation: Sweat glands produce perspiration, evaporating to cool the body and maintain optimal temperature.

Question 117: Which brain region is involved in emotion and memory?

a) Cerebellum
b) Brainstem
c) Limbic system
d) Occipital lobe

Correct Answer: c) Limbic system

Explanation: The limbic system, including the hippocampus and amygdala, processes emotions and forms memories, influencing behavior.

Question 118: What organ stores bile from the liver?

a) Pancreas
b) Gallbladder
c) Spleen
d) Stomach

Correct Answer: b) Gallbladder

Explanation: The gallbladder stores and concentrates bile, releasing it into the small intestine to aid in fat digestion.

Question 119: Which hormone boosts heart rate and blood pressure during stress?

a) Insulin
b) Cortisol
c) Adrenaline (epinephrine)
d) Thyroxine

Correct Answer: c) Adrenaline (epinephrine)

Explanation: Adrenaline, released by the adrenal glands, prepares the body for "fight or flight" by increasing heart rate and energy availability.

Question 120: What is the primary function of red blood cells?

a) To fight infections
b) To transport oxygen
c) To clot blood
d) To store nutrients

Correct Answer: b) To transport oxygen
Explanation: Red blood cells, containing hemoglobin, carry oxygen from the lungs to tissues and return carbon dioxide for exhalation.

Question 121: Which vitamin is vital for forming red blood cells?

a) Vitamin A
b) Vitamin B12
c) Vitamin C
d) Vitamin D

Correct Answer: b) Vitamin B12
Explanation: Vitamin B12 is necessary for red blood cell production and DNA synthesis, with deficiency leading to anemia.

Question 122: Which joint type allows the greatest movement?

a) Hinge joint
b) Pivot joint
c) Ball-and-socket joint
d) Gliding joint

Correct Answer: c) Ball-and-socket joint
Explanation: Ball-and-socket joints, like the shoulder and hip, permit a wide range of motion, including rotation and angular movements.

Question 123: What role does the pancreas play in digestion?

a) To produce bile
b) To secrete digestive enzymes
c) To absorb nutrients
d) To store glycogen

Correct Answer: b) To produce digestive enzymes
Explanation: The pancreas secretes enzymes like amylase and lipase into the small intestine, aiding in the breakdown of carbohydrates, proteins, and fats.

Question 124: Which mineral is crucial for fluid balance in the body?

a) Potassium
b) Calcium
c) Sodium
d) Magnesium

Correct Answer: c) Sodium
Explanation: Sodium regulates fluid balance and blood pressure, facilitating nerve impulse transmission and muscle function.

Question 125: Which brain area is responsible for speech production?

a) Wernicke's area
b) Broca's area
c) Hippocampus
d) Cerebellum

Correct Answer: b) Broca's area
Explanation: Broca's area, located in the frontal lobe, coordinates speech production, enabling articulate verbal communication.

Question 126: What is the main function of the immune system?

a) To produce hormones
b) To protect the body from infections
c) To transport oxygen
d) To digest food

Correct Answer: b) To protect the body from infections
Explanation: The immune system detects and neutralizes pathogens like bacteria and viruses, preventing disease and maintaining health.

Question 127: Which vitamin is essential for healthy bones and teeth?

a) Vitamin A
b) Vitamin B6
c) Vitamin C
d) Vitamin D

Correct Answer: d) Vitamin D
Explanation: Vitamin D facilitates calcium absorption, crucial for strong bones and teeth, and preventing disorders like rickets.

Question 128: Which blood vessels carry oxygenated blood away from the heart?

a) Veins
b) Capillaries
c) Arteries
d) Lymphatics

Correct Answer: c) Arteries
Explanation: Arteries transport oxygen-rich blood from the heart to tissues, with the aorta being the largest artery.

Question 129: What is the liver's primary role in metabolism?

a) To store fat
b) To process nutrients and detoxify substances
c) To produce insulin
d) To absorb water

Correct Answer: b) To process nutrients and detoxify substances
Explanation: The liver metabolizes nutrients from digestion, detoxifies harmful substances, and stores glycogen, supporting metabolic functions.

Question 130: Which vitamin is vital for vision and skin health?

a) Vitamin A
b) Vitamin B12
c) Vitamin C
d) Vitamin E

Correct Answer: a) Vitamin A
Explanation: Vitamin A maintains healthy vision and skin, supporting cell growth and immune function, preventing night blindness and skin issues.

Question 131: Which hormone controls water reabsorption in kidneys?

a) Insulin
b) Adrenaline
c) Antidiuretic hormone (ADH)
d) Cortisol

Correct Answer: c) Antidiuretic hormone (ADH)
Explanation: ADH regulates water balance by increasing kidney water reabsorption, concentrating urine and maintaining blood volume.

Question 132: What does the cerebrum do in the brain?

a) Control voluntary actions and cognitive functions
b) Regulate hormones
c) Maintain balance
d) Control automatic functions

Correct Answer: a) Control voluntary actions and cognitive functions
Explanation: The cerebrum processes sensory information, initiates voluntary movements, and is involved in cognition and reasoning.

Question 133: Which mineral is crucial for enzymes and protein synthesis?

a) Iron
b) Calcium
c) Zinc
d) Magnesium

Correct Answer: c) Zinc
Explanation: Zinc is involved in numerous enzymatic reactions and protein synthesis, essential for growth, immune function, and wound healing.

Question 134: Which digestive system part absorbs nutrients?

a) Stomach
b) Large intestine
c) Small intestine
d) Esophagus

Correct Answer: c) Small intestine
Explanation: The small intestine, with its villi and microvilli, maximizes nutrient absorption, transferring digested nutrients into the bloodstream.

Question 135: Which vitamin is vital for energy metabolism and red blood cell production?

a) Vitamin A
b) Vitamin B6
c) Vitamin C
d) Vitamin D

Correct Answer: b) Vitamin B6
Explanation: Vitamin B6 supports enzymatic reactions in energy metabolism and is crucial for hemoglobin synthesis and red blood cell production.

Question 136: What is the main function of the reproductive system?

a) To produce hormones
b) To produce offspring
c) To transport nutrients
d) To regulate body temperature

Correct Answer: b) To produce offspring
Explanation: The reproductive system generates gametes and facilitates fertilization and development, ensuring species continuation.

Question 137: Which tissue type connects muscles to bones?

a) Ligaments
b) Tendons
c) Cartilage
d) Fascia

Correct Answer: b) Tendons
Explanation: Tendons are robust, fibrous connective tissues that attach muscles to bones, facilitating movement by transmitting the force generated by muscle contractions to the skeletal system.

Question 138: Which stage of Dirofilaria immitis, causing heartworm in dogs, is diagnostic?

a) Adult stage
b) Larval stage
c) Microfilarial stage
d) Egg stage

Correct Answer: c) Microfilarial stage
Explanation: The microfilarial stage is the larval form detectable in the bloodstream, indicating an active heartworm infection in dogs, and is crucial for diagnosis and treatment planning.

Question 139: Which of the following parasites is NOT a potential zoonotic pathogen?

a) Cryptosporidium
b) Giardia
c) Toxoplasma
d) Demodex canis

Correct Answer: d) Demodex canis
Explanation: Demodex canis, a common mite in dogs, is not zoonotic, unlike other parasites like Cryptosporidium, Giardia, Toxoplasma, and Toxocara, which can infect humans.

Question 140: How long should an incision be monitored after uncomplicated surgery?

a) 1 week
b) 2 weeks
c) 3 weeks
d) 4 weeks

Correct Answer: b) 2 weeks
Explanation: Monitoring an incision for two weeks post-surgery ensures proper healing, allowing for early intervention if infection or complications arise, promoting optimal recovery.

Question 141: How many milliliters of a 2.5% solution are needed for a 100-kg patient requiring 50 mg?

a) 1 ml
b) 2 ml
c) 3 ml
d) 4 ml

Correct Answer: b) 2 ml
Explanation: A 2.5% solution equals 25 mg/ml. For a 50 mg dose, divide 50 mg by 25 mg/ml, resulting in 2 ml to be administered, ensuring accurate dosing.

Question 142: A dog has a week-old wound on its side that smells bad and contains dead tissue. What term best describes this wound?

a) Infected
b) Necrotic
c) Inflamed
d) Abrasion

Correct Answer: b) Necrotic
Explanation: Necrotic describes tissue death, characterized by a foul odor and nonviable tissue, necessitating debridement and treatment to prevent further infection.

Question 143: Several Heinz bodies have been identified on a blood smear of a sick dog. What does this indicate?

a) Vitamin deficiency
b) Oxidative damage
c) Bacterial infection
d) Autoimmune disorder

Correct Answer: b) Oxidative damage
Explanation: Heinz bodies form due to oxidative damage to red blood cells, often linked to toxins or disease, potentially leading to hemolytic anemia.

Question 144: What is the name of the triangular-shaped structure behind the sole of a horse's hoof?

a) Sole
b) Frog
c) Wall
d) Bulbs

Correct Answer: b) Frog
Explanation: The frog is a vital shock absorber and traction aid in the horse's hoof, contributing to hoof health and biomechanics.

Question 145: A bulldog regularly eats dirt, toys, and other non-food items. What is this condition known as?

a) Bulimia
b) Anorexia
c) Pica
d) Dyspepsia

Correct Answer: c) Pica
Explanation: Pica is the compulsive ingestion of non-nutritive substances, which may indicate nutritional deficiencies or behavioral issues requiring intervention.

Question 146: A client asks about spironolactone for their pet. What is your response regarding its use?

a) It's an antibiotic for infections
b) It's a pain reliever
c) It's a diuretic for heart issues
d) It's a sedative

Correct Answer: c) It is a diuretic for her pet's congestive heart failure
Explanation: Spironolactone, a diuretic, reduces fluid buildup in congestive heart failure, enhancing heart function and alleviating symptoms.

Question 147: What is another name for the dog's abdominal region?

a) Dorsal region
b) Ventral region
c) Cranial region
d) Caudal region

Correct Answer: b) Ventral region
Explanation: The ventral region encompasses the abdomen's lower surface, opposite the dorsal (back) side, crucial for anatomical orientation.

Question 148: Which feline disease is mainly spread through saliva sharing?

a) Feline Immunodeficiency Virus
b) Feline Panleukopenia
c) Feline Leukemia Virus
d) Feline Calicivirus

Correct Answer: c) Feline Leukemia Virus
Explanation: Feline Leukemia Virus spreads through saliva and bodily fluids, emphasizing the importance of preventing direct contact among cats.

Question 149: What does the Veterinary Technician Code of Ethics include?

a) Sharing client information freely
b) Protecting client confidential information
c) Promoting personal beliefs to clients
d) Encouraging self-medication in animals

Correct Answer: b) Veterinary technicians shall protect confidential information provided by clients.
Explanation: Upholding client confidentiality is a cornerstone of ethical practice, fostering trust and professionalism in veterinary care.

Question 150: What disease can humans contract through contact with infected urine?

a) Rabies
b) Toxoplasmosis
c) Leptospirosis
d) Brucellosis

Correct Answer: c) Leptospirosis
Explanation: Leptospirosis, a zoonotic bacterial infection, spreads via contact with contaminated urine, highlighting the need for protective measures.

Question 151: What would not cause a urine specific gravity lower than 1.020?

a) Renal failure
b) Overhydration
c) Diabetes insipidus
d) Dehydration

Correct Answer: d) Dehydration
Explanation: Dehydration typically results in concentrated urine (high specific gravity), contrasting with causes of dilute urine like renal failure.

Question 152: What is the primary role of the cardiovascular system?

a) To digest food
b) To circulate blood and transport nutrients, oxygen, and waste products
c) To produce hormones
d) To protect against infections

Correct Answer: b) To circulate blood and transport nutrients, oxygen, and waste products
Explanation: The cardiovascular system delivers nutrients and oxygen to cells, removes waste products, and maintains homeostasis through blood circulation.

Question 153: What is the function of hemolymph in insects?

a) To produce energy
b) To transport nutrients and waste products
c) To control movement
d) To regulate temperature

Correct Answer: b) To transport nutrients and waste products
Explanation: Hemolymph in insects circulates nutrients and waste, analogous to blood in vertebrates, crucial for maintaining metabolic processes.

Question 154: Which organ primarily filters and removes blood waste?

a) Liver
b) Kidneys
c) Spleen
d) Lungs

Correct Answer: b) Kidneys
Explanation: Kidneys filter blood, excreting waste as urine, and maintaining fluid and electrolyte balance, critical for homeostasis.

Question 155: Which vitamin is essential for normal blood clotting?

a) Vitamin A
b) Vitamin B12
c) Vitamin D
d) Vitamin K

Correct Answer: d) Vitamin K
Explanation: Vitamin K is vital for synthesizing clotting factors, preventing excessive bleeding and ensuring effective hemostasis.

Question 156: What role does the large intestine play in digestion?

a) To digest proteins
b) To absorb water and electrolytes
c) To produce bile
d) To store vitamins

Correct Answer: b) To absorb water and electrolytes from indigestible food matter
Explanation: The large intestine reabsorbs water and electrolytes, forming solid waste for elimination, completing the digestive process.

Question 157: Which mineral is vital for strong bones and teeth?

a) Iron
b) Sodium
c) Potassium
d) Calcium

Correct Answer: d) Calcium
Explanation: Calcium is crucial for bone and tooth structure, muscle function, and nerve signaling, playing a key role in skeletal health.

Question 158: Which brain part regulates hunger and thirst?

a) Cerebellum
b) Medulla oblongata
c) Hypothalamus
d) Thalamus

Correct Answer: c) Hypothalamus
Explanation: The hypothalamus maintains homeostasis by regulating hunger, thirst, and other autonomic functions through hormonal and neural pathways.

Question 159: Which hormone is released during stress by the adrenal glands?

a) Adrenaline
b) Insulin
c) Cortisol
d) Thyroxine

Correct Answer: c) Cortisol
Explanation: Cortisol, a glucocorticoid, modulates stress responses, metabolism, and immune function, preparing the body for prolonged stressors.

Question 160: What is the primary function of the lymphatic system?

a) To produce red blood cells
b) To digest fats
c) To return excess tissue fluid and protect against infections
d) To regulate body temperature

Correct Answer: c) To return excess tissue fluid to the bloodstream and protect against infections
Explanation: The lymphatic system maintains fluid balance and filters pathogens, supporting immune responses and preventing edema.

Question 161: Which vitamin is known as the "sunshine vitamin"?

a) Vitamin A
b) Vitamin C
c) Vitamin D
d) Vitamin E

Correct Answer: c) Vitamin D
Explanation: Vitamin D, synthesized from sunlight exposure, is essential for calcium absorption and bone health, preventing rickets and osteoporosis.

Question 162: What is the main purpose of the respiratory system?

a) To transport blood
b) To facilitate oxygen and carbon dioxide exchange
c) To produce hormones
d) To regulate body temperature

Correct Answer: b) To facilitate the exchange of oxygen and carbon dioxide
Explanation: The respiratory system ensures efficient oxygen intake and carbon dioxide expulsion, vital for cellular respiration and energy production.

Question 163: Which mineral is necessary for thyroid hormone production?

a) Calcium
b) Iron
c) Iodine
d) Magnesium

Correct Answer: c) Iodine
Explanation: Iodine is integral to thyroid hormone synthesis, regulating metabolism, growth, and development via hormones like thyroxine.

Question 164: Which organelle is known as the "powerhouse" of the cell?

a) Nucleus
b) Endoplasmic reticulum
c) Golgi apparatus
d) Mitochondria

Correct Answer: d) Mitochondria
Explanation: Mitochondria generate ATP through cellular respiration, providing energy for cellular processes and sustaining life functions.

Question 165: Which part of the nervous system manages voluntary movements?

a) Autonomic nervous system
b) Central nervous system
c) Peripheral nervous system
d) Somatic nervous system

Correct Answer: d) Somatic nervous system
Explanation: The somatic nervous system controls voluntary muscle movements and reflex arcs, enabling conscious motor activity and responses.

Question 166: What is the main function of the endocrine system?

a) To transport oxygen
b) To secrete hormones regulating bodily processes
c) To protect against infections
d) To filter blood

Correct Answer: b) To secrete hormones that regulate bodily processes
Explanation: The endocrine system releases hormones into the bloodstream, influencing growth, metabolism, and homeostasis through targeted actions.

Question 167: Which vitamin is essential for collagen synthesis and immune function?

a) Vitamin A
b) Vitamin B12
c) Vitamin C
d) Vitamin D

Correct Answer: c) Vitamin C
Explanation: Vitamin C supports collagen formation, wound healing, and immune defense, protecting against infections and promoting skin health.

Question 168: What is the primary function of red blood cells?

a) To fight infections
b) To transport oxygen from the lungs to the body's tissues
c) To produce hormones
d) To store nutrients

Correct Answer: b) To transport oxygen from the lungs to the body's tissues
Explanation: Red blood cells, rich in hemoglobin, deliver oxygen to tissues and return carbon dioxide to the lungs for exhalation, sustaining cellular metabolism.

Question 169: Which type of joint allows for rotational movement?

a) Ball-and-socket joint
b) Hinge joint
c) Pivot joint
d) Saddle joint

Correct Answer: c) Pivot joint

Explanation: Pivot joints, like those in the neck, enable rotational movement, allowing bones to turn around an axis, crucial for head and limb flexibility.

Question 170: Which gland regulates metabolism and calcium levels?

a) Pituitary gland
b) Adrenal gland
c) Thyroid gland
d) Parathyroid gland

Correct Answer: c) Thyroid gland

Explanation: The thyroid gland produces hormones like thyroxine, which regulate metabolism, and calcitonin, which helps control calcium levels, maintaining metabolic and skeletal balance.

Full Test 7 with Detailed Explanations

Question 1: What is the normal amount of gastric reflux obtained from a healthy horse via nasogastric tube placement?

a) 14-18 liters
b) 10-12 liters
c) 5-8 liters
d) 1-3 liters

Correct Answer: d) 1-3 liters

Explanation: Normally, a healthy horse will have a small amount of gastric reflux, 1-3 liters. If you get back 8-12 or more liters of reflux, the horse likely has an obstructive intestinal disease or ileus of some sort.

Question 2: Which hormone is the trigger for ovulation and development of the corpus luteum?

a) Luteinizing hormone (LH)
b) Progesterone
c) Follicle stimulating hormone (FSH)
d) Testosterone

Correct Answer: a) Luteinizing hormone (LH)

Explanation: Luteinizing hormone is produced by the anterior pituitary gland. The LH surge is the trigger for ovulation and development of the corpus luteum. Progesterone levels increase after ovulation has already occurred.

Question 3: What is the "top" shell of a tortoise called?

a) Choana
b) Patagium
c) Carapace
d) Cloaca
e) Plastron
f) Scute

Correct Answer: c) Carapace

Explanation: The carapace is the dorsal (top) part of a tortoise's shell, providing protection and structural support, essential for its survival.

Question 4: Which of the following is expected from a positive inotropic drug?

a) Increase in cardiac contractility
b) Dramatic decrease in blood pressure
c) Decrease in adrenal gland stimulation
d) Prevention of arrhythmias

Correct Answer: a) Increase in cardiac contractility
Explanation: Positive inotropic drugs increase the force of heart muscle contractions, improving cardiac output in conditions like heart failure.

Question 5: Aside from diabetes, what is another cause for glucosuria in a cat?

a) High carbohydrate diet
b) Estrus
c) Excitement
d) Dehydration

Correct Answer: c) Excitement
Explanation: Excitement, stress, and fear can raise blood glucose levels. If those levels exceed the renal threshold, glucosuria can occur. The other options do not typically result in glucosuria.

Question 6: Assessing which of the following on serum chemistry is most appropriate in the assessment of liver function?

a) Blood Urea Nitrogen (BUN)
b) Bilirubin
c) Creatinine
d) Glucose

Correct Answer: b) Bilirubin
Explanation: Elevated bilirubin levels can indicate liver dysfunction or bile duct obstruction, making it a useful marker for liver health assessment.

Question 7: An "FHO" would most likely be performed on a patient with which of the following problems?

a) Incontinence
b) Arthritic hip
c) Blindness from glaucoma
d) Ovarian cysts

Correct Answer: b) Arthritic hip
Explanation: Femoral Head Ostectomy (FHO) is a surgical procedure often used to address severe hip arthritis or hip dysplasia, alleviating pain and improving mobility.

Question 8: Sulfasalazine is sometimes used in veterinary medicine to treat which chronic condition?

a) Bronchitis
b) Colitis
c) Hepatitis
d) Pancreatitis

Correct Answer: b) Colitis
Explanation: Sulfasalazine acts as an anti-inflammatory in the colon, used to manage chronic colitis by reducing inflammation and controlling symptoms.

Question 9: What is the average gestation length of a horse?

a) Approximately 290 days
b) Approximately 400 days

c) Approximately 230 days
d) Approximately 340 days

Correct Answer: d) Approximately 340 days
Explanation: The average gestation period for a horse is approximately 340 days, or about 11 months, necessary for the full development of the foal.

Question 10: Which is NOT true of cytology?

a) It is read under the microscope
b) It evaluates tissue architecture
c) It can be useful to help differentiate a tumor from inflammatory tissue
d) One method of sample collection is a fine needle aspirate

Correct Answer: b) It evaluates tissue architecture
Explanation: Cytology involves the examination of individual cells and does not assess tissue architecture, which is evaluated through histopathology.

Question 11: How many milliliters of 25% dextrose should be added to 1 L of 0.9% saline to make a 5% dextrose solution?

a) 200 ml
b) 50 ml
c) 20 ml
d) 100 ml

Correct Answer: a) 200 ml
Explanation: To make a 5% dextrose solution, use the formula $C(1)V(1) = C(2)V(2)$. For a solution with 0.25 concentration, 200 ml of 25% dextrose should be added to 1 L of saline.

Question 12: What is the normal heart rate range for a healthy adult dog?

a) 40-60 beats per minute
b) 60-120 beats per minute
c) 70-160 beats per minute
d) 100-180 beats per minute

Correct Answer: c) 70-160 beats per minute
Explanation: The normal heart rate for a healthy adult dog is typically between 70 and 160 beats per minute, varying by size, breed, and activity level.

Question 13: Which of the following is a common sign of feline hyperthyroidism?

a) Weight gain
b) Lethargy
c) Increased appetite
d) Decreased heart rate

Correct Answer: c) Increased appetite
Explanation: Feline hyperthyroidism often leads to increased appetite combined with weight loss due to elevated metabolism, resulting from excessive thyroid hormone production.

Question 14: What type of anesthesia is used to numb a specific area of the body?

a) General anesthesia
b) Local anesthesia
c) Regional anesthesia
d) Conscious sedation

Correct Answer: b) Local anesthesia
Explanation: Local anesthesia involves the administration of anesthetic agents to a specific area of the body, providing temporary loss of sensation without affecting consciousness.

Question 15: What is the primary function of the kidneys?

a) Produce red blood cells
b) Filter and excrete waste products from the blood
c) Regulate body temperature
d) Break down fats

Correct Answer: b) Filter and excrete waste products from the blood
Explanation: The kidneys filter blood, removing waste and excess substances, and excreting them as urine, maintaining fluid and electrolyte balance in the body.

Question 16: Which of the following is a zoonotic disease that can be transmitted from animals to humans?

a) Canine distemper
b) Feline leukemia
c) Rabies
d) Equine influenza

Correct Answer: c) Rabies
Explanation: Rabies is a viral zoonotic disease that affects the nervous system of mammals, including humans, transmitted through bites from infected animals.

Question 17: Which blood vessel carries oxygenated blood from the heart to the rest of the body?

a) Pulmonary artery
b) Vena cava
c) Aorta
d) Pulmonary vein

Correct Answer: c) Aorta
Explanation: The aorta is the largest artery in the body, carrying oxygen-rich blood from the left ventricle of the heart to distribute it throughout the body.

Question 18: What is the most common cause of ear infections in dogs?

a) Viral infection
b) Yeast infection
c) Foreign bodies
d) Bacterial infection

Correct Answer: d) Bacterial infection
Explanation: Bacterial infections are a common cause of canine ear infections, often exacerbated by moisture, allergies, or anatomical factors in certain breeds.

Question 19: Which vitamin is crucial for blood clotting?

a) Vitamin A
b) Vitamin B12
c) Vitamin C
d) Vitamin K

Correct Answer: d) Vitamin K
Explanation: Vitamin K is essential for synthesizing clotting factors, preventing excessive bleeding and ensuring effective blood coagulation processes.

Question 20: Which of the following is a common sign of canine heartworm disease?

a) Increased appetite
b) Weight gain
c) Persistent cough
d) Increased urination

Correct Answer: c) Persistent cough

Explanation: A persistent cough is a common sign of heartworm disease in dogs, caused by the presence of worms in the heart and pulmonary arteries, affecting respiratory function.

Question 21: Which part of the brain is responsible for balance and coordination?

a) Cerebrum
b) Brainstem
c) Cerebellum
d) Thalamus

Correct Answer: c) Cerebellum

Explanation: The cerebellum is responsible for coordinating voluntary movements, maintaining balance, posture, and fine motor skills, essential for smooth and coordinated physical activity.

Question 22: Which hormone is responsible for regulating blood sugar levels?

a) Insulin
b) Adrenaline
c) Cortisol
d) Thyroxine

Correct Answer: a) Insulin

Explanation: Insulin, produced by the pancreas, regulates blood glucose levels by facilitating cellular uptake of glucose, essential for energy production and metabolic balance.

Question 23: Which mineral is important for maintaining a healthy immune system?

a) Iron
b) Calcium
c) Zinc
d) Sodium

Correct Answer: c) Zinc

Explanation: Zinc plays a crucial role in maintaining a healthy immune system, promoting wound healing, and supporting normal growth and development in animals.

Question 24: What is the primary function of red blood cells?

a) To fight infections
b) To transport oxygen from the lungs to the body's tissues
c) To produce hormones
d) To store nutrients

Correct Answer: b) To transport oxygen from the lungs to the body's tissues

Explanation: Red blood cells, rich in hemoglobin, deliver oxygen to tissues and return carbon dioxide to the lungs for exhalation, sustaining cellular metabolism.

Question 25: What is the primary function of the liver?

a) To store calcium
b) To produce red blood cells
c) To filter toxins from the blood
d) To regulate body temperature

Correct Answer: c) To filter toxins from the blood
Explanation: The liver detoxifies blood, metabolizes nutrients, produces bile, and plays a vital role in maintaining metabolic homeostasis and overall health.

Question 26: What is the term for a heart rate that is faster than normal?

a) Bradycardia
b) Tachycardia
c) Arrhythmia
d) Hypertension

Correct Answer: b) Tachycardia
Explanation: Tachycardia refers to a heart rate that exceeds the normal resting rate, which can occur due to stress, fever, or underlying cardiac conditions.

Question 27: Which of the following is a common sign of feline diabetes mellitus?

a) Weight gain
b) Increased thirst and urination
c) Decreased appetite
d) Constipation

Correct Answer: b) Increased thirst and urination
Explanation: Feline diabetes mellitus often presents with increased thirst (polydipsia) and urination (polyuria), as high blood sugar levels affect kidney function.

Question 28: Which gland is responsible for the fight-or-flight response?

a) Thyroid gland
b) Pituitary gland
c) Adrenal gland
d) Pancreas

Correct Answer: c) Adrenal gland
Explanation: The adrenal glands release adrenaline and cortisol during stress, initiating the fight-or-flight response, increasing energy and alertness.

Question 29: What is the function of white blood cells?

a) To transport oxygen
b) To fight infections
c) To produce hormones
d) To store nutrients

Correct Answer: b) To fight infections
Explanation: White blood cells, or leukocytes, are crucial to the immune system, defending the body against infections and foreign invaders.

Question 30: Which vitamin is essential for vision and immune function?

a) Vitamin A
b) Vitamin B6
c) Vitamin C
d) Vitamin D

Correct Answer: a) Vitamin A
Explanation: Vitamin A is crucial for maintaining healthy vision and immune function, supporting cell growth and differentiation, and preventing night blindness.

Question 31: Which type of joint allows for rotational movement?

a) Ball-and-socket joint
b) Hinge joint
c) Pivot joint
d) Saddle joint

Correct Answer: c) Pivot joint

Explanation: Pivot joints, like those in the neck, enable rotational movement, allowing bones to turn around an axis, crucial for head and limb flexibility.

Question 32: What is the primary role of platelets in the blood?

a) To carry oxygen
b) To fight infections
c) To clot blood
d) To transport nutrients

Correct Answer: c) To clot blood

Explanation: Platelets, or thrombocytes, are essential for blood clot formation, preventing excessive bleeding by forming a temporary plug in vessel injuries.

Question 33: Which hormone stimulates milk production in mammals?

a) Estrogen
b) Progesterone
c) Prolactin
d) Oxytocin

Correct Answer: c) Prolactin

Explanation: Prolactin, produced by the anterior pituitary gland, stimulates milk production in mammary glands, essential for nursing offspring.

Question 34: Which part of the eye controls the amount of light entering?

a) Cornea
b) Lens
c) Iris
d) Retina

Correct Answer: c) Iris

Explanation: The iris regulates the size of the pupil, controlling the amount of light entering the eye, crucial for optimal vision and protection against bright light.

Question 35: What is the primary function of the spleen?

a) To produce hormones
b) To store vitamins
c) To filter blood and recycle red blood cells
d) To produce digestive enzymes

Correct Answer: c) To filter blood and recycle red blood cells

Explanation: The spleen filters blood, removes old or damaged red blood cells, and plays a role in immune response by storing white blood cells and platelets.

Question 36: Which mineral is necessary for the production of thyroid hormones?

a) Calcium
b) Iron
c) Iodine
d) Magnesium

Correct Answer: c) Iodine
Explanation: Iodine is integral to thyroid hormone synthesis, regulating metabolism, growth, and development via hormones like thyroxine.

Question 37: Which organelle is known as the "powerhouse" of the cell?

a) Nucleus
b) Endoplasmic reticulum
c) Golgi apparatus
d) Mitochondria

Correct Answer: d) Mitochondria
Explanation: Mitochondria generate ATP through cellular respiration, providing energy for cellular processes and sustaining life functions.

Question 38: Which type of muscle is under voluntary control?

a) Cardiac muscle
b) Skeletal muscle
c) Smooth muscle
d) Involuntary muscle

Correct Answer: b) Skeletal muscle
Explanation: Skeletal muscles are under voluntary control, allowing conscious movement and coordination, attached to bones by tendons.

Question 39: Which part of the nervous system is responsible for voluntary movements?

a) Autonomic nervous system
b) Central nervous system
c) Peripheral nervous system
d) Somatic nervous system

Correct Answer: d) Somatic nervous system
Explanation: The somatic nervous system controls voluntary muscle movements and reflex arcs, enabling conscious motor activity and responses.

Question 40: What is the main function of the endocrine system?

a) To transport oxygen
b) To secrete hormones regulating bodily processes
c) To protect against infections
d) To filter blood

Correct Answer: b) To secrete hormones that regulate bodily processes
Explanation: The endocrine system releases hormones into the bloodstream, influencing growth, metabolism, and homeostasis through targeted actions.

Question 41: Which vitamin is essential for collagen synthesis and immune function?

a) Vitamin A
b) Vitamin B12
c) Vitamin C
d) Vitamin D

Correct Answer: c) Vitamin C
Explanation: Vitamin C supports collagen formation, wound healing, and immune defense, protecting against infections and promoting skin health.

Question 42: Which blood vessels carry blood back to the heart?

a) Arteries
b) Capillaries
c) Veins
d) Lymphatics

Correct Answer: c) Veins

Explanation: Veins transport deoxygenated blood back to the heart, with valves preventing backflow, ensuring efficient circulation.

Question 43: What is the primary function of the lymphatic system?

a) To produce red blood cells
b) To digest fats
c) To return excess tissue fluid and protect against infections
d) To regulate body temperature

Correct Answer: c) To return excess tissue fluid to the bloodstream and protect against infections

Explanation: The lymphatic system maintains fluid balance and filters pathogens, supporting immune responses and preventing edema.

Question 44: Which vitamin is known as the "sunshine vitamin" due to its synthesis in the skin?

a) Vitamin A
b) Vitamin C
c) Vitamin D
d) Vitamin E

Correct Answer: c) Vitamin D

Explanation: Vitamin D, synthesized from sunlight exposure, is essential for calcium absorption and bone health, preventing rickets and osteoporosis.

Question 45: What is the main purpose of the respiratory system?

a) To transport blood
b) To facilitate oxygen and carbon dioxide exchange
c) To produce hormones
d) To regulate body temperature

Correct Answer: b) To facilitate the exchange of oxygen and carbon dioxide

Explanation: The respiratory system ensures efficient oxygen intake and carbon dioxide expulsion, vital for cellular respiration and energy production.

Question 46: What is the primary role of red blood cells?

a) To fight infections
b) To transport oxygen from the lungs to the body's tissues
c) To produce hormones
d) To store nutrients

Correct Answer: b) To transport oxygen from the lungs to the body's tissues

Explanation: Red blood cells, rich in hemoglobin, deliver oxygen to tissues and return carbon dioxide to the lungs for exhalation, sustaining cellular metabolism.

Question 47: Which hormone stimulates the production of red blood cells?

a) Insulin
b) Estrogen
c) Erythropoietin
d) Thyroxine

Correct Answer: c) Erythropoietin
Explanation: Erythropoietin, primarily produced by the kidneys, stimulates the bone marrow to produce red blood cells, especially in response to low oxygen levels in tissues.

Question 48: What is the proper name for the "third eyelid"?

a) Nictitating membrane
b) Tympanic membrane
c) Frenulum
d) Ranula

Correct Answer: a) Nictitating membrane
Explanation: The nictitating membrane, or third eyelid, provides additional protection and moisture to the eye, particularly important in many animals, including cats and dogs.

Question 49: An elevated PCV is considered normal for which of the following breeds?

a) Greyhound
b) Akita
c) Chihuahua
d) Cavalier King Charles Spaniel

Correct Answer: a) Greyhound
Explanation: Greyhounds naturally have higher packed cell volumes (PCV) compared to other breeds, aiding in oxygen transport during their high-speed activities.

Question 50: What is the most common anticoagulant used for hematology?

a) Heparin
b) Ethylenediaminetetracetic acid (EDTA)
c) Sodium citrate
d) Sodium fluoride

Correct Answer: b) Ethylenediaminetetracetic acid (EDTA)
Explanation: EDTA is commonly used in hematology for anticoagulation, preserving blood cell integrity and preventing clotting in samples for complete blood counts.

Question 51: The attending veterinarian asks you to administer 120 mg of enrofloxacin (Baytril) IV slow over 20 minutes to a dog that is hospitalized in your clinic. The strength of injectable enrofloxacin is 2.27%, how many milliliters of drug will you administer?

a) There is not enough information available to calculate the dosage
b) 0.53 mls
c) 5.3 ml
d) 52.8 mls

Correct Answer: c) 5.3 ml
Explanation: A 2.27% solution equates to 22.7 mg/ml. To administer 120 mg, calculate 120 mg ÷ 22.7 mg/ml = 5.3 mls, ensuring accurate dosing.

Question 52: A male ferret is also referred to as which of the following?

a) Jack
b) Boar
c) Hob
d) Jill

Correct Answer: c) Hob
Explanation: In ferret terminology, a male is called a "hob," while a female is known as a "jill," important for understanding gender-specific care needs.

Question 53: A dog presents for stumbling, has a head tilt, and you notice his eyes are moving back and forth rapidly in a horizontal motion. What is the term for this type of eye movement?

a) Nystagmus
b) Ataxia
c) Miosis
d) Hypermetria
e) Mydriasis

Correct Answer: a) Nystagmus
Explanation: Nystagmus refers to involuntary, rhythmic eye movements, often indicating vestibular dysfunction or neurological issues in dogs.

Question 54: A 2-year-old male Golden Retriever has been brought to your facility in cardiac arrest. Obtaining intravenous access will be extremely difficult due to degloving injuries on all legs and additional trauma to the head and neck. What alternate route would be the first choice for atropine and epinephrine administration?

a) Subcutaneous
b) Intratracheal
c) Intramuscular
d) Rectal
e) Intracardiac

Correct Answer: b) Intratracheal
Explanation: In emergency cases where IV access is challenging, intratracheal administration allows rapid drug absorption through the respiratory tract, beneficial in cardiac arrest scenarios.

Question 55: Lactose-fermenting bacteria such as Escherichia coli and Klebsiella appear what color on MacConkey agar?

a) Clear or white
b) Pink or red
c) Blue or green
d) Tan or grey

Correct Answer: b) Pink or red
Explanation: On MacConkey agar, lactose-fermenting bacteria like E. coli and Klebsiella produce acid, turning colonies pink or red, aiding in microbial identification.

Question 56: When collecting blood for a blood transfusion, the maximum recommended amount that can be collected from a donor horse (500 kg) is what volume?

a) 12-14 liters
b) 3-6 liters
c) 6-8 liters
d) 10-12 liters

Correct Answer: c) 6-8 liters
Explanation: Safely, 15-16 ml/kg of blood can be collected from a horse, equating to 6-8 liters for a 500 kg horse, ensuring donor safety and adequate volume for transfusion.

Question 57: A young male cat with symptoms of feline lower urinary tract disease and struvite crystalluria should receive:

a) Diet with low protein
b) Alkalinizing diet
c) Diet with low fat
d) Acidifying diet

Correct Answer: d) Acidifying diet
Explanation: An acidifying diet helps dissolve struvite crystals and prevents recurrence by reducing urinary pH, crucial for managing feline lower urinary tract disease.

Question 58: Some bacteria produce beta-lactamases that destroy or inactivate penicillins. What beta-lactamase inhibitor is added to amoxicillin to prevent this from occurring?

a) Chloride
b) Sulfamethoxazole
c) Clavulanic acid
d) Procaine

Correct Answer: c) Clavulanic acid
Explanation: Clavulanic acid inhibits beta-lactamases, protecting amoxicillin from degradation and extending its antimicrobial spectrum, enhancing treatment efficacy.

Question 59: A dog with hypothyroidism comes in to have his blood drawn to check his thyroid level. He has been on Levothyroxine since he was first diagnosed. How many hours after the thyroid medication is given should the blood be drawn?

a) 1-2 hours
b) 8-10 hours
c) 12 hours just before the next dose is due
d) 4-6 hours
e) 5-7 hours

Correct Answer: d) 4-6 hours
Explanation: Blood should be drawn 4-6 hours post-medication for peak thyroid levels, enabling accurate assessment of Levothyroxine efficacy in managing hypothyroidism.

Question 60: Which of the following drugs is a controlled substance?

a) Hydrocodone
b) Acepromazine
c) Propofol
d) Medetomidine

Correct Answer: a) Hydrocodone
Explanation: Hydrocodone is a controlled opiate agonist with anti-tussive properties, necessitating regulation due to its potential for abuse and dependency.

Question 61: Which of the following is a common symptom of canine distemper?

a) Increased appetite
b) Persistent cough
c) Fever and nasal discharge
d) Weight gain

Correct Answer: c) Fever and nasal discharge
Explanation: Canine distemper presents with fever, nasal discharge, and neurological symptoms, caused by a viral infection that affects multiple body systems in dogs.

Question 62: What is the primary function of the pancreas?

a) To produce red blood cells
b) To secrete insulin and digestive enzymes
c) To filter toxins from the blood
d) To store bile

Correct Answer: b) To secrete insulin and digestive enzymes
Explanation: The pancreas plays a dual role, releasing insulin to regulate blood glucose and producing digestive enzymes to aid nutrient absorption in the intestines.

Question 63: Which electrolyte imbalance is commonly associated with Addison's disease?

a) Hypernatremia
b) Hypercalcemia
c) Hyponatremia
d) Hypokalemia

Correct Answer: c) Hyponatremia
Explanation: Addison's disease, characterized by adrenal insufficiency, often leads to hyponatremia due to decreased aldosterone, affecting sodium balance and fluid regulation.

Question 64: Which of the following is a symptom of feline leukemia virus (FeLV) infection?

a) Hyperactivity
b) Chronic diarrhea
c) Increased thirst
d) Hair loss

Correct Answer: b) Chronic diarrhea
Explanation: Feline leukemia virus can cause chronic diarrhea, immunosuppression, and anemia, impacting overall health and increasing susceptibility to other infections.

Question 65: What is the primary role of the gallbladder?

a) To produce bile
b) To store and concentrate bile
c) To detoxify blood
d) To regulate blood sugar levels

Correct Answer: b) To store and concentrate bile
Explanation: The gallbladder stores and concentrates bile produced by the liver, releasing it into the small intestine to aid fat digestion and absorption.

Question 66: Which of the following is a common effect of hyperthyroidism in cats?

a) Weight gain
b) Lethargy
c) Increased appetite and activity
d) Constipation

Correct Answer: c) Increased appetite and activity
Explanation: Hyperthyroidism in cats often leads to increased appetite and activity due to elevated metabolism, despite weight loss, necessitating dietary and medical management.

Question 67: What is the primary function of the large intestine?

a) To absorb nutrients
b) To absorb water and electrolytes
c) To produce digestive enzymes
d) To filter blood

Correct Answer: b) To absorb water and electrolytes
Explanation: The large intestine absorbs water and electrolytes from indigestible food matter, forming and storing feces until excretion, maintaining fluid balance.

Question 68: Which of the following is an example of an NSAID (Non-Steroidal Anti-Inflammatory Drug)?

a) Prednisone
b) Ibuprofen
c) Morphine
d) Amoxicillin

Correct Answer: b) Ibuprofen
Explanation: Ibuprofen is an NSAID used to reduce inflammation and pain, acting by inhibiting cyclooxygenase enzymes, but must be used cautiously in animals.

Question 69: What is the primary cause of Cushing's disease in dogs?

a) Adrenal gland tumors
b) Viral infection
c) Dietary imbalance
d) Heart failure

Correct Answer: a) Adrenal gland tumors
Explanation: Cushing's disease, or hyperadrenocorticism, often results from adrenal gland tumors, causing excessive cortisol production and presenting with symptoms like PU/PD.

Question 70: Which organ is primarily responsible for detoxification in the body?

a) Spleen
b) Kidney
c) Liver
d) Pancreas

Correct Answer: c) Liver
Explanation: The liver detoxifies chemicals, metabolizes drugs, and produces proteins essential for blood clotting, crucial for maintaining metabolic homeostasis and health.

Question 71: Which of the following is a common cause of anemia in dogs?

a) Excessive exercise
b) Kidney disease
c) Dehydration
d) Obesity

Correct Answer: b) Kidney disease
Explanation: Kidney disease can lead to anemia due to reduced erythropoietin production, impairing red blood cell formation and causing fatigue and weakness.

Question 72: What is the primary function of the small intestine?

a) To store bile
b) To produce insulin
c) To absorb nutrients and minerals
d) To filter blood

Correct Answer: c) To absorb nutrients and minerals
Explanation: The small intestine's primary role is to absorb nutrients and minerals from digested food, facilitated by villi and microvilli increasing surface area.

Question 73: Which of the following is a characteristic of a malignant tumor?

a) Slow-growing and localized
b) Encapsulated and non-invasive
c) Invasive and capable of metastasis
d) Non-invasive and benign

Correct Answer: c) Invasive and capable of metastasis
Explanation: Malignant tumors are characterized by their invasive nature and potential to spread (metastasize) to other parts of the body, posing significant health risks.

Question 74: Which hormone is responsible for regulating the sleep-wake cycle?

a) Melatonin
b) Insulin
c) Cortisol
d) Glucagon

Correct Answer: a) Melatonin
Explanation: Melatonin, produced by the pineal gland, regulates the sleep-wake cycle, influenced by light exposure, playing a crucial role in circadian rhythm.

Question 75: Which of the following is a symptom of rabies in animals?

a) Excessive thirst
b) Aggression and foaming at the mouth
c) Increased appetite
d) Hair loss

Correct Answer: b) Aggression and foaming at the mouth
Explanation: Rabies often presents with aggression, foaming at the mouth, and neurological symptoms due to viral infection affecting the central nervous system.

Question 76: What is the primary function of the thyroid gland?

a) To secrete insulin
b) To regulate metabolism and energy balance
c) To filter blood
d) To produce red blood cells

Correct Answer: b) To regulate metabolism and energy balance
Explanation: The thyroid gland produces hormones like thyroxine, regulating metabolism, energy balance, and growth, essential for maintaining physiological homeostasis.

Question 77: Which vitamin is crucial for blood coagulation?

a) Vitamin A
b) Vitamin B12
c) Vitamin C
d) Vitamin K

Correct Answer: d) Vitamin K
Explanation: Vitamin K is essential for synthesizing proteins required for blood coagulation, preventing excessive bleeding and ensuring effective clotting processes.

Question 78: What is the primary cause of feline infectious peritonitis (FIP)?

a) Bacterial infection
b) Viral infection
c) Fungal infection
d) Parasitic infection

Correct Answer: b) Viral infection
Explanation: Feline infectious peritonitis (FIP) is caused by a mutation of the feline coronavirus, leading to a severe inflammatory response, often fatal in cats.

Question 79: Which of the following is a common symptom of parvovirus in dogs?

a) Increased thirst
b) Vomiting and diarrhea
c) Weight gain
d) Hyperactivity

Correct Answer: b) Vomiting and diarrhea
Explanation: Canine parvovirus typically causes severe vomiting and diarrhea, leading to dehydration and requiring prompt veterinary intervention for survival.

Question 80: What is the primary function of the adrenal glands?

a) To produce bile
b) To secrete hormones like adrenaline and cortisol
c) To filter toxins from the blood
d) To regulate blood sugar levels

Correct Answer: b) To secrete hormones like adrenaline and cortisol
Explanation: Adrenal glands produce hormones like adrenaline and cortisol, crucial for stress response, metabolism, and maintaining homeostasis.

Question 81: Which of the following is an example of a parasitic infection in animals?

a) Feline leukemia
b) Heartworm disease
c) Canine distemper
d) Rabies

Correct Answer: b) Heartworm disease
Explanation: Heartworm disease is a parasitic infection caused by Dirofilaria immitis, transmitted by mosquitoes, affecting the heart and lungs of dogs and cats.

Question 82: Which of the following is a common cause of hypothyroidism in dogs?

a) Iodine deficiency
b) Autoimmune thyroiditis
c) Liver disease
d) Diabetes

Correct Answer: b) Autoimmune thyroiditis
Explanation: Autoimmune thyroiditis, where the immune system attacks the thyroid gland, is a leading cause of hypothyroidism in dogs, impacting hormone production.

Question 83: What is the main function of the pituitary gland?

a) To secrete digestive enzymes
b) To regulate other endocrine glands
c) To filter toxins from the blood
d) To produce red blood cells

Correct Answer: b) To regulate other endocrine glands
Explanation: The pituitary gland, known as the "master gland," regulates other endocrine glands by releasing hormones that influence growth, metabolism, and reproduction.

Question 84: Which of the following is a common symptom of Lyme disease in dogs?

a) Increased appetite
b) Lameness and joint pain
c) Hair loss
d) Vomiting

Correct Answer: b) Lameness and joint pain
Explanation: Lyme disease, transmitted by ticks, often presents with lameness, joint pain, and fever in dogs, requiring prompt antibiotic treatment for recovery.

Question 85: What is the primary function of the hypothalamus?

a) To produce bile
b) To regulate body temperature and hunger
c) To filter blood
d) To produce red blood cells

Correct Answer: b) To regulate body temperature and hunger
Explanation: The hypothalamus maintains homeostasis by regulating body temperature, hunger, thirst, and circadian rhythms, linking the nervous and endocrine systems.

Question 86: Which nutrient is essential for muscle contraction and nerve function?

a) Calcium
b) Iron
c) Zinc
d) Vitamin D

Correct Answer: a) Calcium
Explanation: Calcium is crucial for muscle contraction, nerve transmission, and bone health, playing a vital role in numerous physiological processes and maintaining cellular functions.

Question 87: What is the primary cause of equine colic?

a) Dietary imbalance
b) Viral infection
c) Bacterial infection
d) Parasitic infection

Correct Answer: a) Dietary imbalance
Explanation: Equine colic often results from dietary imbalances, such as abrupt feed changes or inadequate fiber, causing gastrointestinal discomfort and requiring veterinary attention.

Question 88: Which of the following is a common symptom of feline asthma?

a) Increased appetite
b) Coughing and wheezing
c) Weight gain
d) Vomiting

Correct Answer: b) Coughing and wheezing
Explanation: Feline asthma manifests as coughing and wheezing due to airway inflammation and constriction, necessitating management with bronchodilators and corticosteroids.

Question 89: What is a pulse deficit?

a) When some heart beats do not result in a palpable pulse
b) When an extra pulse occurs sporadically
c) When no pulses are palpable in a patient
d) When a pulse is synchronous with a heartbeat

Correct Answer: a) When some heart beats do not result in a palpable pulse
Explanation: A pulse deficit occurs when the heart's ventricular contractions do not produce a palpable pulse, indicating a potential issue with peripheral perfusion or cardiac output.

Question 90: Which of the following should never be given in a bolus to a patient?

a) Hetastarch
b) Lidocaine
c) Potassium chloride
d) Mannitol
e) 0.9% Sodium chloride

Correct Answer: c) Potassium chloride
Explanation: Bolusing potassium chloride can cause fatal cardiac arrest due to rapid changes in serum potassium levels. It must be administered slowly and carefully to avoid complications.

Question 91: Which of the following is an ectoparasite of animals?

a) Feline infectious peritonitis
b) Paragonimus kellicotti
c) Filaroides osleri
d) Ctenocephalides felis
e) Ancylostoma caninum

Correct Answer: d) Ctenocephalides felis
Explanation: Ctenocephalides felis, commonly known as the cat flea, is an ectoparasite that infests the skin and causes discomfort, requiring treatment to eliminate and prevent re-infestation.

Question 92: Giardia is what type of parasite?

a) Coccidial
b) Protozoan
c) Ascarid
d) Cestode
e) Trematode

Correct Answer: b) Protozoan
Explanation: Giardia is a protozoan parasite causing gastrointestinal issues. It exists in motile trophozoite and cyst forms, requiring specific treatment to clear infection.

Question 93: The adrenal glands are closest to what other structure?

a) Brain
b) Bladder
c) Kidneys
d) Pancreas
e) Liver

Correct Answer: c) Kidneys
Explanation: The adrenal glands are located atop the kidneys, playing a crucial role in hormone production, including cortisol and adrenaline, impacting stress response and metabolism.

Question 94: Which intestinal parasite is NOT considered zoonotic to humans?

a) Coccidia
b) Toxocara
c) Giardia
d) Ancylostoma

Correct Answer: a) Coccidia
Explanation: Coccidia, a type of protozoan parasite, primarily affects animals and is not typically considered zoonotic, unlike others that can be transmitted to humans.

Question 95: Which of the following over-the-counter medications is sometimes given for diarrhea?

a) Simethicone
b) Bismuth subsalicylate
c) Famotidine
d) Diphenhydramine

Correct Answer: b) Bismuth subsalicylate
Explanation: Bismuth subsalicylate, found in medications like Pepto-Bismol, is used to treat mild diarrhea by reducing inflammation and protecting the stomach lining.

Question 96: A horse is presented for a surgical procedure. What is the best time to administer perioperative antibiotics to the patient?

a) When the surgeon makes the first cut
b) Within 1 hour of cut time
c) When the incision is being closed
d) 1 hour post-operatively

Correct Answer: b) Within 1 hour of cut time
Explanation: Administering antibiotics within 1 hour of the surgical incision helps achieve optimal tissue concentration, reducing infection risk and improving surgical outcomes.

Question 97: What is true regarding chelonians?

a) They don't have a urinary bladder
b) They don't have a diaphragm
c) They don't have eyelids
d) They don't have a spleen

Correct Answer: b) They don't have a diaphragm
Explanation: Chelonians, such as turtles and tortoises, lack a diaphragm, relying on other muscular structures for respiration, influencing their care and handling.

Question 98: A large dog collapses in the lobby of your veterinary clinic. The dog is taken to the treatment area where an ECG reveals that the patient is in ventricular tachycardia. What drug would be administered intravenously in an attempt to convert the dog to a normal sinus rhythm?

a) Vasopressin
b) Atropine
c) Digoxin
d) 2% lidocaine
e) Ephinephrine

Correct Answer: d) 2% lidocaine
Explanation: 2% lidocaine is used to treat ventricular tachycardia, stabilizing the heart's electrical activity and potentially converting the rhythm to normal sinus.

Question 99: In which situation would perioperative antibiotics NOT be indicated?

a) An orthopedic procedure lasting 1 hour
b) Surgery on a patient with diabetes mellitus
c) Surgery on a patient treated with glucocorticoids
d) Surgery on a patient with hyperadrenocorticism
e) Excisional biopsy of a 2cm mass

Correct Answer: e) Excisional biopsy of a 2cm mass
Explanation: Routine excisional biopsy of a small, uncomplicated mass typically does not require perioperative antibiotics unless additional risk factors for infection are present.

Question 100: Microbiology materials or media that are not in use should be stored where?

a) Freezer
b) Refrigerator
c) In the dark room at room temperature
d) In a lighted cabinet at room temperature

Correct Answer: b) Refrigerator
Explanation: Storing microbiology materials in a refrigerator preserves their integrity and prevents bacterial overgrowth, ensuring accurate results when used for testing.

Question 101: In a horse, what is the most common surgical approach to the abdominal cavity?

a) Transverse incision
b) Parasaggital incision
c) Ventral midline incision
d) Flank incision

Correct Answer: c) Ventral midline incision
Explanation: A ventral midline incision provides optimal access to the equine abdominal cavity, allowing thorough exploration and surgical intervention when necessary.

Question 102: Where would you find Anaplasma marginale?

a) Platelets of horses
b) Erythrocytes of cattle
c) White blood cells of horses
d) Urine of sheep

Correct Answer: b) Erythrocytes of cattle
Explanation: Anaplasma marginale, a tick-borne pathogen, infects cattle's erythrocytes, leading to anaplasmosis characterized by fever, anemia, and jaundice, requiring prompt treatment.

Question 103: The California Mastitis Test (CMT) is an assay that gives a score that corresponds to which of the following?

a) Presence of contagious bacteria in milk
b) Somatic cell count in milk
c) Fat content of milk
d) Presence of environmental bacteria in milk

Correct Answer: b) Somatic cell count in milk
Explanation: The CMT measures somatic cell count, indicating mastitis levels in milk by detecting increased white blood cells, crucial for dairy herd health management.

Question 104: What is the most common anticoagulant used for hematology?

a) Sodium citrate
b) Ethylenediaminetetracetic acid (EDTA)
c) Sodium fluoride
d) Heparin

Correct Answer: b) Ethylenediaminetetracetic acid (EDTA)
Explanation: EDTA is widely used in hematology for anticoagulation, preserving blood cell morphology and preventing clotting in samples for complete blood counts.

Question 105: How many mammary glands does the goat have?

a) 4
b) 6
c) 1
d) 2

Correct Answer: d) 2
Explanation: Goats typically have two mammary glands, or udders, each with a single teat, essential for milk production and nurturing offspring.

Question 106: Which of the following is FALSE regarding the use of Humulin insulin?

a) It can be given intramuscularly
b) Shake well before use
c) Keep refrigerated
d) It causes blood sugar to decrease when administered

Correct Answer: a) It can be given intramuscularly
Explanation: Humulin insulin is typically administered subcutaneously, not intramuscularly, to manage blood sugar levels in diabetic patients, ensuring effective glucose control.

Question 107: What is the primary function of the spleen?

a) To produce bile
b) To filter blood and recycle iron
c) To secrete digestive enzymes
d) To regulate calcium levels

Correct Answer: b) To filter blood and recycle iron
Explanation: The spleen filters blood, recycles iron from old red blood cells, and plays a role in immune response, contributing to overall hematologic and immune health.

Question 108: Which of the following is a symptom of diabetes mellitus in dogs?

a) Increased appetite and weight gain
b) Increased thirst and urination
c) Hair loss and skin irritation
d) Vomiting and diarrhea

Correct Answer: b) Increased thirst and urination
Explanation: Diabetes mellitus often results in polydipsia (increased thirst) and polyuria (increased urination) due to glucose imbalances and osmotic diuresis in dogs.

Question 109: Which of the following is a common symptom of hyperthyroidism in cats?

a) Lethargy and weight gain
b) Increased appetite and weight loss
c) Coughing and wheezing
d) Vomiting and diarrhea

Correct Answer: b) Increased appetite and weight loss
Explanation: Hyperthyroidism in cats typically presents with increased appetite and weight loss due to an elevated metabolic rate, necessitating medical or dietary intervention.

Question 110: What is the primary role of the liver in metabolism?

a) To produce insulin
b) To store glucose as glycogen and metabolize fats
c) To filter waste from the blood
d) To absorb nutrients from the intestine

Correct Answer: b) To store glucose as glycogen and metabolize fats
Explanation: The liver stores glucose as glycogen, metabolizes fats, and regulates blood sugar, playing a crucial role in maintaining energy balance and metabolic functions.

Question 111: Which of the following is a common cause of hepatic lipidosis in cats?

a) Obesity and anorexia
b) Viral infection
c) Parasitic infestation
d) Bacterial infection

Correct Answer: a) Obesity and anorexia
Explanation: Hepatic lipidosis, or fatty liver disease, often arises from obesity followed by anorexia in cats, leading to fat accumulation in the liver and hepatic dysfunction.

Question 112: Which of the following is a common symptom of chronic kidney disease in cats?

a) Increased appetite
b) Hyperactivity
c) Increased thirst and urination
d) Hair loss

Correct Answer: c) Increased thirst and urination
Explanation: Chronic kidney disease often results in increased thirst and urination due to impaired renal function and inability to concentrate urine, impacting fluid balance in cats.

Question 113: Which of the following is a common cause of pancreatitis in dogs?

a) High-fat diet
b) Low-protein diet
c) Viral infection
d) Fungal infection

Correct Answer: a) High-fat diet
Explanation: Pancreatitis in dogs is frequently triggered by a high-fat diet, resulting in inflammation and digestive enzyme leakage, requiring dietary management and veterinary care.

Question 114: Which of the following is a common symptom of Addison's disease in dogs?

a) Hyperactivity
b) Lethargy and weight loss
c) Increased thirst and urination
d) Hair loss

Correct Answer: b) Lethargy and weight loss
Explanation: Addison's disease, or adrenal insufficiency, often presents with lethargy, weight loss, and electrolyte imbalances due to insufficient cortisol production in dogs.

Question 115: Which of the following is a common cause of feline infectious anemia?

a) Bacterial infection
b) Parasitic infection
c) Viral infection
d) Fungal infection

Correct Answer: b) Parasitic infection
Explanation: Feline infectious anemia is typically caused by the parasitic infection Mycoplasma haemofelis, leading to red blood cell destruction and anemia in cats.

Question 116: Which of the following is a symptom of hypothyroidism in dogs?

a) Increased appetite
b) Weight loss
c) Lethargy and weight gain
d) Hyperactivity

Correct Answer: c) Lethargy and weight gain
Explanation: Hypothyroidism in dogs often results in lethargy, weight gain, and skin issues due to decreased thyroid hormone production, affecting metabolism and energy levels.

Question 117: Which of the following is a common cause of feline hyperthyroidism?

a) Iodine deficiency
b) Thyroid adenoma
c) Adrenal tumor
d) Viral infection

Correct Answer: b) Thyroid adenoma
Explanation: Feline hyperthyroidism is commonly caused by a benign thyroid adenoma, leading to excessive thyroid hormone production and increased metabolic rate, requiring treatment.

Question 118: Which of the following is a symptom of Cushing's disease in dogs?

a) Weight loss and increased appetite
b) Increased thirst and urination
c) Hair loss and skin thinning
d) Vomiting and diarrhea

Correct Answer: c) Hair loss and skin thinning
Explanation: Cushing's disease, or hyperadrenocorticism, often presents with hair loss, skin thinning, and increased thirst and urination due to elevated cortisol levels in dogs.

Question 119: What is the primary function of the pancreas?

a) To produce red blood cells
b) To secrete insulin and digestive enzymes
c) To filter toxins from the blood
d) To store bile

Correct Answer: b) To secrete insulin and digestive enzymes
Explanation: The pancreas is crucial for regulating blood sugar through insulin secretion and aiding digestion by producing enzymes, essential for metabolic and digestive health.

Question 120: Which of the following is a common symptom of feline leukemia virus (FeLV) infection?

a) Hyperactivity
b) Chronic diarrhea
c) Increased thirst
d) Hair loss

Correct Answer: b) Chronic diarrhea
Explanation: Feline leukemia virus can cause chronic diarrhea, immunosuppression, and anemia, impacting overall health and increasing susceptibility to other infections.

Question 121: What is the primary role of the gallbladder?

a) To produce bile
b) To store and concentrate bile
c) To detoxify blood
d) To regulate blood sugar levels

Correct Answer: b) To store and concentrate bile
Explanation: The gallbladder stores and concentrates bile produced by the liver, releasing it into the small intestine to aid fat digestion and absorption.

Question 122: Which of the following is a common effect of hyperthyroidism in cats?

a) Weight gain
b) Lethargy
c) Increased appetite and activity
d) Constipation

Correct Answer: c) Increased appetite and activity
Explanation: Hyperthyroidism in cats often leads to increased appetite and activity due to elevated metabolism, despite weight loss, necessitating dietary and medical management.

Question 123: What is the primary function of the large intestine?

a) To absorb nutrients
b) To absorb water and electrolytes
c) To produce digestive enzymes
d) To filter blood

Correct Answer: b) To absorb water and electrolytes
Explanation: The large intestine absorbs water and electrolytes from indigestible food matter, forming and storing feces until excretion, maintaining fluid balance.

Question 124: Which of the following is an example of an NSAID (Non-Steroidal Anti-Inflammatory Drug)?

a) Prednisone
b) Ibuprofen
c) Morphine
d) Amoxicillin

Correct Answer: b) Ibuprofen
Explanation: Ibuprofen is an NSAID used to reduce inflammation and pain, acting by inhibiting cyclooxygenase enzymes, but must be used cautiously in animals.

Question 125: What is the primary cause of Cushing's disease in dogs?

a) Adrenal gland tumors
b) Viral infection
c) Dietary imbalance
d) Heart failure

Correct Answer: a) Adrenal gland tumors
Explanation: Cushing's disease, or hyperadrenocorticism, often results from adrenal gland tumors, causing excessive cortisol production and presenting with symptoms like PU/PD.

Question 126: Which organ is primarily responsible for detoxification in the body?

a) Spleen
b) Kidney
c) Liver
d) Pancreas

Correct Answer: c) Liver
Explanation: The liver detoxifies chemicals, metabolizes drugs, and produces proteins essential for blood clotting, crucial for maintaining metabolic homeostasis and health.

Question 127: Which of the following is a common cause of anemia in dogs?

a) Excessive exercise
b) Kidney disease
c) Dehydration
d) Obesity

Correct Answer: b) Kidney disease
Explanation: Kidney disease can lead to anemia due to reduced erythropoietin production, impairing red blood cell formation and causing fatigue and weakness.

Question 128: What is the primary function of the small intestine?

a) To store bile
b) To produce insulin
c) To absorb nutrients and minerals
d) To filter blood

Correct Answer: c) To absorb nutrients and minerals
Explanation: The small intestine's primary role is to absorb nutrients and minerals from digested food, facilitated by villi and microvilli increasing surface area.

Question 129: Which of the following is a characteristic of a malignant tumor?

a) Slow-growing and localized
b) Encapsulated and non-invasive
c) Invasive and capable of metastasis
d) Non-invasive and benign

Correct Answer: c) Invasive and capable of metastasis
Explanation: Malignant tumors are characterized by their invasive nature and potential to spread (metastasize) to other parts of the body, posing significant health risks.

Question 130: Which hormone is responsible for regulating the sleep-wake cycle?

a) Melatonin
b) Insulin
c) Cortisol
d) Glucagon

Correct Answer: a) Melatonin
Explanation: Melatonin, produced by the pineal gland, regulates the sleep-wake cycle, influenced by light exposure, playing a crucial role in circadian rhythm.

Question 131: How many milliliters of 25% dextrose should be added to 1 L of 0.9% saline to make a 5% dextrose solution?

a) 20 ml
b) 50 ml
c) 100 ml
d) 200 ml

Correct Answer: d) 200 ml
Explanation: Using the formula $C(1)V(1) = C(2)V(2)$, where C is the concentration and V is the volume, solve for V(1): $(0.25)V(1) = (0.05)(1000)$, resulting in V(1) = 200 ml. Thus, 200 ml of 25% dextrose is required.

Question 132: An elevated PCV is considered normal for which of the following breeds?

a) Cavalier King Charles Spaniel
b) Akita
c) Chihuahua
d) Greyhound

Correct Answer: d) Greyhound
Explanation: Greyhounds naturally have a higher packed cell volume (PCV) compared to other breeds, which is normal and attributed to their athletic physiology and increased oxygen-carrying capacity.

Question 133: This canine patient presents following his neuter surgery. He was neutered at the local animal shelter and the owner did not follow instructions to use an E-collar. He now has an open wound and a swollen scrotum. The scrotum is filled with blood due to self-trauma. This could be called which of the following?

a) Scrotal atrophy
b) Scrotal ablation
c) Scrotal torsion
d) Scrotal hematoma

Correct Answer: d) Scrotal hematoma
Explanation: A scrotal hematoma is a collection of blood within the scrotum due to injury or trauma, often caused by self-inflicted damage post-surgery, requiring medical evaluation.

Question 134: Which essential amino acid is a requirement in the feline diet?

a) Lysine
b) Leucine
c) Arginine
d) Taurine

Correct Answer: d) Taurine
Explanation: Taurine is critical for feline health, supporting heart muscle function, vision, and reproduction, and must be included in their diet to prevent deficiencies and related health issues.

Question 135: Mannitol Salt Agar, or MSA, selects for growth of which species of organism?

a) Campylobacter
b) Staphylococcus
c) Clostridium
d) Streptococcus
e) Escherichia coli

Correct Answer: b) Staphylococcus
Explanation: Mannitol Salt Agar contains a high salt concentration, inhibiting most bacteria except Staphylococci, which are salt-tolerant, making it selective for these organisms.

Question 136: Purkinje fibers are found in which of the following organs?

a) Bladder
b) Stomach
c) Duodenum
d) Pancreas
e) Heart

Correct Answer: e) Heart
Explanation: Purkinje fibers are specialized conductive fibers in the heart's ventricular walls, essential for coordinating contractions by relaying impulses to cardiac muscle cells.

Question 137: What purpose is the administration of the drug Guaifenesin typically used for in horses?

a) Muscle relaxation
b) Intestinal Prokinetic
c) Antimicrobial
d) Expectorant
e) Anti-inflammatory

Correct Answer: a) Muscle relaxation
Explanation: Guaifenesin is used intravenously in horses to relax skeletal muscles during anesthesia

induction, aiding in smooth and controlled anesthesia management, distinct from its expectorant use in other species.

Question 138: A 3-month old kitten presents for mucoid diarrhea and anemia. The clinic where you work has recently seen several other puppies and kittens with similar clinical signs that were infected with Strongyloides stercoralis. You look up and find that this parasite is passed in the feces in the L1 larval form. What is the best way to recover and identify this parasite?

a) Fecal flotation
b) Baermann fecal technique
c) Direct fecal smear
d) Fecal sedimentation

Correct Answer: b) Baermann fecal technique
Explanation: The Baermann technique is optimal for recovering larvae like Strongyloides stercoralis from fecal samples, using water to encourage larval migration and facilitating identification.

Question 139: A surgeon is asking for any non-absorbable suture to close a skin defect. Which of the following sutures would NOT be appropriate for you to give the surgeon?

a) Nylon
b) Polydioxanone
c) Polypropylene
d) Silk

Correct Answer: b) Polydioxanone
Explanation: Polydioxanone is an absorbable suture known as PDS, unsuitable for non-absorbable requirements, whereas nylon, polypropylene, and silk are non-absorbable options for skin closure.

Question 140: Which bacterium is gram-positive?

a) Campylobacter
b) Streptococcus
c) E. coli
d) Salmonella

Correct Answer: b) Streptococcus
Explanation: Streptococcus species are gram-positive bacteria, identifiable by their thick peptidoglycan cell wall, differentiating them from gram-negative bacteria like E. coli and Salmonella.

Question 141: What is commonly done to get a mare to cycle out of season?

a) Manual manipulation of the ovaries via rectal palpation
b) Keep a stallion in the same barn
c) Administration of oxytocin
d) Artificial lighting

Correct Answer: d) Artificial lighting
Explanation: Artificial lighting extends daylight hours, simulating longer days, encouraging mares to cycle out of season by influencing their reproductive physiology and hormone production.

Question 142: A young male cat with symptoms of feline lower urinary tract disease and struvite crystalluria should receive:

a) Acidifying diet
b) Diet with low protein
c) Diet with low fat
d) Alkalinizing diet

Correct Answer: a) Acidifying diet
Explanation: An acidifying diet lowers urine pH, helping dissolve struvite crystals, preventing recurrence, and managing feline lower urinary tract disease (FLUTD).

Question 143: What is the vertebral formula for dogs and cats?

a) Cervical 7, Thoracic 13, Lumbar 7, Sacral 3
b) Cervical 3, Thoracic 12, Lumbar 6, Sacral 7
c) Cervical 6, Thoracic 10, Lumbar 7, Sacral 7
d) Cervical 6, Thoracic 12, Lumbar 5, Sacral 13

Correct Answer: a) Cervical 7, Thoracic 13, Lumbar 7, Sacral 3
Explanation: The vertebral formula for dogs and cats is C7, T13, L7, S3, reflecting their spinal anatomy, essential for understanding their musculoskeletal structure.

Question 144: What is the primary function of hemoglobin in the blood?

a) To transport nutrients
b) To transport oxygen
c) To remove waste products
d) To fight infections

Correct Answer: b) To transport oxygen
Explanation: Hemoglobin is a protein in red blood cells responsible for transporting oxygen from the lungs to tissues and returning carbon dioxide from tissues to the lungs for exhalation.

Question 145: Which of the following is a common cause of ear infections in dogs?

a) Parasitic infestation
b) Fungal infection
c) Allergies
d) Vitamin deficiency

Correct Answer: c) Allergies
Explanation: Allergies often lead to ear infections in dogs, causing inflammation that predisposes the ear to secondary bacterial or yeast infections, necessitating veterinary intervention.

Question 146: Which of the following is a symptom of heartworm disease in dogs?

a) Increased appetite
b) Coughing and exercise intolerance
c) Vomiting and diarrhea
d) Hair loss

Correct Answer: b) Coughing and exercise intolerance
Explanation: Heartworm disease causes respiratory distress and exercise intolerance due to worms residing in pulmonary arteries, impacting cardiac and pulmonary function in dogs.

Question 147: Which of the following is a common symptom of feline asthma?

a) Increased thirst
b) Hair loss
c) Coughing and wheezing
d) Vomiting

Correct Answer: c) Coughing and wheezing
Explanation: Feline asthma is characterized by coughing and wheezing due to airway inflammation and constriction, requiring management to prevent exacerbations and respiratory distress.

Question 148: What is the primary function of insulin in the body?

a) To increase blood sugar levels
b) To decrease blood sugar levels
c) To regulate blood pressure
d) To promote protein synthesis

Correct Answer: b) To decrease blood sugar levels

Explanation: Insulin, produced by the pancreas, lowers blood sugar by facilitating glucose uptake into cells, essential for energy production and metabolic regulation.

Question 149: Which of the following is a symptom of hypothyroidism in dogs?

a) Increased energy and weight loss
b) Lethargy and weight gain
c) Increased thirst and urination
d) Hyperactivity

Correct Answer: b) Lethargy and weight gain

Explanation: Hypothyroidism in dogs manifests as lethargy, weight gain, and skin changes due to reduced thyroid hormone levels, impacting metabolism and overall energy levels.

Question 150: Which of the following is a common cause of pancreatitis in dogs?

a) Low-fat diet
b) High-fat diet
c) High-protein diet
d) High-fiber diet

Correct Answer: b) High-fat diet

Explanation: A high-fat diet can trigger pancreatitis in dogs, leading to inflammation of the pancreas, requiring dietary management and medical treatment to prevent recurrence.

Question 151: What is the primary role of the kidneys?

a) To produce insulin
b) To filter and excrete waste products from the blood
c) To store bile
d) To absorb nutrients

Correct Answer: b) To filter and excrete waste products from the blood

Explanation: The kidneys filter blood, excreting waste and excess substances as urine, maintaining fluid and electrolyte balance, and supporting overall metabolic functions.

Question 152: Which of the following is a symptom of Cushing's disease in dogs?

a) Weight loss and increased appetite
b) Increased thirst and urination
c) Hair loss and skin thinning
d) Vomiting and diarrhea

Correct Answer: c) Hair loss and skin thinning

Explanation: Cushing's disease, or hyperadrenocorticism, presents with hair loss, skin thinning, and increased thirst and urination due to excess cortisol production in dogs.

Question 153: What is a common treatment for hyperthyroidism in cats?

a) High-fat diet
b) Methimazole medication
c) Corticosteroid therapy
d) Insulin injections

Correct Answer: b) Methimazole medication
Explanation: Methimazole is used to manage hyperthyroidism in cats, inhibiting thyroid hormone production and alleviating symptoms, with other options like surgery or radioactive iodine available.

Question 154: Which of the following is a symptom of feline leukemia virus (FeLV) infection?

a) Hyperactivity
b) Chronic diarrhea
c) Increased thirst
d) Hair loss

Correct Answer: b) Chronic diarrhea
Explanation: Feline leukemia virus can cause chronic diarrhea, immunosuppression, and anemia, impacting overall health and increasing susceptibility to other infections.

Question 155: What is the primary function of the liver in metabolism?

a) To produce insulin
b) To store glucose as glycogen and metabolize fats
c) To filter waste from the blood
d) To absorb nutrients from the intestine

Correct Answer: b) To store glucose as glycogen and metabolize fats
Explanation: The liver stores glucose as glycogen, metabolizes fats, and regulates blood sugar, playing a crucial role in maintaining energy balance and metabolic functions.

Question 156: Which of the following is a common symptom of chronic kidney disease in cats?

a) Increased appetite
b) Hyperactivity
c) Increased thirst and urination
d) Hair loss

Correct Answer: c) Increased thirst and urination
Explanation: Chronic kidney disease often results in increased thirst and urination due to impaired renal function and inability to concentrate urine, impacting fluid balance in cats.

Question 157: Which of the following is the primary function of bile in digestion?

a) To emulsify fats
b) To digest carbohydrates
c) To absorb proteins
d) To neutralize stomach acid

Correct Answer: a) To emulsify fats
Explanation: Bile emulsifies fats, breaking them into smaller droplets, aiding in digestion and absorption in the small intestine, crucial for lipid metabolism.

Question 158: What is the primary cause of feline infectious peritonitis (FIP)?

a) Bacterial infection
b) Coronavirus infection
c) Parasitic infection
d) Fungal infection

Correct Answer: b) Coronavirus infection
Explanation: FIP is caused by a mutation of the feline coronavirus, leading to a systemic inflammatory response, often fatal, with no effective treatment currently available.

Question 159: Which of the following is a common cause of urinary tract infections in cats?

a) Viral infection
b) Bacterial infection
c) Fungal infection
d) Parasitic infection

Correct Answer: b) Bacterial infection
Explanation: Urinary tract infections in cats are primarily caused by bacterial infection, requiring antimicrobial treatment and sometimes dietary management to prevent recurrence.

Question 160: What is the primary function of red blood cells?

a) To transport oxygen and carbon dioxide
b) To fight infections
c) To produce hormones
d) To digest food

Correct Answer: a) To transport oxygen and carbon dioxide
Explanation: Red blood cells transport oxygen from the lungs to tissues and return carbon dioxide from tissues to the lungs, essential for respiratory and metabolic processes.

Question 161: Which of the following is a symptom of diabetes mellitus in cats?

a) Increased thirst and urination
b) Weight gain
c) Decreased appetite
d) Hyperactivity

Correct Answer: a) Increased thirst and urination
Explanation: Diabetes mellitus in cats often results in polydipsia (increased thirst) and polyuria (increased urination) due to glucose imbalances and osmotic diuresis.

Question 162: Which of the following is a common treatment for heartworm disease in dogs?

a) Antifungal medication
b) Melarsomine injections
c) Insulin therapy
d) Antibiotic treatment

Correct Answer: b) Melarsomine injections
Explanation: Melarsomine injections are used to treat heartworm disease in dogs, targeting adult worms in the heart and lungs, often alongside other supportive therapies.

Question 163: Which of the following is a common cause of anemia in cats?

a) Dehydration
b) Parasites
c) Kidney disease
d) Obesity

Correct Answer: b) Parasites
Explanation: Parasitic infections, such as fleas or intestinal worms, can cause anemia in cats by blood loss or destruction, requiring treatment to address the underlying cause.

Question 164: What is the primary function of the endocrine system?

a) To transport oxygen
b) To produce hormones
c) To fight infections
d) To digest food

Correct Answer: b) To produce hormones
Explanation: The endocrine system produces hormones regulating body functions, including growth, metabolism, and reproduction, maintaining homeostasis and physiological balance.

Question 165: Which of the following is a common symptom of hyperthyroidism in cats?

a) Lethargy and weight gain
b) Increased appetite and weight loss
c) Vomiting and diarrhea
d) Coughing and wheezing

Correct Answer: b) Increased appetite and weight loss
Explanation: Hyperthyroidism in cats typically presents with increased appetite and weight loss due to an elevated metabolic rate, necessitating medical or dietary intervention.

Question 166: What is the primary function of the respiratory system?

a) To transport nutrients
b) To exchange gases
c) To produce hormones
d) To filter blood

Correct Answer: b) To exchange gases
Explanation: The respiratory system facilitates gas exchange, providing oxygen to the blood and removing carbon dioxide, essential for cellular respiration and energy production.

Question 167: Which of the following is a common cause of liver disease in dogs?

a) High-protein diet
b) Viral infection
c) Obesity
d) Toxic ingestion

Correct Answer: d) Toxic ingestion
Explanation: Toxic substances, including certain medications and plants, can cause liver disease in dogs by damaging liver cells, requiring prompt veterinary intervention.

Question 168: Which of the following is a symptom of Addison's disease in dogs?

a) Hyperactivity
b) Lethargy and weight loss
c) Increased thirst and urination
d) Hair loss

Correct Answer: b) Lethargy and weight loss
Explanation: Addison's disease, or adrenal insufficiency, often presents with lethargy, weight loss, and electrolyte imbalances due to insufficient cortisol production in dogs.

Question 169: What is the primary function of the immune system?

a) To produce energy
b) To fight infections
c) To transport oxygen
d) To digest food

Correct Answer: b) To fight infections
Explanation: The immune system defends against infections through a network of cells and organs, identifying and neutralizing pathogens to maintain health and prevent disease.

Question 170: Which of the following is a common symptom of feline immunodeficiency virus (FIV) infection?

a) Hyperactivity
b) Weight gain
c) Decreased appetite and weight loss
d) Hair loss

Correct Answer: c) Decreased appetite and weight loss
Explanation: Feline immunodeficiency virus leads to immunosuppression, resulting in decreased appetite, weight loss, and increased susceptibility to secondary infections, impacting overall health.

Full Test 8 with Detailed Explanations

Question 1: Where is the standard tuberculosis test administered in the bovine species?

a) Ear pinna
b) Caudal tail fold
c) Proximal axilla
d) Eye lid

Correct Answer: b) Caudal tail fold
Explanation: The caudal tail fold is the standard site for administering the tuberculosis test in bovines. This location is chosen due to its accessibility and because it allows for easy observation of the reaction, which is crucial for interpreting test results.

Question 2: Which of the following would be elevated in a pet with regenerative anemia?

a) Reticulocyte count
b) Lymphocyte count
c) Hematocrit
d) Hemoglobin concentration

Correct Answer: a) Reticulocyte count
Explanation: In regenerative anemia, the bone marrow responds to the decreased red blood cell count by releasing more reticulocytes, which are immature red blood cells. An increased reticulocyte count indicates active red blood cell production as the body attempts to compensate for the anemia.

Question 3: You are performing a urinalysis and identify this six-sided crystal (see image). What type of crystal is this?

a) Calcium oxalate
b) Struvite
c) Cystine
d) Urate

Correct Answer: c) Cystine
Explanation: Cystine crystals are identifiable by their characteristic hexagonal shape. These crystals typically form due to a genetic defect in renal tubular amino acid reabsorption, leading to cystinuria, a condition that requires monitoring and management.

Question 4: You are assisting with an exploratory surgery, and the dog has a septic peritonitis from a perforated bowel. Before closure, the veterinarian lavages the abdomen with what?

a) Sterile physiologic saline with betadine
b) Sterile physiologic saline infused with antibiotics
c) Sterile physiologic saline
d) Sterile Lactated Ringer's solution

Correct Answer: c) Sterile physiologic saline
Explanation: In cases of septic peritonitis, sterile physiologic saline is used to lavage the abdomen to reduce bacterial load and remove contaminants. This helps to minimize postoperative complications and supports the healing process.

Question 5: A 2-year old male Golden Retriever has been brought to your facility in cardiac arrest. Obtaining intravenous access will be extremely difficult due to degloving injuries on all legs and additional trauma to the head and neck. What alternate route would be the first choice for atropine and epinephrine administration?

a) Rectal
b) Intracardiac
c) Subcutaneous
d) Intratracheal
e) Intramuscular

Correct Answer: d) Intratracheal
Explanation: Intratracheal administration of atropine and epinephrine is effective in emergency situations when intravenous access is not feasible. These medications can be delivered via the endotracheal tube, allowing for rapid absorption and action during resuscitation efforts.

Question 6: Schnauzers are notorious for having hyperlipidemia, and when their blood is spun down, the serum often appears milky. This is due to a high level of what in the serum?

a) Lymph
b) Chyme
c) Leukocytes
d) Triglycerides

Correct Answer: d) Triglycerides
Explanation: Hyperlipidemia in Schnauzers is characterized by elevated triglyceride levels, which cause the serum to appear milky. This condition requires dietary management and regular monitoring to prevent associated health issues.

Question 7: Which of the following scenarios describes the proper care of surgical instruments?

a) Place instruments in surgical milk. Remove from surgical milk and rinse to remove any debris and residue. Place instruments in ultrasonic cleaner for 10 minutes. Let instruments dry.
b) Place instruments in ultrasonic cleaner for approximately 10 minutes. Rinse instruments with distilled water and scrub as necessary. Place instruments in surgical milk. Remove from surgical milk and let instruments dry.
c) Pre-rinse the instruments immediately after surgery to remove residues. Place in ultrasonic cleaner for approximately 10 minutes. Place in surgical milk. Remove from surgical milk and let instruments dry.
d) Rinse the instruments to remove the debris and residue. Place in an ultrasonic cleaner for 30 minutes. Then place the instruments in surgical milk. After removing instruments from the surgical milk rinse them again.

Correct Answer: c) Pre-rinse the instruments immediately after surgery to remove residues. Place in ultrasonic cleaner for approximately 10 minutes. Place in surgical milk. Remove from surgical milk and let instruments dry.
Explanation: Proper care involves pre-rinsing to remove residues, followed by cleaning in an ultrasonic cleaner to ensure thorough decontamination. Surgical milk is used to lubricate and protect instruments, enhancing their longevity.

Question 8: Which of the following is a reason why a tick should not be removed without an effective removal device?

a) Mouthparts may be left embedded and create a focus for infection
b) Improperly squeezing the tick may cause the animal to have an anaphylactic reaction
c) Partial removal of the tick may increase the risk of transmission of certain rickettsial diseases
d) Ticks should never be removed manually and should be allowed to fall off in time or killed with an acaricide

Correct Answer: a) Mouthparts may be left embedded and create a focus for infection
Explanation: If a tick is removed improperly, its mouthparts can remain embedded in the skin, leading to

irritation and infection. Using a proper removal tool ensures complete removal and reduces the risk of secondary complications.

Question 9: Which of the following would you use to induce emesis in cats?

a) Activated charcoal
b) Xylazine
c) Apomorphine
d) Naltrexone

Correct Answer: b) Xylazine
Explanation: Xylazine is effective for inducing emesis in cats, stimulating the central emetic center. While apomorphine is used for dogs, it is less effective in cats, making xylazine the preferred choice for this purpose.

Question 10: Johne's disease is an intestinal infection that can lead to clinical signs of diarrhea and weight loss. It affects cattle, sheep, goats, and other species. What is the Genus of the causative agent of Johne's disease?

a) Fusobacterium
b) Mycobacterium
c) Listeria
d) Brucella

Correct Answer: b) Mycobacterium
Explanation: Johne's disease is caused by Mycobacterium avium subspecies paratuberculosis, leading to chronic intestinal inflammation and malabsorption, significantly impacting the health and productivity of affected animals.

Question 11: An owner calls your vet clinic in a panic because her epileptic dog is currently having a seizure. She says that the vet at your hospital had given her a drug to give rectally to help. She starts to list off the medications in her medicine cabinet. Which of these is the appropriate drug for this instance?

a) Diazepam
b) Clomipramine
c) Potassium bromide
d) Naloxone
e) Ketamine

Correct Answer: a) Diazepam
Explanation: Diazepam is a benzodiazepine used to control seizures in dogs, often administered rectally when immediate intervention is required. It acts quickly to stabilize the dog and prevent further convulsions.

Question 12: One of the most common incisional complications encountered in veterinary surgery is the formation of a seroma. Which of the following is a poor treatment choice for an incision diagnosed with a seroma?

a) Exercise restriction
b) Antibiotics
c) Warm compress
d) Placement of a drain

Correct Answer: b) Antibiotics
Explanation: Seromas are fluid-filled swellings that are non-infectious and thus do not require antibiotics. Management typically involves exercise restriction, warm compresses, and possibly drainage if necessary.

Question 13: What is the optimal method of sampling if a urine culture is to be performed in a dog?

a) Cystocentesis
b) Free catch
c) Urinary catheterization
d) Bladder expression

Correct Answer: a) Cystocentesis

Explanation: Cystocentesis is the preferred method for urine culture collection as it provides a sterile sample directly from the bladder, minimizing contamination and ensuring accurate culture results.

Question 14: Which of the following instruments would be LEAST effective at cutting or removing bone from a patient?

a) Osteotome
b) Gigli wire
c) Curette
d) Periosteal elevator
e) Michel trephine

Correct Answer: d) Periosteal elevator

Explanation: Periosteal elevators are designed to lift periosteum or soft tissues from bone surfaces, not for cutting or removing bone. They are essential in orthopedic surgeries for tissue separation.

Question 15: The attending veterinarian asks you to administer 120 mg of enrofloxacin (Baytril) IV slow over 20 minutes to a dog that is hospitalized in your clinic. The strength of injectable enrofloxacin is 2.27%, how many milliliters of drug will you administer?

a) 5.3 ml
b) 52.8 ml
c) There is not enough information available to calculate the dosage
d) 0.53 ml

Correct Answer: a) 5.3 ml

Explanation: A 2.27% solution of enrofloxacin contains 22.7 mg/ml. To administer 120 mg, divide 120 mg by 22.7 mg/ml, which equals approximately 5.3 ml, ensuring precise dosage delivery.

Question 16: What is the primary function of hemoglobin in the blood?

a) To transport nutrients
b) To transport oxygen
c) To remove waste products
d) To fight infections

Correct Answer: b) To transport oxygen

Explanation: Hemoglobin is a protein found in red blood cells responsible for carrying oxygen from the lungs to tissues and returning carbon dioxide from tissues to the lungs for exhalation, vital for cellular respiration.

Question 17: Which of the following is a common cause of ear infections in dogs?

a) Parasitic infestation
b) Fungal infection
c) Allergies
d) Vitamin deficiency

Correct Answer: c) Allergies

Explanation: Allergies often lead to ear infections in dogs by causing inflammation and irritation in the ear canal, predisposing the area to secondary bacterial or yeast infections, necessitating veterinary care.

Question 18: Which of the following is a symptom of heartworm disease in dogs?

a) Increased appetite
b) Coughing and exercise intolerance
c) Vomiting and diarrhea
d) Hair loss

Correct Answer: b) Coughing and exercise intolerance

Explanation: Heartworm disease causes respiratory distress and exercise intolerance due to worms residing in the pulmonary arteries, impacting the heart and lungs, necessitating prompt treatment.

Question 19: Which of the following is a common symptom of feline asthma?

a) Increased thirst
b) Hair loss
c) Coughing and wheezing
d) Vomiting

Correct Answer: c) Coughing and wheezing

Explanation: Feline asthma is characterized by coughing and wheezing due to airway inflammation and constriction, requiring management to prevent exacerbations and respiratory distress.

Question 20: What is the primary function of insulin in the body?

a) To increase blood sugar levels
b) To decrease blood sugar levels
c) To regulate blood pressure
d) To promote protein synthesis

Correct Answer: b) To decrease blood sugar levels

Explanation: Insulin is a hormone produced by the pancreas that facilitates glucose uptake into cells, reducing blood sugar levels and playing a crucial role in energy metabolism and homeostasis.

Question 21: Which of the following is a symptom of hypothyroidism in dogs?

a) Increased energy and weight loss
b) Lethargy and weight gain
c) Increased thirst and urination
d) Hyperactivity

Correct Answer: b) Lethargy and weight gain

Explanation: Hypothyroidism in dogs leads to reduced metabolism, causing symptoms like lethargy and weight gain, often accompanied by skin changes, requiring hormone replacement therapy for management.

Question 22: Which of the following is a common cause of pancreatitis in dogs?

a) Low-fat diet
b) High-fat diet
c) High-protein diet
d) High-fiber diet

Correct Answer: b) High-fat diet

Explanation: A high-fat diet can trigger pancreatitis in dogs by causing inflammation of the pancreas, necessitating dietary management and medical intervention to alleviate symptoms and prevent recurrence.

Question 23: What is the primary role of the kidneys?

a) To produce insulin
b) To filter and excrete waste products from the blood
c) To store bile
d) To absorb nutrients

Correct Answer: b) To filter and excrete waste products from the blood
Explanation: The kidneys filter blood, removing waste and excess substances, maintaining fluid and electrolyte balance, and supporting overall metabolic and homeostatic functions.

Question 24: Which of the following is a symptom of Cushing's disease in dogs?

a) Weight loss and increased appetite
b) Increased thirst and urination
c) Hair loss and skin thinning
d) Vomiting and diarrhea

Correct Answer: c) Hair loss and skin thinning
Explanation: Cushing's disease, or hyperadrenocorticism, results in excess cortisol production, leading to symptoms like hair loss, skin thinning, and increased panting, requiring medical management.

Question 25: What is a common treatment for hyperthyroidism in cats?

a) High-fat diet
b) Methimazole medication
c) Corticosteroid therapy
d) Insulin injections

Correct Answer: b) Methimazole medication
Explanation: Methimazole is commonly used to manage hyperthyroidism in cats by inhibiting thyroid hormone production, alleviating symptoms, and stabilizing the cat's metabolic state.

Question 26: Which of the following is a symptom of feline leukemia virus (FeLV) infection?

a) Hyperactivity
b) Chronic diarrhea
c) Increased thirst
d) Hair loss

Correct Answer: b) Chronic diarrhea
Explanation: Feline leukemia virus can cause chronic diarrhea, immunosuppression, and anemia, significantly impacting the cat's health and making them prone to secondary infections.

Question 27: What is the primary function of the liver in metabolism?

a) To produce insulin
b) To store glucose as glycogen and metabolize fats
c) To filter waste from the blood
d) To absorb nutrients from the intestine

Correct Answer: b) To store glucose as glycogen and metabolize fats
Explanation: The liver stores glucose as glycogen, metabolizes fats, and regulates blood sugar, playing a crucial role in maintaining energy balance and metabolic homeostasis.

Question 28: Which of the following is a common symptom of chronic kidney disease in cats?

a) Increased appetite
b) Hyperactivity
c) Increased thirst and urination
d) Hair loss

Correct Answer: c) Increased thirst and urination
Explanation: Chronic kidney disease often results in increased thirst and urination due to impaired renal function and inability to concentrate urine, impacting fluid balance and overall health in cats.

Question 29: Which of the following is the primary function of bile in digestion?

a) To emulsify fats
b) To digest carbohydrates
c) To absorb proteins
d) To neutralize stomach acid

Correct Answer: a) To emulsify fats

Explanation: Bile emulsifies fats, breaking them into smaller droplets, aiding in digestion and absorption in the small intestine, crucial for lipid metabolism and nutrient absorption.

Question 30: What is the primary cause of feline infectious peritonitis (FIP)?

a) Bacterial infection
b) Coronavirus infection
c) Parasitic infection
d) Fungal infection

Correct Answer: b) Coronavirus infection

Explanation: FIP is caused by a mutation of the feline coronavirus, leading to a systemic inflammatory response, often fatal, with no effective treatment currently available, requiring supportive care.

Question 31: Which of the following is a common cause of urinary tract infections in cats?

a) Viral infection
b) Bacterial infection
c) Fungal infection
d) Parasitic infection

Correct Answer: b) Bacterial infection

Explanation: Urinary tract infections in cats are primarily caused by bacterial infection, requiring antimicrobial treatment and sometimes dietary management to prevent recurrence and promote recovery.

Question 32: What is the primary function of red blood cells?

a) To transport oxygen and carbon dioxide
b) To fight infections
c) To produce hormones
d) To digest food

Correct Answer: a) To transport oxygen and carbon dioxide

Explanation: Red blood cells transport oxygen from the lungs to tissues and return carbon dioxide from tissues to the lungs, essential for respiratory and metabolic processes, maintaining cellular function.

Question 33: Which of the following is a symptom of diabetes mellitus in cats?

a) Increased thirst and urination
b) Weight gain
c) Decreased appetite
d) Hyperactivity

Correct Answer: a) Increased thirst and urination

Explanation: Diabetes mellitus in cats often results in polydipsia (increased thirst) and polyuria (increased urination) due to glucose imbalances and osmotic diuresis, requiring insulin therapy and dietary management.

Question 34: Which of the following is a common treatment for heartworm disease in dogs?

a) Antifungal medication
b) Melarsomine injections
c) Insulin therapy
d) Antibiotic treatment

Correct Answer: b) Melarsomine injections
Explanation: Melarsomine injections are used to treat heartworm disease in dogs, targeting adult worms in the heart and lungs, often alongside other supportive therapies to manage the condition.

Question 35: Which of the following is a common cause of anemia in cats?

a) Dehydration
b) Parasites
c) Kidney disease
d) Obesity

Correct Answer: b) Parasites
Explanation: Parasitic infections, such as fleas or intestinal worms, can cause anemia in cats by blood loss or destruction, requiring treatment to address the underlying cause and restore health.

Question 36: What is the primary function of the endocrine system?

a) To transport oxygen
b) To produce hormones
c) To fight infections
d) To digest food

Correct Answer: b) To produce hormones
Explanation: The endocrine system produces hormones regulating body functions, including growth, metabolism, and reproduction, maintaining homeostasis and physiological balance across the body.

Question 37: Which of the following is expected from a positive inotropic drug?

a) Increase in cardiac contractility
b) Prevention of arrhythmias
c) Dramatic decrease in blood pressure
d) Decrease in adrenal gland stimulation

Correct Answer: a) Increase in cardiac contractility
Explanation: Positive inotropic drugs are designed to increase the force of heart muscle contractions. This can be beneficial in treating heart failure by improving cardiac output and ensuring adequate blood circulation throughout the body.

Question 38: Sulfasalazine is sometimes used in veterinary medicine to treat which chronic condition?

a) Pancreatitis
b) Colitis
c) Bronchitis
d) Hepatitis

Correct Answer: b) Colitis
Explanation: Sulfasalazine is an anti-inflammatory drug used in the treatment of chronic intestinal conditions such as ulcerative colitis. It helps reduce inflammation in the colon, improving symptoms and enhancing the quality of life for affected animals.

Question 39: Approximately how much urine should a 40-pound dog produce in a 24-hour period if the dog is drinking and urinating normal amounts and is not dehydrated?

a) About 2.2 Liters of urine
b) Between 450 and 850 mL of urine
c) About 1.5 Liters of urine
d) Between 150 to 300 mL of urine

Correct Answer: b) Between 450 and 850 mL of urine

Explanation: A 40-pound dog, which is approximately 18 kg, typically produces urine at a rate of 1-2 mL/kg/hour. Over a 24-hour period, this equates to 432-864 mL, reflecting normal hydration and renal function.

Question 40: You are asked to start a dog on maintenance fluids. The dog weighs 80 pounds. What fluid rate do you start on this dog?

a) 25 mL/hr
b) 90 mL/hr
c) 45 mL/hr
d) 150 mL/hr

Correct Answer: b) 90 mL/hr

Explanation: For maintenance fluid therapy, the standard rate is approximately 60 mL/kg/day. An 80-pound dog (about 36 kg) would require 2160 mL/day, which calculates to a fluid rate of 90 mL/hr to maintain hydration and physiological balance.

Question 41: A six-month-old Collie comes into your clinic for a technician exam and deworming. What antiparasitic drug should be used with caution in this breed?

a) Propofol
b) Pyrantel pamoate
c) Sulfadimethoxine
d) Ivermectin
e) Fenbendazole

Correct Answer: d) Ivermectin

Explanation: Collies and similar breeds have a genetic sensitivity to Ivermectin due to a mutation affecting the blood-brain barrier. This can lead to toxicity even at standard doses, requiring cautious use and monitoring.

Question 42: When using the ultrasonic cleaner, it is important to do which of the following?

a) Add surgical milk to the solution
b) Lay the instruments in an open position
c) Run the clean cycle for at least 27 minutes
d) Scrub the instruments while the ultrasonic cleaner is running

Correct Answer: b) Lay the instruments in an open position

Explanation: Instruments should be laid open in the ultrasonic cleaner to ensure thorough cleaning. This allows the ultrasonic waves to effectively reach all surfaces, removing debris and ensuring sterility.

Question 43: After which procedure is it most important that you immediately wash your hands as soon as the procedure is complete?

a) Restraining a cat that has Feline Immunodeficiency Virus (FIV)
b) Skin scraping on a dog with Demodex
c) Fluoroscopy
d) Holding a dog that may have Microsporum canis

Correct Answer: d) Holding a dog that may have Microsporum canis

Explanation: Microsporum canis is a zoonotic fungus causing ringworm, which can spread to humans. Immediate handwashing prevents transmission and maintains hygiene, safeguarding both human and animal health.

Question 44: What is the most common blood type in cats in the United States?

a) Type O
b) Type AB

c) Type A
d) Type B

Correct Answer: c) Type A
Explanation: Most domestic cats in the United States have type A blood. Blood typing is crucial before transfusions to prevent acute hemolytic reactions, especially in type B cats with strong anti-A alloantibodies.

Question 45: How many pairs of cranial nerves are there?

a) 12
b) 15
c) 8
d) 10

Correct Answer: a) 12
Explanation: There are 12 pairs of cranial nerves, each with specific functions related to sensation, movement, and autonomic control. These nerves are essential for various physiological activities, including smell, sight, and facial expressions.

Question 46: Which of the following medications requires special handling because it can cause aplastic anemia in humans?

a) Chlorpheniramine
b) Famotidine
c) Chloramphenicol
d) Metronidazole
e) Phenylpropanolamine

Correct Answer: c) Chloramphenicol
Explanation: Chloramphenicol is an antibiotic that can cause aplastic anemia in humans through bone marrow suppression. Proper handling and precautions are necessary to minimize exposure and ensure safety.

Question 47: What is colic in a horse?

a) Abdominal pain secondary to intestinal volvulus
b) Abdominal pain secondary to intestinal strangulation
c) Abdominal pain that can be secondary to multiple etiologies
d) Abdominal pain secondary to gastrointestinal gas

Correct Answer: c) Abdominal pain that can be secondary to multiple etiologies
Explanation: Colic in horses refers to abdominal pain from various causes, including gas, impaction, or intestinal torsion. It requires prompt diagnosis and treatment to prevent serious complications.

Question 48: Which of the following is an abnormal finding in a free catch of urine in a dog?

a) Bilirubin
b) Calcium oxalate crystals
c) Bacteria
d) Ketones

Correct Answer: d) Ketones
Explanation: Ketones in urine indicate abnormal fat metabolism, often due to diabetes mellitus or starvation. This finding requires further investigation and management to address underlying metabolic issues.

Question 49: All the following inhaled anesthetic drugs should be used with a rebreathing system except:

a) Halothane
b) Isoflurane

c) Nitrous oxide
d) Desflurane

Correct Answer: c) Nitrous oxide

Explanation: Nitrous oxide is typically used with a non-rebreathing system because it is less soluble and requires rapid exhalation to prevent accumulation in the body, ensuring safe and effective anesthesia.

Question 50: You should bury the needle in the vein of which of the following animals when taking a blood sample?

a) Persian cat
b) Golden retriever
c) Oriental cat
d) Pomeranian

Correct Answer: b) Golden retriever

Explanation: For larger dogs like Golden Retrievers, the needle should be fully inserted into the vein to ensure a stable and secure blood draw, preventing movement and ensuring accurate sampling.

Question 51: Which of the following would contraindicate the administration of morphine as a preanesthetic agent?

a) Preexisting tachycardia
b) Liver disease
c) Gastrointestinal obstruction
d) Respiratory disease

Correct Answer: c) Gastrointestinal obstruction

Explanation: Morphine can exacerbate gastrointestinal issues by decreasing motility and increasing the risk of ileus, making it contraindicated in cases of gastrointestinal obstruction.

Question 52: All the following pieces of information would be subject to the confidentiality requirements of patients' medical records except a:

a) Report of injuries sustained as a result of abuse
b) Report of a contagious or zoonotic disease
c) Record of a patient's vaccination history
d) Record of abnormal behavior

Correct Answer: b) Report of a contagious or zoonotic disease

Explanation: Reporting of contagious or zoonotic diseases is mandated by public health authorities to prevent outbreaks, thus excluded from confidentiality rules to ensure community safety and disease control.

Question 53: An abscess is best described as a/an:

a) Abnormal communication between the oral and nasal cavities
b) Collection of material from a bacterial infection in the tooth
c) Tooth that can't break past the gum surface
d) Hole or chip in the tooth

Correct Answer: b) Collection of material from a bacterial infection in the tooth

Explanation: An abscess is a localized collection of pus due to bacterial infection, often causing pain and swelling, requiring drainage and antibiotic therapy to resolve the infection and alleviate symptoms.

Question 54: Which medication would be given to a patient experiencing constipation?

a) Oxazepam
b) Ranitidine
c) Bisacodyl
d) Apomorphine

Correct Answer: c) Bisacodyl

Explanation: Bisacodyl is a stimulant laxative that promotes bowel movements by increasing intestinal motility, effectively relieving constipation in patients with gastrointestinal stasis or impaction.

Question 55: A cholinergic is a drug that:

a) Decreases pain sensations
b) Blocks the action of adrenaline at beta-adrenergic receptors
c) Causes pupil dilation
d) Stimulates the parasympathetic nervous system

Correct Answer: d) Stimulates the parasympathetic nervous system

Explanation: Cholinergic drugs mimic the action of acetylcholine, activating the parasympathetic nervous system, which can decrease heart rate, enhance digestion, and promote relaxation.

Question 56: When disposing of a used needle, you should:

a) Destroy the needle and dispose of it in the appropriate container
b) Separate the needle and syringe and dispose of it in the appropriate container
c) Recap the needle and dispose of it in the appropriate container
d) Handle the needle carefully and dispose of it in the appropriate container

Correct Answer: d) Handle the needle carefully and dispose of it in the appropriate container

Explanation: Used needles should be handled with care and disposed of in designated sharps containers to prevent needle-stick injuries and ensure safe, compliant waste management.

Question 57: You are treating a dehydrated dog that presents with sunken eyes, increased CRT, and dry mucus membranes. What is the patient's estimated degree of dehydration?

a) 5-6% dehydration
b) 8% dehydration
c) 10-12% dehydration
d) 12-15% dehydration

Correct Answer: c) 10-12% dehydration

Explanation: Clinical signs such as sunken eyes and dry mucous membranes indicate moderate to severe dehydration, typically around 10-12%, requiring aggressive fluid therapy to restore hydration and support recovery.

Question 58: A veterinary technician receives a frantic call from a pet owner. From what the owner says, the technician concludes the owner's dog is experiencing gastric dilation and volvulus. In which of the following categories of emergency should the technician place the patient?

a) Nonemergency
b) Minor
c) Serious
d) Life threatening

Correct Answer: d) Life threatening

Explanation: Gastric dilation and volvulus (GDV) is a critical emergency requiring immediate veterinary intervention to prevent shock, tissue necrosis, and death, necessitating rapid stabilization and surgical correction.

Question 59: Barium is considered a/an:

a) Soluble positive contrast medium
b) Insoluble negative contrast medium
c) Soluble negative contrast medium
d) Insoluble positive contrast medium

Correct Answer: d) Insoluble positive contrast medium

Explanation: Barium is an insoluble positive contrast medium used in radiography to enhance the visibility of gastrointestinal structures, aiding in the diagnosis of conditions like blockages or abnormalities.

Question 60: Trichiasis most commonly affects which breed of canine?

a) English bulldog
b) Poodle
c) Pug
d) Cocker spaniel

Correct Answer: b) Poodle

Explanation: Trichiasis, where eyelashes grow abnormally and irritate the eye, is commonly seen in Poodles. This condition requires veterinary attention to prevent corneal damage and maintain ocular health.

Question 61: A surgeon uses Jacobs chucks to:

a) Break up and remove bone
b) Hold bone fragments in reduction
c) Cut through bone
d) Advance pin placement

Correct Answer: d) Advance pin placement

Explanation: Jacobs chucks are surgical tools used to hold and advance pins in orthopedic procedures, ensuring precise placement and stabilization during fracture repair or bone alignment.

Question 62: Which of the following is a common cause of ear infections in dogs?

a) Parasitic infestation
b) Fungal infection
c) Allergies
d) Vitamin deficiency

Correct Answer: c) Allergies

Explanation: Allergies often lead to ear infections in dogs by causing inflammation and irritation in the ear canal, predisposing the area to secondary bacterial or yeast infections.

Question 63: Which of the following is a symptom of heartworm disease in dogs?

a) Increased appetite
b) Coughing and exercise intolerance
c) Vomiting and diarrhea
d) Hair loss

Correct Answer: b) Coughing and exercise intolerance

Explanation: Heartworm disease causes respiratory distress and exercise intolerance due to worms residing in the pulmonary arteries, impacting the heart and lungs, necessitating prompt treatment.

Question 64: Which of the following is a common symptom of feline asthma?

a) Increased thirst
b) Hair loss
c) Coughing and wheezing
d) Vomiting

Correct Answer: c) Coughing and wheezing

Explanation: Feline asthma is characterized by coughing and wheezing due to airway inflammation and constriction, requiring management to prevent exacerbations and respiratory distress.

Question 65: What is the primary function of insulin in the body?

a) To increase blood sugar levels
b) To decrease blood sugar levels
c) To regulate blood pressure
d) To promote protein synthesis

Correct Answer: b) To decrease blood sugar levels
Explanation: Insulin is a hormone produced by the pancreas that facilitates glucose uptake into cells, reducing blood sugar levels and playing a crucial role in energy metabolism and homeostasis.

Question 66: Which of the following is a symptom of hypothyroidism in dogs?

a) Increased energy and weight loss
b) Lethargy and weight gain
c) Increased thirst and urination
d) Hyperactivity

Correct Answer: b) Lethargy and weight gain
Explanation: Hypothyroidism in dogs leads to reduced metabolism, causing symptoms like lethargy and weight gain, often accompanied by skin changes, requiring hormone replacement therapy for management.

Question 67: Which of the following is a common cause of pancreatitis in dogs?

a) Low-fat diet
b) High-fat diet
c) High-protein diet
d) High-fiber diet

Correct Answer: b) High-fat diet
Explanation: A high-fat diet can trigger pancreatitis in dogs by causing inflammation of the pancreas, necessitating dietary management and medical intervention to alleviate symptoms and prevent recurrence.

Question 68: What is the primary role of the kidneys?

a) To produce insulin
b) To filter and excrete waste products from the blood
c) To store bile
d) To absorb nutrients

Correct Answer: b) To filter and excrete waste products from the blood
Explanation: The kidneys filter blood, removing waste and excess substances, maintaining fluid and electrolyte balance, and supporting overall metabolic and homeostatic functions.

Question 69: Which of the following is a symptom of Cushing's disease in dogs?

a) Weight loss and increased appetite
b) Increased thirst and urination
c) Hair loss and skin thinning
d) Vomiting and diarrhea

Correct Answer: c) Hair loss and skin thinning
Explanation: Cushing's disease, or hyperadrenocorticism, results in excess cortisol production, leading to symptoms like hair loss, skin thinning, and increased panting, requiring medical management.

Question 70: What is a common treatment for hyperthyroidism in cats?

a) High-fat diet
b) Methimazole medication
c) Corticosteroid therapy
d) Insulin injections

Correct Answer: b) Methimazole medication
Explanation: Methimazole is commonly used to manage hyperthyroidism in cats by inhibiting thyroid hormone production, alleviating symptoms, and stabilizing the cat's metabolic state.

Question 71: Which of the following is a symptom of feline leukemia virus (FeLV) infection?

a) Hyperactivity
b) Chronic diarrhea
c) Increased thirst
d) Hair loss

Correct Answer: b) Chronic diarrhea
Explanation: Feline leukemia virus can cause chronic diarrhea, immunosuppression, and anemia, significantly impacting the cat's health and making them prone to secondary infections.

Question 72: What is the primary function of the liver in metabolism?

a) To produce insulin
b) To store glucose as glycogen and metabolize fats
c) To filter waste from the blood
d) To absorb nutrients from the intestine

Correct Answer: b) To store glucose as glycogen and metabolize fats
Explanation: The liver stores glucose as glycogen, metabolizes fats, and regulates blood sugar, playing a crucial role in maintaining energy balance and metabolic homeostasis.

Question 73: Which of the following is a common symptom of chronic kidney disease in cats?

a) Increased appetite
b) Hyperactivity
c) Increased thirst and urination
d) Hair loss

Correct Answer: c) Increased thirst and urination
Explanation: Chronic kidney disease often results in increased thirst and urination due to impaired renal function and inability to concentrate urine, impacting fluid balance and overall health in cats.

Question 74: Which of the following is the primary function of bile in digestion?

a) To emulsify fats
b) To digest carbohydrates
c) To absorb proteins
d) To neutralize stomach acid

Correct Answer: a) To emulsify fats
Explanation: Bile emulsifies fats, breaking them into smaller droplets, aiding in digestion and absorption in the small intestine, crucial for lipid metabolism and nutrient absorption.

Question 75: Which of the following would be considered a poor inventory control practice?

a) Using control cards or a computer system for inventory control
b) Closely monitoring expiration dates of the stored products
c) Purchasing the most affordable medications possible
d) Arranging medications based on frequency of use

Correct Answer: c) Purchasing the most affordable medications possible
Explanation: While cost management is important, prioritizing the cheapest options can compromise quality and efficacy, leading to potential treatment failures. Effective inventory control balances cost with quality and safety.

Question 76: Which of the following drugs would be used to reduce intracranial pressure?

a) Atropine
b) Pimobendan
c) Mannitol
d) Prazosin

Correct Answer: c) Mannitol
Explanation: Mannitol is an osmotic diuretic that reduces intracranial pressure by drawing fluid out of the brain tissue, used in conditions like traumatic brain injury to prevent further damage.

Question 77: Which of the following statements would be true of the anesthetic agent guaifenesin?

a) It crosses the placental barrier but has no effect on the fetus.
b) It crosses the placental barrier but has little effect on the fetus.
c) It doesn't cross the placental barrier and has no effect on the fetus.
d) It doesn't cross the placental barrier and has little effect on the fetus.

Correct Answer: b) It crosses the placental barrier but has little effect on the fetus.
Explanation: Guaifenesin is an anesthetic muscle relaxant that minimally affects the fetus despite crossing the placental barrier, making it relatively safe for use in pregnant animals.

Question 78: A healthy horse should have a white blood cell count ranging from:

a) 3-10
b) 6-12
c) 6-17
d) 7-14

Correct Answer: b) 6-12
Explanation: The normal range for a horse's white blood cell count is $6\text{-}12 \times 10^3/\mu L$, reflecting a healthy immune system capable of responding to infections and diseases.

Question 79: Which of the following should be used to detect external odontoclastic resorptive lesions in a cat?

a) Periodontal probe
b) Shepherd's hook
c) Curette
d) Sickle scaler

Correct Answer: b) Shepherd's hook
Explanation: A Shepherd's hook is a dental instrument used to detect subtle dental lesions and abnormalities, such as external odontoclastic resorptive lesions, by feeling for irregularities in the tooth surface.

Question 80: Which physical factor might result in diminished radiographic detail in an X-ray?

a) Ineffective filtration
b) Low subject contrast
c) Patient movement
d) Negative contrast use

Correct Answer: c) Patient movement
Explanation: Patient movement during X-ray imaging can blur the image, reducing detail and diagnostic accuracy, emphasizing the need for proper restraint and sedation when necessary.

Question 81: Canine patients should be placed in lateral recumbency when extracting a blood sample from which vein?

a) Jugular vein
b) Cephalic vein

c) Saphenous vein
d) Femoral vein

Correct Answer: c) Saphenous vein

Explanation: For blood collection from the saphenous vein, dogs are typically placed in lateral recumbency, allowing optimal access to the vein on the hind limb for a smooth and effective procedure.

Question 82: When preparing a patient for a blood sample collection from the cephalic vein, the restrainer should:

a) Hold the patient's front legs with one hand and its head with the other while extending the neck.
b) Place the fingers of one hand behind the patient's elbow to extend the front leg.
c) Hold the patient's distal thigh or proximal tibia to compress the vein while extending the stifle.
d) Compress the vein by placing one hand on the medial side of the upper thigh.

Correct Answer: b) Place the fingers of one hand behind the patient's elbow to extend the front leg.
Explanation: This technique helps expose the cephalic vein by extending the front leg, facilitating easier and more precise access for blood collection or intravenous injections.

Question 83: Which cardiovascular drug serves to provide long-term maintenance of contractibility?

a) Dobutamine
b) Hydralazine
c) Propranolol
d) Digoxin

Correct Answer: d) Digoxin
Explanation: Digoxin enhances cardiac contractility and is used for long-term management of heart conditions like heart failure and atrial fibrillation, helping maintain normal heart function.

Question 84: Tissue forceps with multiple fine, intermeshing teeth on the edges are known as:

a) Brown-Adson tissue forceps
b) Rat-tooth thumb forceps
c) Adson tissue forceps
d) Russian tissue forceps

Correct Answer: a) Brown-Adson tissue forceps
Explanation: Brown-Adson tissue forceps have fine, interlocking teeth ideal for grasping delicate tissues during surgery without causing damage, ensuring precise manipulation and control.

Question 85: A feline blood donor must weigh no less than:

a) 5 pounds
b) 8 pounds
c) 10 pounds
d) 12 pounds

Correct Answer: c) 10 pounds
Explanation: A minimum weight of 10 pounds ensures the feline donor is healthy and large enough to safely donate blood without adverse effects, maintaining donor and recipient safety.

Question 86: You are treating a dog with itchy patches around the ears, chest, abdomen, and front legs. Which of the following is most likely to be the correct diagnosis?

a) Demodectic mange
b) Walking dandruff
c) Sarcoptic mange
d) Fleas

Correct Answer: c) Sarcoptic mange
Explanation: Sarcoptic mange, caused by the Sarcoptes scabiei mite, typically presents with intense itching and patchy hair loss in dogs, requiring treatment to eradicate the mites and alleviate symptoms.

Question 87: You are experiencing a conflict with a colleague. Which of the following approaches to the situation would be least likely to lead to a positive outcome?

a) Have a face-to-face conversation
b) Bring up the issue at a staff meeting
c) File a formal, written complaint
d) Allow the problem to resolve itself

Correct Answer: d) Allow the problem to resolve itself
Explanation: Ignoring conflicts rarely resolves them and can lead to ongoing tension. Addressing issues directly or through formal channels encourages resolution and maintains a harmonious workplace.

Question 88: Azaperone is most often used as a preanesthetic for:

a) Pigs
b) Dogs
c) Cats
d) Birds

Correct Answer: a) Pigs
Explanation: Azaperone is a sedative commonly used in pigs to calm them before procedures, reducing stress and facilitating safer handling and anesthesia administration.

Question 89: When developing an X-ray, what is the primary purpose of the rinse bath?

a) To begin the development process on the film
b) To convert the exposed silver halide crystals to metallic silver
c) To clear away the underexposed silver halide crystals
d) To stop the process of development and prevent contamination of the fixer

Correct Answer: d) To stop the process of development and prevent contamination of the fixer
Explanation: The rinse bath halts the development process and removes excess chemicals, preventing contamination of the fixer and ensuring clear, accurate radiographic images.

Question 90: Which anesthetic agent would be most appropriate for use with a greyhound?

a) Etomidate
b) Cyclohexamine
c) Propofol
d) Fentanyl

Correct Answer: c) Propofol
Explanation: Propofol is suitable for greyhounds due to its rapid onset and short duration of action, minimizing prolonged recovery times associated with their unique metabolic rates.

Question 91: How much hair should be removed from either side of the midline in a large dog being prepared for surgery?

a) 2 inches
b) 3 inches
c) 4 inches
d) 5 inches

Correct Answer: c) 4 inches
Explanation: Removing 4 inches of hair on either side of the midline ensures a clean surgical field, reducing infection risk and allowing clear access for incisions and procedures.

Question 92: Which term refers to the tooth surface area that faces towards the cheek?

a) Buccal
b) Labial
c) Rostral
d) Occlusal

Correct Answer: a) Buccal
Explanation: The buccal surface of a tooth is the side that faces the cheeks, important in dental assessments and procedures for identifying and treating oral health issues.

Question 93: When protected with wrapping material and kept on an open shelf, up to how long can a surgical instrument remain sterile?

a) One week
b) Two weeks
c) Three weeks
d) Four weeks

Correct Answer: c) Three weeks
Explanation: Properly wrapped surgical instruments can maintain sterility for up to three weeks on an open shelf, ensuring they remain safe and effective for use in procedures.

Question 94: Which of the following would be a normal sulcus depth for a cat?

a) Less than 0.5 millimeters
b) Less than 1 millimeter
c) More than 1 millimeter
d) More than 1.5 millimeters

Correct Answer: b) Less than 1 millimeter
Explanation: A sulcus depth of less than 1 millimeter is normal for cats, indicating healthy gums and periodontal structures, crucial for maintaining overall oral health.

Question 95: Which of the following would be a sign of overhydration?

a) Lowered blood pressure
b) Decreased lung sounds
c) Fatigue
d) Chemosis

Correct Answer: d) Chemosis
Explanation: Chemosis, or swelling of the conjunctiva, is a sign of fluid overload in the body, suggesting overhydration and necessitating adjustments to fluid therapy to maintain balance.

Question 96: Which substance commonly used in wound lavage may result in tissue damage?

a) Isotonic saline
b) Hydrogen peroxide
c) Chlorhexidine diacetate solution
d) Povidone-iodine solution

Correct Answer: b) Hydrogen peroxide
Explanation: Hydrogen peroxide can cause tissue damage due to its oxidative properties, potentially delaying healing. Alternatives like isotonic saline are safer for wound cleansing.

Question 97: A veterinary technician has a question about whether a certain practice is ethical. Which of the following resources would be the best place to find answers to an ethical problem in the veterinary workplace?

a) The technician's own sense of morality and ethics
b) The technician's state laws and codes about veterinary medicine
c) A veterinary medicine professional organization
d) A friend of the technician who doesn't work in veterinary medicine

Correct Answer: c) A veterinary medicine professional organization
Explanation: Professional organizations offer guidelines and resources tailored to veterinary ethics and standards, providing reliable and industry-specific advice for ethical dilemmas.

Question 98: Which of the following is the most commonly used anticoagulant for blood testing?

a) Oxalate
b) Heparin
c) EDTA
d) Sodium citrate

Correct Answer: c) EDTA
Explanation: EDTA is widely used in blood testing due to its effectiveness in preserving blood samples by preventing clotting, ensuring accurate hematological analyses.

Question 99: Which of the following drugs is used as an immunosuppressant agent?

a) Dextran
b) Lactulose
c) Interferon
d) Auranofin

Correct Answer: d) Auranofin
Explanation: Auranofin is an immunosuppressant used to treat autoimmune conditions by reducing immune system activity, helping manage symptoms and prevent organ damage.

Question 100: On an X-ray, denser body parts will appear:

a) Darker
b) Whiter
c) Grayer
d) Foggier

Correct Answer: b) Whiter
Explanation: Denser tissues absorb more X-rays, appearing whiter on radiographs, providing contrast that aids in identifying structures and abnormalities.

Question 101: Which of the following dog breeds is at a higher risk for hip dysplasia?

a) Chihuahua
b) Mastiff
c) Jack Russell terrier
d) Greyhound

Correct Answer: b) Mastiff
Explanation: Mastiffs, being large breed dogs, are predisposed to hip dysplasia due to their size and rapid growth, necessitating monitoring and preventive measures.

Question 102: In order to achieve the most accurate diagnosis, an X-ray should always be taken from at least how many angles?

a) One
b) Two
c) Three
d) Four

Correct Answer: b) Two
Explanation: Taking X-rays from at least two angles provides comprehensive views, crucial for detecting issues that may not be visible from a single perspective, enhancing diagnostic accuracy.

Question 103: Which of the following barbiturates has a lethal dosage only two to three times its normal anesthetic dosage?

a) Thiopental
b) Pentobarbital
c) Methohexital
d) Phenobarbital

Correct Answer: c) Methohexital
Explanation: Methohexital is a potent barbiturate with a narrow safety margin, making precise dosing critical to avoid overdose and ensure patient safety during anesthesia.

Question 104: When using a non-rebreathing system during anesthesia, the fresh gas flow rate should be set between:

a) 85 to 115 mL/kg/min
b) 100 to 130 mL/kg/min
c) 130 to 300 mL/kg/min
d) 300 to 400 mL/kg/min

Correct Answer: c) 130 to 300 mL/kg/min
Explanation: This flow rate ensures adequate oxygen delivery and removal of exhaled gases, maintaining patient safety and optimal anesthetic conditions in a non-rebreathing system.

Question 105: Which of the following is a synthetic absorbable suture material?

a) Polydioxanone
b) Polypropylene
c) Polyamide
d) Polymerized caprolactam

Correct Answer: a) Polydioxanone
Explanation: Polydioxanone is a synthetic absorbable suture material known for its tensile strength and predictable absorption, used for internal tissue suturing.

Question 106: A dog presents with a dental malocclusion in which two of the maxillary incisors are displaced so that they are lingual to the mandibular incisors. This condition is referred to as:

a) Posterior crossbite
b) Anterior crossbite
c) Distoclusion
d) Mesiocclusion

Correct Answer: b) Anterior crossbite
Explanation: An anterior crossbite involves the misalignment of anterior teeth, where maxillary incisors are positioned behind mandibular incisors, impacting oral function and requiring correction.

Question 107: Which of the following species develops only one set of teeth during its lifetime?

a) Horse
b) Sheep
c) Rabbit
d) Swine

Correct Answer: c) Rabbit
Explanation: Rabbits are monophyodonts, developing one set of teeth that continuously grow throughout their lives, necessitating regular dental care to prevent overgrowth.

Question 108: A medication delivered intraosseously is injected into:

a) The skin
b) The bone cavity
c) A muscle
d) A blood vessel

Correct Answer: b) The bone cavity
Explanation: Intraosseous injection involves delivering medication directly into the bone marrow, providing rapid drug absorption and circulation, especially in emergency situations.

Question 109: Veterinary technicians are sometimes the first people in a veterinary office to see a patient. As this is a major responsibility, they must be able to categorize the patient into the appropriate emergency group. An example of a patient with a serious emergency would be a:

a) Dog with a bee sting
b) Cat with a minor burn
c) Bird with a gaping wound
d) Ferret with an abscess

Correct Answer: c) Bird with a gaping wound
Explanation: A gaping wound in a bird is a critical emergency, as birds have limited blood volume and rapid metabolism, requiring prompt treatment to prevent severe complications.

Question 110: Which of the following should a veterinary technician do in case of an accidental perivascular administration of diazepam?

a) Rapidly inject sterile saline into the injection site
b) Slowly inject sterile saline into the injection site
c) Rapidly inject lidocaine to numb the injection site
d) Slowly inject lidocaine to numb the injection site

Correct Answer: b) Slowly inject sterile saline into the injection site
Explanation: Slow saline injection helps dilute the diazepam, minimizing tissue irritation and potential necrosis, ensuring patient comfort and preventing further complications.

Question 111: Catgut, a commonly used absorbable suture material, is made from the submucosal layer of the intestines of which animal?

a) Cats
b) Sheep
c) Dogs
d) Cattle

Correct Answer: b) Sheep
Explanation: Catgut is derived from sheep intestines, not cats, and is favored for its natural absorbability, used in surgical procedures requiring temporary tissue support.

Question 112: Which of the following antimicrobial drug types functions by interfering with DNA/RNA synthesis?

a) Penicillin
b) Ketoconazole
c) Tetracycline
d) Amoxicillin

Correct Answer: b) Ketoconazole

Explanation: Ketoconazole interferes with fungal DNA/RNA synthesis, disrupting cell function and reproduction, effective in treating fungal infections by inhibiting growth.

Question 113: Which of the following drugs is a nonsteroidal anti-inflammatory drug (NSAID)?

a) Betamethasone
b) Hyaluronate
c) Methocarbamol
d) Etodolac

Correct Answer: d) Etodolac

Explanation: Etodolac is an NSAID that reduces inflammation and pain by inhibiting cyclooxygenase enzymes, commonly used for managing arthritis and other inflammatory conditions.

Question 114: Which of the following X-ray processing errors would result in a yellow radiograph?

a) Marks left by fingerprints
b) Exhausted fixer solution
c) Low developing solution
d) High drying temperature

Correct Answer: b) Exhausted fixer solution

Explanation: An exhausted fixer solution fails to adequately remove unexposed silver halide crystals, leading to yellowing of the radiograph, indicating improper processing.

Question 115: Which top color indicates a Vacutainer containing only EDTA and no other additives?

a) Red
b) Lavender
c) Light blue
d) Dark blue

Correct Answer: b) Lavender

Explanation: Lavender-top Vacutainers contain EDTA as an anticoagulant, ideal for hematological tests, preserving the integrity of blood cells for accurate analysis.

Question 116: The most common type of oral tumor among dogs is:

a) Fibrosarcoma
b) Melanoma
c) Osteosarcoma
d) Squamous cell carcinoma

Correct Answer: b) Melanoma

Explanation: Melanoma is a frequent oral tumor in dogs, aggressive in nature and often requiring surgical intervention alongside adjunctive therapies for management.

Question 117: A cat with type AB blood may receive:

a) Type A blood
b) Type B blood
c) Type AB blood
d) Any feline blood type

Correct Answer: d) Any feline blood type

Explanation: Cats with type AB blood can safely receive blood from any feline blood type due to the lack of anti-A or anti-B antibodies, making them universal recipients.

Question 118: Which anesthetic agent may result in an increase in cerebrospinal fluid pressure?

a) Halothane
b) Guaifenesin
c) Isoflurane
d) Sevoflurane

Correct Answer: a) Halothane
Explanation: Halothane can elevate cerebrospinal fluid pressure, posing risks for patients with conditions like intracranial hypertension, necessitating careful monitoring.

Question 119: Which size needle is most commonly used for venipuncture in cats and small dogs?

a) 18 gauge
b) 20 gauge
c) 22 gauge
d) 24 gauge

Correct Answer: c) 22 gauge
Explanation: A 22-gauge needle balances ease of blood draw with minimal discomfort, commonly used for venipuncture in cats and small dogs due to its appropriate size.

Question 120: You are treating a cat that has consumed a non-caustic toxin. Which of the following drugs would you administer in order to induce vomiting?

a) Chlorpromazine
b) Xylazine
c) Metoclopramide
d) Aminopentamide

Correct Answer: b) Xylazine
Explanation: Xylazine is effective in inducing emesis in cats after toxin ingestion, facilitating removal of the substance from the stomach, though its use must be monitored.

Question 121: After a surgery on a dog, you are asked to disinfect. On which surface could you safely use bleach to disinfect?

a) The dog's skin and wounds
b) The metal operating table
c) The steel surgical instruments
d) The linoleum floors

Correct Answer: d) The linoleum floors
Explanation: Bleach is suitable for disinfecting non-porous surfaces like linoleum floors, providing effective microbial control without damaging the material.

Question 122: Which of the following antiemetic drugs would be prescribed for an animal experiencing chemotherapy sickness?

a) Dimenhydrinate
b) Meclizine
c) Metoclopramide
d) Ondansetron

Correct Answer: d) Ondansetron
Explanation: Ondansetron is used to manage nausea and vomiting associated with chemotherapy, blocking serotonin receptors to alleviate symptoms and improve patient comfort.

Question 123: Which type of chew toy can lead to gingival trauma?

a) Nylon rope toys
b) Dried hooves

c) Nylon chew bones
d) Rawhide strips

Correct Answer: a) Nylon rope toys
Explanation: Nylon rope toys can cause gingival injuries due to their abrasive texture, necessitating careful selection of toys to prevent oral damage in pets.

Question 124: Radiographic detail can be increased by:

a) Increasing the source-image distance
b) Decreasing the source-image distance
c) Increasing the object-film distance
d) Increasing the kVp level

Correct Answer: a) Increasing the source-image distance
Explanation: Increasing the source-image distance reduces magnification and distortion, enhancing radiographic detail and clarity for accurate diagnostics.

Question 125: Which of the following is the definitive means of diagnosing a malignant tumor?

a) Cytology
b) Radiography
c) Histopathology
d) Serum chemistry profile

Correct Answer: c) Histopathology
Explanation: Histopathology involves microscopic examination of tissue samples, providing definitive diagnosis and characterization of malignant tumors for effective treatment planning.

Question 126: Which of the following is a negative effect of an improperly applied bandage?

a) Wound drainage
b) Immobilization of a limb
c) Tissue necrosis
d) Wound debridement

Correct Answer: c) Tissue necrosis
Explanation: Improperly applied bandages can restrict circulation, leading to tissue necrosis, emphasizing the importance of proper technique to ensure healing and prevent complications.

Question 127: The minimum weight for a canine blood donor is:

a) 25 pounds
b) 45 pounds
c) 55 pounds
d) 65 pounds

Correct Answer: c) 55 pounds
Explanation: Canine blood donors must weigh at least 55 pounds to ensure they can safely donate blood without adverse effects, providing sufficient volume for transfusions.

Question 128: Which of the following species requires sedation or anesthesia for venipuncture?

a) Mongolian gerbil
b) Mouse
c) Rat
d) Guinea pig

Correct Answer: d) Guinea pig
Explanation: Guinea pigs often require sedation or anesthesia for venipuncture due to their small size and stress response, ensuring accurate and safe blood collection.

Question 129: All the following antimicrobial medications can be administered to rabbits except:

a) Clindamycin
b) Lincomycin
c) Erythromycin
d) Tylosin

Correct Answer: a) Clindamycin
Explanation: Clindamycin is contraindicated in rabbits due to the risk of severe gastrointestinal disturbances, including enterotoxemia, making it unsafe for use in this species.

Question 130: During a surgical procedure, a canine patient develops malignant hyperthermia. With what drug should the patient be treated?

a) Calcium EDTA
b) Dantrolene
c) Pamidronate
d) Atropine

Correct Answer: b) Dantrolene
Explanation: Dantrolene is the treatment of choice for malignant hyperthermia, a life-threatening condition, as it helps to relax muscles and reduce excessive heat production.

Question 131: In an induction that does not go smoothly, which normally bypassed stage is experienced?

a) Stage 1
b) Stage 2
c) Stage 3
d) Stage 4

Correct Answer: b) Stage 2
Explanation: Stage 2, or the excitement stage, may be experienced during a poorly managed induction, characterized by involuntary movement and irregular breathing patterns.

Question 132: When using a Bard-Parker scalpel handle during a small animal surgical procedure, which blade would you use with a Number 3 handle to sever ligaments?

a) Number 10
b) Number 11
c) Number 12
d) Number 15

Correct Answer: b) Number 11
Explanation: The Number 11 blade, with its sharp, pointed tip, is ideal for precise incisions and cutting ligaments during surgical procedures, offering control and accuracy.

Question 133: A high dose of which of the following preanesthetic agents could be dangerous for a ruminant?

a) Droperidol
b) Xylazine
c) Azaperone
d) Acepromazine

Correct Answer: b) Xylazine
Explanation: Xylazine, at high doses, can cause severe cardiovascular and respiratory depression in ruminants, necessitating careful dose management and monitoring.

Question 134: An excessively high level of what vitamin is thought to be a possible contributing factor in the development of feline odontoclastic resorptive lesions?

a) Vitamin A
b) Vitamin B12
c) Vitamin C
d) Vitamin D

Correct Answer: d) Vitamin D
Explanation: High levels of Vitamin D have been linked to odontoclastic resorptive lesions in cats, affecting dental health by altering calcium metabolism and bone resorption.

Question 135: Veterinary technicians sometimes use tourniquets to immobilize limbs and stop blood. The recommended maximum amount of time a tourniquet should be used is:

a) 5 minutes
b) 20 minutes
c) 40 minutes
d) 60 minutes

Correct Answer: b) 20 minutes
Explanation: Tourniquets should not exceed 20 minutes of application to prevent tissue damage and ensure adequate blood flow, critical for limb health and function.

Question 136: Which teeth are absent in lagomorphs?

a) Incisors
b) Canines
c) Premolars
d) Molars

Correct Answer: b) Canines
Explanation: Lagomorphs, such as rabbits, lack canine teeth, having a dental formula adapted for their herbivorous diet, consisting mainly of incisors and molars.

Question 137: In guinea pigs, what dental condition is associated with vitamin C deficiency?

a) Malocclusion
b) Caries
c) Overgrowth
d) Periodontal disease

Correct Answer: c) Overgrowth
Explanation: Vitamin C deficiency in guinea pigs can lead to dental overgrowth, as it affects collagen synthesis, crucial for maintaining healthy periodontal structures.

Question 138: An accurate statement concerning slow speed screens would be that they:

a) Produce average quality resolution radiographs with relatively low exposures
b) Are used when increased patient penetration is needed
c) Are designed to produce optimum detail with little regard to exposure time
d) Normally have a thicker phosphor layer

Correct Answer: c) Are designed to produce optimum detail with little regard to exposure time
Explanation: Slow speed screens prioritize image detail quality over exposure time, requiring longer exposures but yielding superior radiographic resolution.

Question 139: Which of the following is a cause of sinus bradycardia?

a) Hyperthyroidism
b) Anemia

c) Increased cerebrospinal fluid pressure
d) Reduced cardiac output

Correct Answer: c) Increased cerebrospinal fluid pressure
Explanation: Elevated cerebrospinal fluid pressure can stimulate the vagus nerve, resulting in sinus bradycardia, a decreased heart rate, affecting cardiac function.

Question 140: Manual compression of the bladder would be an appropriate method for:

a) Examining solute concentration in urine
b) Relieving bladder distention due to obstruction
c) Collecting a sterile urine sample for urinalysis and culture
d) Clearing a urethral obstruction

Correct Answer: a) Examining solute concentration in urine
Explanation: Manual bladder compression can help obtain urine samples to assess solute concentration, crucial for evaluating kidney function and hydration status.

Question 141: Halsted mosquito forceps have:

a) Distal transverse grooves
b) Transverse serrations covering the entire jaw length
c) Complete transverse grooves
d) Longitudinal grooves and distal transverse grooves

Correct Answer: b) Transverse serrations covering the entire jaw length
Explanation: Halsted mosquito forceps feature full-length transverse serrations, designed for precise grasping and hemostasis of small blood vessels during surgery.

Question 142: When cutting and dissecting dense tissue, a veterinary surgeon would most likely use:

a) Metzenbaum scissors
b) Iris scissors
c) Spencer scissors
d) Mayo scissors

Correct Answer: d) Mayo scissors
Explanation: Mayo scissors, with their sturdy design, are ideal for cutting dense tissues, providing the necessary leverage and precision for effective dissection.

Question 143: Miconazole is used to treat:

a) Gastrointestinal and skin Candida infections
b) Dermatophytosis or avian mycoses
c) Fungal ophthalmic infections
d) Inflammatory bowel disease

Correct Answer: c) Fungal ophthalmic infections
Explanation: Miconazole is an antifungal agent effective against fungal infections in the eyes, helping clear infections and restore ocular health.

Question 144: Which inhaled anesthetic has the highest rate of metabolization?

a) Halothane
b) Sevoflurane
c) Nitrous oxide
d) Desflurane

Correct Answer: a) Halothane
Explanation: Halothane undergoes significant hepatic metabolism compared to other inhaled anesthetics, impacting its pharmacokinetics and potential for side effects.

Question 145: Which of the following is a common side effect of corticosteroid use in animals?

a) Hypertension
b) Hypoglycemia
c) Polyuria
d) Bradycardia

Correct Answer: c) Polyuria
Explanation: Corticosteroid therapy can lead to increased urine production (polyuria) due to its effects on kidney function and electrolyte balance, necessitating monitoring.

Question 146: What is the most appropriate first aid treatment for a dog experiencing heat stroke?

a) Administering activated charcoal
b) Applying ice packs to the head and neck
c) Immersing the dog in cold water
d) Offering a high-protein meal

Correct Answer: c) Immersing the dog in cold water
Explanation: Rapid cooling by immersing in cold water helps reduce body temperature efficiently during heat stroke, crucial for preventing organ damage and stabilizing the patient.

Question 147: Which diagnostic test is most suitable for detecting heartworms in dogs?

a) Fecal flotation
b) SNAP test
c) Blood smear
d) Urinalysis

Correct Answer: b) SNAP test
Explanation: The SNAP test detects heartworm antigens quickly and accurately, providing essential information for diagnosis and management of heartworm disease in dogs.

Question 148: What is a common complication of untreated diabetes mellitus in cats?

a) Hypercalcemia
b) Ketoacidosis
c) Hypoglycemia
d) Hyperthyroidism

Correct Answer: b) Ketoacidosis
Explanation: Untreated diabetes can lead to ketoacidosis, a life-threatening condition where high ketone levels cause systemic acidosis, requiring immediate medical intervention.

Question 149: Which of the following is an example of a zoonotic disease?

a) Canine distemper
b) Feline leukemia
c) Rabies
d) Parvovirus

Correct Answer: c) Rabies
Explanation: Rabies is a zoonotic disease transmissible between animals and humans, necessitating vaccination and control measures to prevent outbreaks and ensure public safety.

Question 150: Which vitamin is crucial for blood clotting?

a) Vitamin A
b) Vitamin B12
c) Vitamin C
d) Vitamin K

Correct Answer: d) Vitamin K
Explanation: Vitamin K is essential for synthesizing clotting factors, playing a critical role in preventing bleeding disorders and ensuring proper hemostasis.

Question 151: What is the primary function of red blood cells?

a) Carrying oxygen
b) Fighting infections
c) Clotting blood
d) Producing antibodies

Correct Answer: a) Carrying oxygen
Explanation: Red blood cells transport oxygen from the lungs to body tissues and return carbon dioxide for exhalation, vital for cellular respiration and energy production.

Question 152: Which organ is primarily responsible for detoxifying chemicals in the body?

a) Kidney
b) Liver
c) Spleen
d) Pancreas

Correct Answer: b) Liver
Explanation: The liver plays a central role in detoxifying harmful substances, metabolizing drugs, and producing essential proteins, crucial for maintaining homeostasis.

Question 153: Which type of cell is involved in producing antibodies?

a) T cells
b) B cells
c) Red blood cells
d) Platelets

Correct Answer: b) B cells
Explanation: B cells, a type of lymphocyte, produce antibodies in response to antigens, forming a key component of the adaptive immune system for pathogen defense.

Question 154: What is the normal range of respiration rate for a healthy adult dog?

a) 5-10 breaths per minute
b) 10-30 breaths per minute
c) 30-50 breaths per minute
d) 50-70 breaths per minute

Correct Answer: b) 10-30 breaths per minute
Explanation: A normal respiration rate for adult dogs ranges from 10 to 30 breaths per minute, indicating healthy respiratory function and effective gas exchange.

Question 155: Which electrolyte imbalance is commonly associated with Addison's disease?

a) Hyperkalemia
b) Hypernatremia
c) Hypomagnesemia
d) Hypercalcemia

Correct Answer: a) Hyperkalemia
Explanation: Addison's disease results in hyperkalemia due to adrenal insufficiency, leading to decreased aldosterone production and impaired potassium regulation.

Question 156: Which part of the eye is responsible for focusing light?

a) Cornea
b) Retina
c) Iris
d) Optic nerve

Correct Answer: a) Cornea

Explanation: The cornea refracts and focuses incoming light onto the retina, playing a critical role in vision by contributing to the eye's optical power.

Question 157: What is the primary role of platelets in the body?

a) Transporting oxygen
b) Fighting infection
c) Blood clotting
d) Producing hormones

Correct Answer: c) Blood clotting

Explanation: Platelets are essential for hemostasis, aggregating at injury sites to form clots and prevent excessive bleeding, crucial for wound healing and maintaining vascular integrity.

Question 158: Which hormone regulates calcium levels in the blood?

a) Insulin
b) Cortisol
c) Parathyroid hormone
d) Thyroid hormone

Correct Answer: c) Parathyroid hormone

Explanation: Parathyroid hormone regulates calcium homeostasis by increasing calcium absorption and release from bones, vital for maintaining stable blood calcium levels.

Question 159: What is the main structural protein found in skin and connective tissues?

a) Elastin
b) Collagen
c) Keratin
d) Fibrin

Correct Answer: b) Collagen

Explanation: Collagen provides structural support and strength to skin and connective tissues, essential for maintaining the integrity and elasticity of various body structures.

Question 160: Which organ filters blood to remove old or damaged blood cells?

a) Liver
b) Kidney
c) Spleen
d) Pancreas

Correct Answer: c) Spleen

Explanation: The spleen filters blood, removing old or damaged red blood cells and recycling iron, playing a vital role in maintaining healthy blood composition.

Question 161: Which part of the brain is responsible for coordinating movement and balance?

a) Cerebrum
b) Cerebellum
c) Medulla oblongata
d) Hypothalamus

Correct Answer: b) Cerebellum
Explanation: The cerebellum coordinates voluntary movements and maintains balance and posture, integrating sensory inputs for smooth and precise motor activity.

Question 162: What is the normal body temperature range for a healthy adult cat?

a) 96.0-98.0°F
b) 98.1-100.0°F
c) 100.5-102.5°F
d) 103.0-105.0°F

Correct Answer: c) 100.5-102.5°F
Explanation: The normal body temperature for adult cats ranges from 100.5°F to 102.5°F, reflecting their metabolic processes and thermoregulation efficiency.

Question 163: Which vitamin is essential for vision and skin health?

a) Vitamin A
b) Vitamin D
c) Vitamin E
d) Vitamin K

Correct Answer: a) Vitamin A
Explanation: Vitamin A is crucial for maintaining healthy vision, skin, and immune function, supporting retinal health and cellular differentiation processes.

Question 164: Which blood vessel carries oxygenated blood from the heart to the body?

a) Pulmonary artery
b) Aorta
c) Vena cava
d) Carotid artery

Correct Answer: b) Aorta
Explanation: The aorta is the main artery that distributes oxygenated blood from the heart to the rest of the body, supporting systemic circulation and tissue oxygenation.

Question 165: What is the function of the pancreas in digestion?

a) Absorbing nutrients
b) Producing bile
c) Secreting digestive enzymes
d) Breaking down carbohydrates

Correct Answer: c) Secreting digestive enzymes
Explanation: The pancreas secretes digestive enzymes into the small intestine, aiding in the breakdown of carbohydrates, proteins, and fats for absorption.

Question 166: Which type of joint allows for the greatest range of motion?

a) Hinge joint
b) Ball-and-socket joint
c) Pivot joint
d) Saddle joint

Correct Answer: b) Ball-and-socket joint
Explanation: Ball-and-socket joints, like the shoulder and hip, allow multidirectional movement and rotation, providing the greatest range of motion among joint types.

Question 167: Which component of the blood is primarily responsible for fighting infections?

a) Red blood cells
b) White blood cells
c) Platelets
d) Plasma

Correct Answer: b) White blood cells

Explanation: White blood cells, or leukocytes, are key players in the immune system, defending the body against infections and foreign invaders through various mechanisms.

Question 168: What is the primary function of the large intestine in the digestive process?

a) Absorbing nutrients
b) Absorbing water
c) Digesting proteins
d) Producing bile

Correct Answer: b) Absorbing water

Explanation: The large intestine absorbs water and electrolytes from indigestible food matter, forming stool and maintaining fluid balance in the body.

Question 169: Which hormone is primarily involved in regulating metabolism and energy balance?

a) Insulin
b) Thyroid hormone
c) Adrenaline
d) Melatonin

Correct Answer: b) Thyroid hormone

Explanation: Thyroid hormones regulate metabolism, influencing energy production, growth, and development, crucial for maintaining overall metabolic homeostasis.

Question 170: Which structure in the ear is responsible for detecting sound vibrations?

a) Cochlea
b) Eustachian tube
c) Semicircular canals
d) Tympanic membrane

Correct Answer: a) Cochlea

Explanation: The cochlea, a spiral-shaped organ in the inner ear, converts sound vibrations into neural signals, facilitating hearing by transmitting information to the brain.

EXTRA CONTENTS

Audiobook

With the audiobook included, you can listen to the contents of your book even while going about your daily activities, maximizing your time. This bonus provides a flexible learning experience, perfectly tailored to your needs.

Digital Flashcards

The digital flashcards included in your purchase allow you to quickly memorize key concepts wherever you are, thanks to their practical and intuitive format. With this bonus, you'll be able to review and reinforce your knowledge effectively and efficiently.

WAKEUPMEMORY Technique

The WAKEUPMEMORY technique offers five innovative strategies to enhance memory, a crucial aspect of VTNE preparation. These techniques include the use of mnemonics, visualization, spaced repetition, association, and the method of loci. By implementing these strategies, students can significantly improve information retention, making the study process more efficient and less stressful. These techniques are particularly useful for memorizing complex and specific details, such as those required in pharmacology and anatomy.

6 Online Tests

We offer 6 online tests that each include 15 VTNE practice questions, providing additional opportunities for practice and self-assessment.

Scan the QR CODE or link and access the bonuses

https://vtnev2.infinityquillpublishing.com/home-page310586-7156-3975-5383-2987-5411-8443-9644-4570-5999-3728-9957-2662

www.ingramcontent.com/pod-product-compliance
Lightning Source LLC
Chambersburg PA
CBHW062348220526
45472CB00008B/1738